T0270654

How to Be a Healthy Human

How to Be a Healthy Human

WHAT YOUR DOCTOR DOESN'T KNOW ABOUT HEALTH AND LONGEVITY

EMMA TEKSTRA, FIA

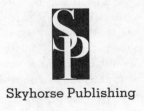

Skyhorse Publishing

Skyhorse Publishing books may be purchased in bulk at special discounts for sales promotion, corporate gifts, fund-raising, or educational purposes. Special editions can also be created to specifications. For details, contact the Special Sales Department, Skyhorse Publishing, 307 West 36th Street, 11th Floor, New York, NY 10018 or info@skyhorsepublishing.com.

Skyhorse® and Skyhorse Publishing® are registered trademarks of Skyhorse Publishing, Inc.®, a Delaware corporation.

Visit our website at www.skyhorsepublishing.com.
Please follow our publisher Tony Lyons on Instagram @tonylyonsisuncertain.

10 9 8 7 6 5 4 3 2 1

Library of Congress Cataloging-in-Publication Data is available on file.

Cover design by Kai Texel
Cover and interior illustrations by Milena Salieri

Print ISBN: 978–1-5107–7950-1
Ebook ISBN: 978–1-5107–7951-8

Printed in the United States of America

This book provides information for educational purposes only. Any medical information included is presented as general information and should not be used to diagnose, treat, cure, or prevent any disease. The information in this book should only be used to supplement rather than replace the advice of your doctor or other trained health professional. Although efforts have been made to ensure the accuracy of the information as of the date of publication, neither the author nor the publisher bears any responsibility for the accuracy or content of the sites, books, or resources listed or for any medical outcomes that may occur as a result of applying the methods suggested in this book.

Contents

Introduction

So there I was: holding my head in my hands, wondering what to do. On the desk was the formal diagnosis. After a tough pregnancy and required C-section my firstborn, Ethan, had been a sickly and complicated child. He was only five years old and was now diagnosed with both Asperger's and attention deficit hyperactivity disorder (ADHD). The long written assessment of his behavior problems had been given to me by a child psychologist who we'd gone to see at the request of Ethan's school. Deep down I already knew Ethan was likely on the autism spectrum, from the discussions I'd been having with the psychologist at the series of visits we'd had, but it was still a shock to see it in black and white. I didn't know it at the time but that moment has defined the trajectory of my life, career, and passion for health.

As a baby, Ethan had had severe gastrointestinal issues and constant ear infections. At just three months old, his reflux was so bad that the pediatrician put him on proton pump inhibitors (Prilosec and Nexium). These medications affected his nervous system so much that he would go rigid and tense his muscles when lying on his back. He had also had multiple rounds of antibiotics before he was two years old. He was my firstborn, what did I know? I put my blind trust in the pediatrician. I was a mathematician and a nervous new mom. Even though Ethan wasn't doing well, I believed that the doctor knew best. As a toddler he was hyperactive and obsessive. At age three, he would throw tantrums if we drove back to our house via a different route or if a toy was left in a spot other than its "home." By age five, Ethan was having such a tough time at school that the principal asked us to have him evaluated. Along with the diagnoses came a recommendation for medication and a bleak prognosis for his life. Red flags started to flare in my head.

Ethan's teacher then introduced me to another mom at the school whose son had been diagnosed with autism at age three. Five years later, though, her son was "almost normal." This mom took me out for coffee and for two hours she carefully educated me on the problems with conventional pediatric care, the ingredients included in child-hood vaccines that certain kids can be particularly sensitive to, and the antibiotics and other medications that can damage the gut. All this, she said, can result in a perfect storm that destroys a child's health. She detailed every intervention she had done with her son, from diet changes and supplements to weekly occupational therapy and a stead-fast commitment to avoiding further toxic exposures.

I listened so closely to what this mom was telling me that my coffee went untouched. Everything she shared made so much sense. I could have sat with her all day, but we had to get back to our lives. Mine had already changed forever. Her story made me determined to find out the truth of what had caused my son's health and behavior problems and how to fix them. My younger son, Max, was three at the time, and I was not going to let him suffer the same fate. Our adventure had begun.

Today Ethan is a happy healthy eighteen-year-old just starting at a major four-year college to study aerospace engineering. You may not believe me when I tell you that he's in such robust good health that in the last ten years he hasn't missed a single day of school, but it's true. Max hasn't either. When other kids are felled by colds and flu, both my boys barely have a sniffle. The only time they visit a doctor is for their annual checkups, and the only pharmaceutical product they have since taken was light anesthetic and a day's worth of ibuprofen the day they each had their wisdom teeth removed.

However, as I sought to recover my son's health back then, my own health suffered. I had an intense global job in corporate America, and the boys' dad was taking drugs and abusing alcohol. With a husband unable to hold down any kind of paid work, the burden of making a living and doing all the parenting fell on my shoulders. There was a lot of time spent researching and testing various therapies, and being Mom and Dad to two growing boys took up any waking hours I wasn't working. On the outside, I seemed to be managing it all. I had a good job, we lived in a nice house, I rarely missed a soccer game or talent show. But on the inside, the stress, anxiety, and unrelenting marital problems were destroying my health.

Every female in my family of origin, including my mom, her two sisters, and my first cousin, had been diagnosed with breast cancer before age fifty. My two aunts both died of the disease, one at forty-seven, the other fifty-two. I was exhausted and unwell. I knew I couldn't ignore my own health problems any longer.

The last straw came when a mom at our small elementary school died of breast cancer leaving three kids under the age of ten. I knew I didn't want to leave my sons motherless; I was the only stable parent they had, and we had no other family around. I made the painful decision to divorce their dad. At the same time, I embarked on a personal journey of healing, both physically and mentally.

A few years earlier, I had started attending a nondenominational Bible-teaching church. I'd been digging into the information presented there week after week hungry to learn more. I was raised Jewish but always felt there was something missing. Growing up, there was no explanation for the way we led our lives and the festivals and ceremonies we celebrated. The more I learned about God, the more I became convinced that our amazing human body is intelligently designed to live in harmony with this world. These two threads of health and faith have weaved themselves throughout my story ever since. The common theme being the search for the truth in every bit of detail, making me one of the most intense people you have ever met!

My life as a single mom became much more stable as I developed close friendships at church. I continued my corporate work and focused on healing my own health and that of my precious boys. I researched tirelessly what to eat and how to address our different symptoms one by one using natural means. While my sons may not have been happy about me switching out Halloween candy for healthy alternatives, we had a lot of fun along the way.

One of our passions was (and still is!) go-karting. On a particular Monday in 2014 my boys had the day off school for some sort of teacher training. I bribed them to behave all day while I worked by promising to take them to K1 Speed, our nearest go-kart track. We ended up there in the early afternoon when there were no other adults around. My boys were able to race each other on the junior karts while I watched. In walked a tall lanky guy with his own helmet to get a few laps in while on a break from work. I was excited to have someone to race myself so joined him on the track. Less than two years later that speed freak became my new husband and my boys' much-loved stepdad.

We all share a love of motor sports, especially Formula One racing. It may seem counterintuitive for a Bible-loving health-conscious math nerd but I love the adrenaline rush of speed. Formula One (F1) is the absolute pinnacle of racing: there are only twenty professional drivers in the world who are skilled enough to compete for one of the ten teams in any given year. F1 is international: the season stretches most of the calendar year and includes races in twenty different countries across all continents. I've been following Max Verstappen since he was seventeen years old and the youngest race car driver to be signed to a major F1 team. My youngest son is also called Max. He was about seven when Verstappen came on the scene, and we've been diehard fans ever since.

Coming into the 2022 season Verstappen was the reigning world champion, winning the 2021 season at age twenty-three. But 2022 got off to a rocky start. Max didn't finish two of the first three races due to technical problems. Now, in a season of just 22 races, not finishing two out of three is pretty concerning. The winner of an F1 race gets 25 points, coming in second gets you just 18, down to 1 point if you place 10th. Not finishing a race at all is a big problem, you get far behind in the leaderboard quickly.

A saying began to crop up: *"It's great to finish first, but first you've got to finish!"* Fans no longer shouted for Max Verstappen to win the following races, they just wanted him to finish the race and get some points on the board. There's a happy ending to this story: Max came back from being so far behind and went on to win a record-breaking 15 races in 2022 and became world champion again for the second time. But the saying that had cropped up makes me think of the best approach to living a healthy life and being a healthy human. So many of us power through life wanting to reap the rewards of all that this life has to offer: the places to see, the houses to buy, the children to raise, the money to be made. Most of us are focusing on the next race, the next achievement, the next bonus at work, the next vacation. And, of course, it is great to finish first and achieve that promotion, that new house, that comfortable retirement. . . . But first you have to finish. In order to live a fulfilled life, you need to avoid the pitfalls of a cancer diagnosis, a heart attack, an autoimmune condition that curtails your travels or your hobbies, or the health problems of a family member that consumes all of your attention. I want you to stay in the race and to make sure you finish well.

Maybe Formula One racing doesn't resonate with you. Or maybe you're not looking to get ahead or win a race. You just want to live a quiet, godly life. You know that God has already numbered your days and that if He has determined to give you a health challenge to deal with it's just part of His plan. But I'd like to gently suggest that you expand your view. After all, think about how much more useful you can be to God and others if you don't need to worry about your health. Think about how much more of God's work you could accomplish if the second half of your life was not filled with doctors' appointments and managing your health symptoms. Ill-health at any age can get in the way of what God has purposed for your life. He's put this book in your hands, after all!

I have written this book to empower you to live the healthiest life possible and discover that you are a unique individual truly known only by yourself and God. While healthcare professionals and other types of practitioners have their gifts, you are the only one inhabiting your body and only you know what it needs. Now, I'm not saying you don't need to get checkups, take a test, or get a diagnosis if you have a problem, but the paradigm of the pedigreed person in the white coat knowing more than you about your body needs to shift. Your doctors spent many years in medical school learning the nuts and bolts of human health, but here's the thing: There is so much more we don't know about the miracle of the human body than is in the typical medical school textbook. It's the very science, particularly of the human body, that has deepened my faith over the years as I will share with you as we go.

This is not a diet or exercise book. I won't be giving you a definitive step-by-step program. There is no silver bullet to being a healthy human, but you've heard the expression—*give a man a fish and he'll eat for a day, but teach a man to fish and he'll never go hungry the rest of his life.* That's my hope for you, that not only will you not go hungry (we're going to talk a LOT about food, real food!), but that you will understand more about the human body than you ever did, and what it takes to get it healthy and keep it healthy so that you can enjoy a long, productive, happy life. You'll stop saying, "I'm just getting old," or making excuses as to why you can't do an activity with your BFF, spouse, children, or grandchildren. Your poor health will no longer limit you. Instead, you'll be able to travel the world, take on that new project or hobby, and make a difference in your little corner of the planet.

I include plenty of ideas for you to try as well as a ton of resources for further reading on your particular needs. My goal is to empower you to take ownership of your health and your body. I want you to be able to see past the myths and marketing and seek the truth. I'll save you a lot of money in the process, which you can put toward all the new activities you'll try once you start feeling better!

In Part I we're going to understand the world we're living in, the complexity of the human body, and why conventional medicine misses the mark for so much of what ails us. It touches on some history of the medical profession and why the industry puts profits before your health. We'll browse through various "alternative" treatment options and the evidence for how well they work without the risks and side effects of conventional approaches that often make matters worse. And we'll look at what causes so many health problems and how you can reduce your risks.

We'll wrap up Part I with a look at the single biggest impact on your health—what you put in your mouth. Even though most of us know junk food isn't healthy, food marketing companies are winning the war against common sense these days. It's likely that your doctor has even scoffed when you asked for nutrition guidance to combat your chronic health condition. You need to know why they roll their eyes, and what a disservice that is to you, their patient. *Let Food Be Thy*

Medicine is not just a cute phrase, I would venture it to be one of the most important principles you can live by.

Have you been diagnosed with a chronic disease? Maybe a heart or lung condition, maybe an autoimmune disease or diabetes? Do you have high cholesterol and a doctor has labeled you with "hyperlipid-emia" and put you on a statin drug, thus medicalizing you for the rest of your life? Or maybe you've been told you have a "sluggish" or an "overactive" thyroid? Part II looks at common health issues many of us are facing and how to put the principles in Part I into practice.

An entire chapter is dedicated to mental health in Part II, as conventional medicine has failed this aspect of our wellbeing more than any other with the most disastrous results. Your brain and emotions cannot be separated from the rest of your body; it is all connected. If you have a condition that would typically be put in the mental health category (depression, anxiety, autism, attention deficit, schizophrenia, bipolar disorder, or obsessive-compulsive disorder, to name a few) you may get some counseling but typically are being labeled and medicated with no hope for reversal or cure. However, your doctors are mislead-ing you. The research is increasingly clear that the majority of mental health problems have their foundations in nutritional deficiencies and/or toxins that can be eliminated. There is hope.

Lastly, we'll look at our later years where the typical adult over sixty is taking four or five prescription medications and spends a large proportion of their income on healthcare. There is another way. There is no reason a human in the twenty-first century cannot live to be a centenarian (see their 100th birthday) with minimal disability or cognitive decline. You've worked hard all your life and now you have wisdom to share and bucket lists to work through. I'll give you tips and recommendations for these twilight years.

I want to give you as many tools and resources as possible. Again, my aim is to empower you to follow your own health journey and figure out what works for you and your unique body and lifestyle. I have provided a list of further reading in key areas you might want to pursue by chapter as well as resources and websites with information and products that I recommend. I may not agree with everything on every page, but they are generally good sources of truth.

In today's world of censorship, you cannot trust your health to a Google search or Amazon recommendation, so I've provided updated resources, information, and products on my website, **EmmaTekstra.com**.

One last word of advice: don't skip ahead! I know you want to get to the tips for your particular ailment but remember: *knowledge is power*. In order to take control of your health, you need to understand the foundations and how it all fits together, which I will walk you through chapter by chapter. If all this information seems scary to you, just absorb what you can and keep going. You're on a journey and there's definitely a lot to learn. But don't worry, I'll summarize the key points to remember at the end of each chapter to help you.

So, are you ready to change your life and improve your health? Let's get started!

PART I

FOUNDATIONS

The greatest medicine of all is to teach people not to need it.

—Hippocrates

CHAPTER 1

The Human Eyeball

How does a Jewish girl from Leeds, England, the daughter of a pharmacist and an accountant, wind up living in Southern California as a Bible-believing Christian writing a book on health?

I planned to be a neurosurgeon as a teenager. I watched every weekly drama on TV that involved doctors and relished close-ups of surgery. My favorite show back then was *St. Elsewhere*. One of the doctors in charge of the hospital, Dr. Donald Westphall, had a son named Tommy who was autistic. A really good-looking kid who struggled immensely and couldn't connect with the outside world. What was going on inside his brain? I wondered this week after week as I watched intently, face fixed on the screen. The fact that I ended up with a son on the autism spectrum is what I think of as a "God shot," a time when God is reminding me that He's in charge.

My traditional Jewish dad did not support me going into medicine. He felt a hospital was no place for a nice Jewish girl who should focus on getting married and settling down with a regular schedule. He would have liked me to become an accountant and take over his practice, but it seemed boring to me. Still, in a Jewish household like ours, parental respect was paramount. I didn't want to disappoint my dad. So, I became the next best thing to an accountant: an actuary. I find people fall into two camps: those who haven't a clue what an actuary is and those who put an actuary into the stereotypical "nerd" bucket. An actuary is a person who assesses risk; insurance risks, health risks, or the risk that a retirement plan will not have enough money to pay out the specified pensions in forty years. Okay so, yes, it's kind of nerdy. But basically, an actuary is a person who is very good at math and at applying mathematical calculations to real life.

But even after I qualified as an actuary, I remained fascinated with medical science and epidemiology, which is the study of the cause of disease. Though I started my career working with cold hard numbers in a pensions consulting firm, in my spare time I loved learning about the medical profession, medicine, and what makes the human body tick or break down.

When you're an actuary in the pensions field you focus a lot on mortality. We are the people who figure out how many years an employee who is retiring in good health will need to receive a pension. We also calculate how much a company or individual needs to save today to make sure there is enough money to last for all your tomorrows. I prefer the science of health rather than death, but there is just as much mathematics involved in both. How do we know what interventions extend life expectancy or improve health? We have to measure them. This requires a lot of math and data science.

The problem is that most doctors are not very good at math. Some scientists aren't either. Journalists, too, are often mathematically challenged. Me, I am a data junkie. Not because I love being buried in spreadsheets, but because I love learning what the data tells us. I can hear anecdotal stories all day long, but anecdotal information is always biased. What you choose to read, or who you choose to talk to, will color what you learn. But data is fact. Not the interpretation of the data, mind you, *that* can always be manipulated. But the data itself, if you understand every aspect of how it was gathered and its limitations, gives you something real and tangible to work with.

By the time I was twenty-seven, my friends had all moved to London. But I didn't want to live in a big city. Instead, in 1998, I decided to move to the United States. I had my eyes set on the outdoor lifestyle of California. I also wanted to expand professionally beyond the narrow field of pensions. So, I joined a large global consulting firm, initially as an actuary and benefits consultant working with multinational companies on their employee benefit plans around the world. My first job, based out of New York City, was a bit of a shock to the system for this country girl from Leeds! But two years later I was able to move out west to set up our international practice on the West Coast.

I met my sons' dad on the beach the month I arrived in California. We were married two years later, in 2002, and had our first son Ethan in 2005. Following Ethan's diagnosis, I took an unpaid leave to understand better his challenges in school and start researching if and how we could recover his health. When I went back to work, I was able to move into a different position with more of an emphasis on health and wellbeing.

In my new specialty, I helped employers understand healthcare around the world and how to support their own employees to be healthy and productive. This job allowed me a front-row seat to witness in real time how healthcare is practiced in different countries and people's differing attitudes to medicine, be it conventional or alternative therapies, Eastern or Western approaches. I also saw how people receive care or get advice for medical problems, and the impact of big business on the whole industry.

In March 2020 everything changed. The announcement that we were in a global pandemic highlighted the limitations of working for big business. When you're a seeker of truth and want to help people lead healthier lives, you want to educate clients and colleagues about clinical trials, actual risk, and safety data. Right from the beginning of Covid, there was high-quality information that safe, simple treatments were effective against this new virus.[1] But my corporate bosses would not allow me to share this knowledge with our employees or clients. Instead, they wanted me to repeat status quo talking points, even though there was no evidence for them. In other words, there was one narrative and one narrative only—one based on fear and industry profits, not on any of the major principles of lasting good health.

The couple of years following the announcement of the pandemic also saw huge cultural change in the US and UK. As my firm embraced this cultural shift unilaterally, making a big show of being a modern employer, it left those of us close to the real science more adrift than ever and unable to be ourselves at work. Speaking truth—that obesity is one of the biggest risks of a bad outcome if you contract Covid, for example, or that a simple regimen of supplements, fresh air, and stress-reducers like socializing would help keep you healthy—became taboo. My employer's only focus was getting everyone masked up and locked down, socially distanced, and on screens full-time.

We are social beings. Human interaction is critical to many aspects of our health not only our mental state but the robustness of our immune system.[2] Confining us to isolation was entirely contrary to what the Bible teaches about human interaction. As a person with a deep faith in God, I felt even more alienated. The response to the pandemic by the US and many other countries was evidence for just how much God has been silenced in our society.

I feel the knowledge of God exists inside every human being but is typically drowned out by the busyness and secular noise of this world. Another way to think of what I call a deep-down knowledge of God is our conscience. Whether we choose to listen to it or not says more about who we are than our family of origin, what political party we vote for, or what we do for a living. This knowledge—that we humans are part of this natural world we inhabit—is important to understanding how to keep ourselves healthy.

While the Bible is not a science text, you will be amazed how much scientific truth is in it. In fact, when it comes to our health, it is sometimes explanations from the Bible that offer us the most exacting truth. These truths will never be superseded by a new study or updated science. Even if you don't necessarily believe in the Christian Bible, I hope to show you how reassuring it is to have this rock-solid foundation as a reference for all of us.

Nature and Your Health

To get started on your health journey, take a walk around your neighborhood or a local park. Even better, if you have time, head to a wilderness area. Bring some paper or a journal with you and a pen, some art supplies so you can doodle, and a camera or your smartphone, if you have one. Now, take a really good look at what you see. Look at the contrasts, the colors, the shapes, and the textures. Appreciate the natural beauty. It is uniquely human to appreciate beauty. I'm not talking about those tropical birds where the male struts his stuff and the female picks the one with the brightest plumage; but where have you seen an animal hang a leaf on the wall of its burrow because they like the shape of it, or just sit and gaze at a sunset or a great view?

Now close your eyes. Inhale the fresh air and pay attention to how it feels as it enters your lungs. As you exhale the stress and tension of your day, listen to the sounds around you. In Japan they call this *Shinrin-yoku*—forest-bathing. Terpenes are the aromatic compounds inside plants that give many of them distinctive smells like lavender or citrus orange. When you walk among the trees—or anywhere in nature—you inhale these terpenes. These "forest aerosols," as botanists call them, are good for your mental and physical well-being.[3] Indeed, there are many scientific studies showing how therapeutic immersing yourself in nature is for your health.[4]

I recently went camping up in the Sierra mountains, at Inyo National Park, where I hiked some of the John Muir Trail with my younger son Max and his Boy Scout buddies. I was awestruck by the beauty and the diversity all around us. The unusual shapes and formation of the mountains; the vibrant colors of the vegetation contrasting with the various types of rocks and the snowy peaks; the brightly colored birds and the dragonflies dancing across the streams. These sights all tingled my senses and took my mind off the stress of my busy life. I wished I had a way to capture everything I was seeing—to bring that nature back with me to my office.

Taking a moment to appreciate nature or beauty of any kind can reduce your blood pressure and your stress levels in an instant. According to one 2020 review, forest bathing actually lowers your pulse rate, improves your heart's efficiency, and lowers levels of harmful hormones that can cause you anxiety and increase your chances of metabolic dysfunction.[5] "Stop and smell the roses" is a really important principle. Most people plan to take time to travel, visit National Parks or go for long leisurely hikes after they retire. But, as busy as we all are, we need to slow down now, get outside today, play in the dirt—not wait until our twilight years.

Nourished by Our Sun

Have you ever seen an eclipse? A solar eclipse is when the moon passes in front of the sun totally obscuring our view of the sun and plunging us into darkness momentarily. Would it surprise you to know that the sun is four hundred times bigger than the moon? The sun is also four hundred times farther away from Earth. This exacting setup turns out to be critical to our health. If the sun were any closer to the Earth, the temperature would not be sustainable for humans, and we would die of heat. If it were any farther away, we would freeze.

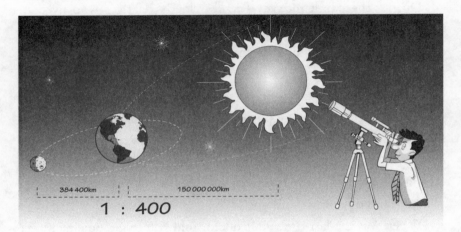

The sun is our life force. It feeds every life-form on the planet, including us humans. Vitamin D is the only vitamin that we can manufacture in our own bodies and only when our skin is exposed to natural sunlight. It is very difficult to obtain vitamin D from food. Vitamin D is critical for many biological functions affecting nearly every system in the body. The vitamin D we get from the sun is essential for bone health. It helps to modulate immune function, reduces inflammation, and affects how your body regulates cell growth and apoptosis (appropriate cell death—cancer grows when this system is not working properly).

Studies have shown that rates of cancer, autoimmune disease such as multiple sclerosis, and poor outcomes of viral infections all increase the farther away from the equator one goes and the fewer hours of sunlight enjoyed.[6, 7, 8] This may all be connected to levels of vitamin D, but is likely a far more complex relationship, which also depends on the body's ability to produce melatonin (another hormone tied to sunlight that regulates your sleep cycle amongst other functions) and the impact of sunlight on your microbiome. I will explain all of this in more detail in later chapters.

During the pandemic, my friend's elderly relatives who lived in Oakland, California, stayed inside. They were afraid to go on their daily walks: they thought they might catch Covid. The one day that her aunt ventured out she came home furious. A group of young men were playing basketball together, with their shirts off, enjoying the sunlight. She felt they were putting her and her husband at risk. But the truth is completely opposite. Scaring people away from going out in nature, taking their daily walks, and getting sunlight on their skin during the pandemic was a quantifiably terrible public health measure. The human body needs sunlight!

When was the last time your doctor told you to get outside more? A walk outside, preferably where you can see some nature, will do more for your health than anything that comes in a bottle or packet—and it is free! Some of the very best healing modalities are actually the cheapest. Many of these remedies have been known for hundreds of years. We'll look at some of them in Chapter 2.

It is a common misconception, fueled by the healthcare industry itself, that natural healing modalities are not scientific and not studied for efficacy. This is simply not true. I've shared my insatiable appetite for the truth and for the data to reveal at least some piece of the truth. Science is not necessarily the whole truth; it is *the quest for truth* and for a better understanding. Science needs to be driven by curiosity and never silenced or censored.

In the 1950s doctors were recommending cigarettes as being good for your health.[9] Later studies proved this to be blatantly wrong. If you are going to take control of your health, you need to keep an open mind and engage your critical thinking. It was the government's top doctors that recommended we stay indoors when fighting a viral infection. Yet now the scientific literature is teeming with studies that show what people who followed God's design for human beings were already aware of: optimizing vitamin D levels helps humans more effectively and efficiently fight off disease, including Covid.[10] The disconnect between common sense and the government's mandates should have raised red flags immediately!

The Complexity of Life

We all want to live our best, healthiest, most interesting life. But what is "life"? How do we know if something is alive? What is the difference between a tree blowing in the wind happily planted by a stream and the log sitting by a fireplace? What about your favorite family member when they were imparting words of wisdom to you compared to when they were lying in a casket at their funeral? Both the tree and the log contain the same set of molecules, but one is alive and one is dead.

Shortly after the turn of this century, the US president at the time, Bill Clinton, held an international press conference with Prime Minister Tony Blair of the UK on satellite. Dr. Francis Collins, then head of the National Human Genome Research Institute, was by his side. Dr. Collins announced that the first draft of the human genome had been assembled. President Clinton's speech, carefully crafted by his speechwriters with Dr. Collins's input, included the words: "Today we are learning the language in which God created life. We are gaining ever more awe for the complexity, the beauty, and the wonder of God's most divine and sacred gift." Dr. Collins added "It is humbling for me, and awe-inspiring, to realize that we have caught the first glimpse of our own instruction book, previously known only to God."[11] Next time a doctor glances at your blood test results or listens to an explanation of your ailments and authoritatively pronounces a diagnosis and a remedy, remember the amazement in Dr. Collins' words. Your body is way more complex than that doctor is giving it credit for.

DNA (deoxyribonucleic acid) is a molecule essential to life. DNA is complicated, yet beautifully simple. It is a long thin molecule that under a microscope has a specific shape we call the double helix. DNA is often compared to a computer program. But I prefer to think of it as a recipe holding the instructions that tell our bodies how to function and develop. DNA exists in every cell in our bodies (and in all living organisms). It consists of sequences of nucleotides we call bases, arranged in pairs. There are only four different bases: adenine (A), guanine (G), cytosine (C) and thymine (T),

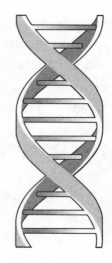

but there are three billion base pairs in the DNA code within each cell. Isn't it amazing that a code with only four letters can lead to something as complex as a person, with every one of us completely unique?

DNA can be thought of as the chemical unit of genetic inheritance while genes are a section of the DNA sequence that can express a specific genetic trait. Chromosomes contain a number of genes, and each human cell has twenty-three pairs of chromosomes (one from each parent). The DNA is so compressed within each cell that if all the DNA in your body's thirty trillion cells were put end to end, it would reach the sun (93 million miles away) and back over six hundred times. The Human Genome Project[12] identified around 22,000 genes that are arranged in the same order in all humans; in fact, 99.9 percent of the sequence is identical from person to person. The few differences found in specific base-pairs are enough to make us entirely distinct.

We are also made up of lots of different types of cells. A liver cell needs to perform very different functions than a nerve cell or bone cell. How is this possible when every cell has the same set of instructions? Quite incredibly, different sets of genes can be turned on or off by specific enzymes. Enzymes are proteins. Proteins are large, complex molecules made up of amino acids. We're going to look at genetics briefly in Chapter 3 but—spoiler alert—their significance matters less than you think! There is so much of life itself that we don't understand and probably never will. What's important to realize is that humans are part of all life on this planet and are beautifully designed to operate in conjunction with it. When we nourish our cells with activities like forest-bathing, dwelling on the beauty of the natural world, spending time with friends and family, and eating real, healthy, whole foods, they know what to do and will always be working together to get the body back in balance.

If reading about DNA is out of your usual comfort zone, I don't blame you. But in addition to needing critical thinking skills, which I mentioned earlier, to take control of your health you have to understand a little bit about the human body. The marketing machine of Big Pharma and the healthcare industry is assuming you won't dig into their claims. They are assuming you haven't bothered to understand some basic elements of the human body, the interconnectedness of its parts, and how little scientists and doctors actually know about how it works. They make claims and cite statistics with great authority. But they have no insight into this vessel you are living in, as you are an individual, not a data figure. When you apply your God-given critical thinking skills to your health, you already have all the context, knowledge, and background information you need. You are the best person—not your doctor, and certainly not Big Pharma—to make the best individual health decisions for yourself and your family.

The Amazing Human Body

When I was in high school taking Biology, we got to dissect a pig's heart and lungs. I was so enthralled by the experience I asked if I could take the pig organs home to study them further. My teacher said yes. The look on my mother's face was a mixture of horror and disgust when she found me wrist-deep in pig cadaver in my bedroom! But the ability to expand the pig's lungs by blowing air into them through a straw, and the interconnectedness of the pig's arteries and veins, ignited my fascination with what was inside, how it all worked, and why it sometimes breaks down. My combined study of health and faith over many years has convinced me that what was once alive but is now dead, like the pig I dissected or a human cadaver in the morgue, bears little resemblance. It's not our physical body that makes us human. We are more than molecules and chemicals. There are electrical impulses in our body that can be measured but we are not computers. The intricate dance of living processes, self-limiting and self-healing, is what makes the human body so incredible. It makes us, frankly, hard to kill. Unless it's a blunt force accident, an overwhelming toxin, or a genetic breakdown at the DNA level, we humans are surprisingly resilient.

The human body has sixty thousand miles of blood vessels in it. Traveling along those vessels are estimated to be over twenty trillion red blood cells—that's four to five million in every cubic centimeter of blood. Red blood cells are the most common cells in the body, estimated to make up about 80 percent of our thirty trillion human cells![13] I say "human" cells because, as we'll see in later chapters, our bodies contain a symbiotic soup of other organisms. Traditionally it's been estimated that the ratio of bacteria and other microscopic organisms, also known as the microbiome, to human cells is ten to one (ten times more microbes than human cells in our bodies). A more recent and perhaps more accurate estimate puts the number of microbial cells in the typical human body more in line with human cells, around the forty trillion mark.[14] These numbers are astounding when you think about them. Realizing we are teeming with nonhuman cohabitants puts into question the very nature of what it means to be human. In fact, there is a whole new avenue of science these days dedicated to looking at us as "holobionts."

A *holobiont* is a host heavily influenced by the complex microbial community that lives in and on it.[15] Our microbial cohabitants are critical to our good health in ways we have barely started to understand. They are not the pesky germs we have been led to believe by Western medicine.

Our bodies are wondrously complex. At a purely chemical level, there are about as many atoms in a single human cell as there are cells in the entire human body. If you remember from your high school chemistry class, an atom is the most basic unit of any matter. It consists of a nucleus of protons and neutrons surrounded by a cloud of electrons. Protons are positively charged, neutrons are electrically neutral, while electrons are negatively charged. The number of protons dictates the chemical properties of the atom which we have named as "elements." The periodic table lists out the elements in order of the number of protons they contain in their nucleus.

Hydrogen is the simplest element at the top of the periodic table. It consists of just one proton and one electron. It is critical for many processes in the body but most often you'll find two hydrogen atoms connected to an oxygen atom, denoted H_2O, otherwise known as water. Over 85 percent of the atoms in our body are hydrogen or oxygen. If you include carbon and nitrogen in the list, you'll be accounting for nearer 99 percent of atoms in our body. The other 1 percent includes 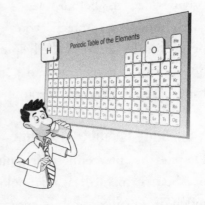 some forty other elements such as calcium, phosphorus, sodium, potassium, magnesium, zinc, and iodine. These are elements that your body needs for optimal health. Even beyond the cellular level, we are all made up of the same elements that exist in any matter in the universe. But we humans, somehow, are able to think and feel and make decisions!

All of our trillions of cells, which are actually made up of just a few simple elements, play very different roles and have different responsibilities in the body. The nerve fibers in our skin send signals to your brain at over 100 mph to make sure when your hand gets too close to the flame you remove it as quickly as possible. The nails on your fingers and toes formed from keratin provide protection and contribute to the dexterity and feeling in your digits. The perfectly designed hair on the top of your head is weight-for-weight comparable to steel in strength yet also elastic, able to stretch one and a half times its original length before breaking. Your hair protects your brain from radiation while helping keep the heat in and the cold out. Something to appreciate and ponder when you next find yourself in front of the mirror with a comb!

> **Oxygen and Free Radicals**
>
> Oxygen is an element in the periodic table with 8 protons (atomic number 8) but only 6 electrons. This makes it rather unstable and reactive. We more typically refer to oxygen in its molecular form O_2. This is when two oxygen atoms bond together by sharing electrons to make them stable.
>
> You may have heard of free radicals in your body. These are essentially unstable oxygen molecules looking to react.

Your Body Is Not a Machine

Despite the interconnected, multispecies, and miraculous nature of our bodies, in medical textbooks the body is treated as a machine, much like a car, with different systems like a drive train, engine, suspension or temperature control. When something goes wrong with a car you want the system specialist to work on it.

Machine metaphors for the human body are everywhere. Our metabolism is compared to an engine, our nervous system to electrical

circuitry, and our knees to hinges. The modern medical model continues to focus on separate systems. Doctors have become ever more
specialized. When something goes wrong in the human body, we
rely on skilled surgeons to switch out our hips, cardiologists to fix our
hearts, and endocrinologists to prescribe medication to improve our
hormones. Doctors are almost like automotive mechanics, replacing
parts much like a grease monkey replaces a faulty fuel pump.

But this medical, mechanized view of the human body is
completely wrong. The body is not the sum of its parts. Your body
is a single amazing entity with all sorts of complicated and graceful
systems that work together, as one, to keep you alive and operational.
There is no need to rely on man-made substances to keep it functioning, and if we treat our body well, there is no reason to expect it to
wear out too soon.

Medical doctors typically focus only on a single issue, set of symptoms or scores on a blood test. They assume your health problems can
be fixed by resolving that single issue or change it with a man-made
modality. In America this is called the "standard of care." This term
has arisen mainly in connection with malpractice lawsuits to establish
whether the doctor was negligent in their care. In the UK it's called
the "duty of care." It determines what the appropriate course of action
should be under certain circumstances. But reducing an individual's
body to a generalized "standard of care" is not only arrogant but akin
to playing God. God is sovereign over everything that is happening in
this world, from pandemics to pollution. He has chosen the time and
place to put you on Earth and provided healthcare options to fit your
particular needs as the unique human that you are. Your job is to be
open to learning about these options, understanding your own body,
and to trust that no professional in a white coat knows more about
your body than you do.

A basic grasp of the marvelous complexity of the human body will help you understand why your medical professional doesn't have all the answers and why only you, living with your body every moment of every day, can be the best person to be in charge of your health. Once you have some fundamental knowledge, you will find that you will often instinctively know what your body needs. This knowledge will help you navigate a broken healthcare industry to use what is helpful and avoid the rest.

I've therefore picked three of the most amazing parts of the human body to introduce you to. I've chosen to highlight these features for their diversity, elements of mystery, and, most of all, how they contribute to your good health.

Let's start with **the human eyeball**. The eye is one of the best examples of "irreducible complexity." This term can be applied to any system of interacting parts in which the removal of any one part destroys the function of the entire system. It lends weight to the logic that complex organisms could not have developed gradually over time through slight modifications but instead were created instantly as a whole. We can think of the entire human body in this way but will focus on just the eye to make the point. Charles Darwin even admitted the complexity of the eye in *The Origin of Species*:

> *To suppose that the eye, with all its inimitable contrivances for adjusting the focus to different distances, for admitting different amounts of light and for the correction of spherical and chromatic aberration could have been formed by natural selection, seems, I freely confess, absurd in the highest degree.*[16]

Our best engineers have never developed a camera lens anywhere near the intricacy of the human eye. If you stood on a mountain on a dark night, a typical human eyeball could see a match lit fifty miles away! Your eye is actually not a single organ but an amazing system of interrelated parts including the retina, iris, pupil, cornea, lens, and optic nerve.

The eye includes two types of special light-sensitive cells called rods and cones. There are about seven million cones packed into a small area behind the retina that are responsible for color vision and seeing tiny details in sharp focus. There are about 130 million rod-shaped cells which are 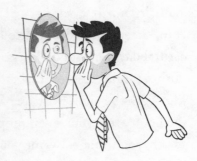 used for seeing in black and white, particularly in darker conditions. When light hits the eye, it is focused by the cornea and enters through the pupil. The iris controls how much light is let in. It passes through the lens, which further focuses the light onto the retina at the back of the eye. There it strikes the rods or cones and is converted into an electrical signal that is sent to the brain via the optic nerve. A special section of the brain called the visual cortex then interprets the electrical pulses to enable us to see images. But what images they are! Filled with depth, contrast, and texture.

Did you take that walk outside yet? Did you focus through your eyes on what you saw, and marvel at the beauty and diversity? As we've discussed, science is only just starting to wake up to the benefits to our health and wellbeing of being outdoors in nature.[17] Much of the benefit is gained through what we see through our eyes. It's actually our incredible brains that do most of the seeing. Think about when you saw a silhouette in the dark but knew instantly who it was, or a flash of movement in the sky and knew it was a bird. Your eyeballs wouldn't work without your brain. Plus, it's been found that there are vitamin D receptor sites in various structures of the eyeball so don't be too quick to put on your sunglasses.[18]

Doctors have only recently realized the indirect effects of losing your sight. It is not just that you cannot see and become a higher risk of having accidents and injuries; your body cannot regulate its circadian rhythm if it cannot tell the difference between night and day. Your circadian rhythm is your internal body clock that is tuned to natural daylight and darkness. Disrupting it has been linked to risks of cardiovascular disease, diabetes, depression, and even cancer.[19] Those who work the night shift are particularly susceptible. The blind are too.

Look after your eyes; proper nutrition is key. But my point here goes beyond that—I want you to look at your eyeballs in a new way. No pun intended! They are not just the spheres at the top of your head that enable you to navigate your surroundings. And your eye health doesn't belong only to the realm of an ophthalmologist (eye doctor). Your eyes are an integral part of the amazing human body and a prime example of its wondrous complexity.

It's easy to appreciate how incredible our eyes are. After all, when you're attracted to someone, you often notice the intelligence in their eyes, or the tint of violet, or sparkle when they laugh. But most of us don't spend a lot of time pondering the most hardworking organ in the human body, **the liver**. Now you thought I was going to land on the brain or the heart next and not the unphotogenic lump of meat that dominates the right side of our internal cavity, but the liver is truly remarkable and deserves recognition.

Your liver is the largest organ in your body (after your skin) and carries out at least five hundred different functions. One of its main jobs is to process the nutrients in the food that you eat so they are available to the rest of your body, storing some of them for future use. It makes bile, a yellowish fluid that helps break down food, particularly fats, with excess bile stored in your gallbladder for later use.

Your liver is the filter and waste disposal crew for your whole body. It metabolizes external chemicals, like alcohol or drugs, that can cause harm to your body. It also removes stuff your body no longer needs, such as damaged cells, proteins, and excess hormones. It produces new proteins, which are constantly being used in your body to repair and create muscles, skin, and bones. Some of these proteins are responsible for blood clotting, so a damaged liver can result in uncontrolled bleeding or bruising. The liver is also in charge of balancing your blood sugar to provide you with energy and is the chief blood recycling factory breaking down old or damaged red blood cells and creating new ones. The liver plays a major role in regulating hormones such as estrogen, testosterone, cortisol, adrenaline, and thyroid hormone.

This is just a simplified sample of what this incredible organ does for you. Not to mention it is the only organ in the human body that can regenerate itself!

Knowing this, you can see why a myriad of individual symptoms can result from an impaired liver. As an example, one of the health challenges I had to address when I took control of my own health at age forty was chronic eczema. My eczema was so severe on my arms that I couldn't wear sleeves when traveling to Europe in the depths of winter. Any fabric would irritate my skin and cause bleeding and intense discomfort. I went to the dermatologist I had used in the past. But the topical creams she recommended only made the situation worse. Another doctor recommended anti-inflammatories such as Aleve (naproxen). But that didn't help. It was only after I found my way to acupuncture and learned about energy medicine that I found relief. The acupuncturist was able to use the tools at his disposal to diagnose that my liver was compromised, and this was affecting my skin. I was skeptical at first. How could an acupuncturist even know that I had a liver issue? And how could that liver issue be connected to skin issues? Still, I followed this naturopathic doctor's protocol, which focused on improving liver function. He promised it would heal my skin, and it did! The first step was cutting out medications, such as the creams and anti-inflammatories prescribed by my doctors—these prescriptions can put undue stress on the liver. The second step was cleaning up my diet and better managing my stress.

The liver is such a resilient powerhouse, it can continue working even when two-thirds of it has been damaged. Often no symptoms are felt until beyond even this critical level. It is estimated that up to 25 percent of individuals in the US and worldwide have nonalcoholic fatty liver disease (NAFLD) and it is rising exponentially with each passing decade. NAFLD is principally caused by excess sugar and processed foods but may have no obvious abdominal symptoms until it has progressed to nonalcoholic steatohepatitis (NASH) causing cirrhosis (scarring) which is much harder to reverse and often leads to liver cancer. This is why it is so important to understand how to care for this magnificent organ. And it gives you a glimpse as to why a symptom-focused approach to health often leads to unintended negative side effects without optimizing your health or your body's abilities, as God designed them.

From the sense of sight to the powerhouse of biological processes I want to wrap up this mini-tour of the body with the highway of our electrical network, the **vagus nerve**. Vagus is Latin for "wandering" as this nerve meanders throughout the body from the head and neck throughout your torso connecting all of your organs to your brain. It is the largest nerve system in the human body after the spinal column.

The vagus nerve is responsible for those butterflies in your stomach when you're experiencing stress, fear, or excitement. It connects to the tongue, the vocal cords, lungs, heart, and even down to the genitals. It influences digestion, metabolism, your breathing, your heartbeat, swallowing, and your overall response to stress. The vagus nerve may not have as many admirers as the eye or the liver but that's probably because scientists are only just starting to understand its amazing significance to our health.

The vagus nerve works hand in glove with the Enteric Nervous System (ENS), which is embedded in the walls of your intestines and stomach and known as your "second brain" due to the estimated five hundred million neurons it comprises. The ENS is pretty cool in itself as it controls your digestion, through muscle contractions, as well as maintaining an optimal chemical environment so digestive enzymes can do their job. Plus, it protects against potential invaders like pathogenic bacteria, signaling for diarrhea, if needed, or alerting 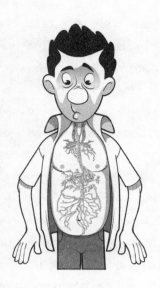 the head brain to initiate vomiting. But it's the vagus nerve that carries those messages to the brain. It is the two-way communication system between your brain and most of your other organs.

While more traditional approaches to health and wellbeing have always sought to understand the interconnectedness of the organs of the body with each other and the brain, research into the vagus nerve has only taken off in the last decade or so. One of these initiatives is known as SPARC which stands for Stimulating Peripheral Activity to Relieve Conditions and was launched in 2016.[20] Some of the vagus nerve stimulation techniques have shown great promise to treat a variety of conditions and we'll meet it again in Part II. For now I want you to think about the implications for your health of this interconnectedness and how little doctors and scientists really know about the self-regulating power of the human body.

Your vagus nerve (also referred to as the parasympathetic nervous system) can be thought of as the chief "calmer" or "brake" in the body. It is the polar opposite to the sympathetic nervous system which revs you up and is responsible for that fight-or-flight response. When your body is working well it moves between these two states easily. Functional medicine practitioners diagnose patients with *low vagal tone* when the vagus nerve is not functioning well. Low vagal tone can have a variety of root causes but is indicated by prolonged stress often coupled with anxiety or depression and the inability to self-calm even when the stressor is no longer present.

Symptoms of low vagal tone can be very wide-ranging, affecting different organs in unexpected ways. But this syndrome of symptoms most commonly includes gastrointestinal problems as the ultimate cause of vagus irritation often begins in the gut. Excess alcohol or spicy foods, for example, aggravate the vagus nerve, and even poor posture (anyone sitting at their desk all day like me?) can enflame it. Stress and fatigue are common culprits too and may be why prolonged stress has been found to be so damaging to our bodies.

Keeping your magnificent, interconnected, and elegantly designed vagus nerve happy and healthy is critical to your long-term health and wellbeing. A compromised vagus nerve just may be the under-lying cause of weight gain, inflammation, emotional ups and downs or other weird symptoms nagging at you. By understanding what the vagus nerve is and how it affects your health you can understand the non-invasive treatment options open to you that would be considered "alternative" by conventional medicine and why they work. We'll look at some of these in Chapter 2.

The Big Picture

When your hand gets too close to a fire, you feel pain so you know that fire is bad for your skin, and you instinctively pull your hand away. When you put contaminated food in your body, your body knows that rotten food is harmful and acts to get the bad bacteria out as quick as possible, which sends you running to the bathroom. When your body has a problem, it tells you. We call that a "symptom." But when your head aches, your body is not telling you its deficient in Tylenol or Advil. Instead, it is signaling to you that something is wrong: Perhaps you've been staring at a computer screen too long without a break, perhaps you haven't drunk enough water and are dehydrated, perhaps you forgot to have lunch. Or maybe that headache is because you are worried about a loved one who is in the hospital, or you've had an argument with your spouse.

God has created the world we live in and has perfectly designed humans to live in harmony with that world. Our intelligently designed bodies are incredibly complex, supernaturally so, and capable of staggering feats of mental and physical prowess. But they are also astoundingly simple. If we treat our bodies well, they will carry us far. Our bodies will self-regulate and self-heal, but only if we treat them right. This kind of healing was well known to past generations but has been all but lost, mostly due to the marketing machine of the modern medical and pharmaceutical industry.

Points to Remember

1. God has perfectly designed our bodies in harmony with the beautifully designed universe.
2. We cannot separate ourselves or our health from the other living organisms on the planet. Plants, animals, and microbes are all part of the same synergistic ecosystem we are.
3. Doctors and researchers have only scratched the surface of how the amazing human body functions.
4. Your body does not operate as separate systems or organs but an integrated whole so only a holistic approach to health will optimize longevity and function.

CHAPTER 2

Medicine for the Soul

Growing up Jewish, it was the in-joke that your parents wanted you to be either a lawyer or a doctor. But in my family's case an accountant would be acceptable. My dad founded an accounting firm that he eventually sold to another company, as none of us kids wanted to follow in his footsteps. While being a lawyer is generally considered a respectable profession, even admired, there is a known downside. In divorces or corporate takeovers, only the lawyers win with their exorbitant fees. Becoming a doctor, on the other hand, seems to convey a kind of halo effect. I often wonder why MDs, perhaps more than any other professionals, are put on such a pedestal. After all, healthcare is an industry just like any other. There needs to be money made. And when you think about it, what incentivizes doctors or any other healthcare practitioners to make you fully well? When you are in vibrant good health, you don't need the system anymore. Why should doctors help you find lifestyle and nutritional cures that do not necessitate payment to the medical establishment?

The healthcare industry was estimated to be $4.2 trillion in the US in 2021[1] (that is twelve zeros!) and growing exponentially every year. This industry includes hospitals, doctors, pharmaceutical companies, medical device makers, as well as the equipment, like disposable masks, gloves, and gowns, and the technology that supports it all. In 2020 the amount spent by the pharmaceutical industry on direct-to-consumer TV advertising alone in the US was $4.6 billion (nine zeros), which was 75 percent of all TV advertising spending.[2]

The US is one of only two countries in the world that allow direct-to-consumer marketing of pharmaceutical drugs. New Zealand is the other one. I find it so strange, and incredibly off-putting, to see adverts for serious and potentially dangerous drugs or surgical procedures on regular TV and billboards as if they were selling candy or the latest skincare product. The push to normalize the daily use of pharmaceutical drugs is nothing more than great marketing by a hugely profitable industry. As America's health declines, big business profits soar.[3]

Doctors are the front men of this business. You trust them to assess what your health problem is and direct you to the services and products that will solve it. To earn this privilege a typical medical doctor goes to college for several years and enters medical residency where they work long hours for basic pay. By then the aspiring doctor often has an enormous amount of debt. The students who manage to pass their medical school studies excel at understanding biology, chemistry, many different diseases, body parts, drug names, and procedures. No wonder we respect and revere them. Graduating from medical school is an academic feat, one that requires perseverance, determination, and hard work. But even though it is difficult to become a qualified doctor, their course of study and subsequent work experience doesn't make them all-knowing and infallible as to what ails you as an individual.

A Less-than-Noble Profession

Before the twentieth century, doctors struggled to make a reasonable living. Other than a few who attended to the very wealthy, the medical profession was considered a low-grade occupation. Surgeons and the old-style apothecaries were viewed even lower. Surgery was considered a trade rather than a profession, akin to a butcher! Most people in the 1900s believed that common sense and their native intelligence could help them resolve their health problems with more success than a medical professional.

Doctors often held wildly different views on how to address various ailments. In fact, there was very little uniformity among medical doctors. This is one of the factors that led to a general distrust of medical authority. That distrust was in large part well-founded. Consider the case of Dr. Ignaz Semmelweis.[4] In the mid-1800s Semmelweis, a Hungarian physician, noticed that women attended to by medical doctors during childbirth, rather than by midwives, more often succumbed to what was called puerperal fever (also known as childbed fever). Some records indicate numbers as high as 50 percent of mothers who gave birth under doctor supervision died. Dr. Semmelweis noted that doctors often came straight to the delivery room after dissecting corpses in the cadaver lab as they sought to learn about the human body or practice surgery. Once he instigated handwashing with a chlorinated lime solution in the hospital where he worked, the maternal mortality rate dropped to zero. Instead of embracing basic hygiene, his contemporaries dismissed his methods. They found the idea that they should wash their hands offensive and insulting. Semmelweis endured years of ridicule before finally dying in a mental asylum in 1865 at age forty-seven shortly after being beaten by guards when he tried to escape. His methods weren't fully adopted until the 1940s with the full understanding of antiseptic conditions and the invention of antibiotics.

Another example of this discord amongst doctors and scientists of the nineteenth and early twentieth centuries is still raging today. Louis Pasteur was a French scientist who died in 1895 and is known as the "Father of Germ Theory." He gave his name to the process of Pasteurization, heating milk products to kill any harmful bacteria. However, a colleague of Pasteur's in the French Academy of Science, Antoine Béchamp, had a competing theory called the Terrain Theory. While Pasteur asserted that microorganisms in the environment spread and caused disease (with every disease the result of a specific germ), Béchamp argued that a specific germ cannot create an infection or a disease unless the state of the body (the terrain) allowed it. A weak immune system or malnutrition can provide a breeding ground for pathogens to cause illness while a healthy body will remain unaffected.

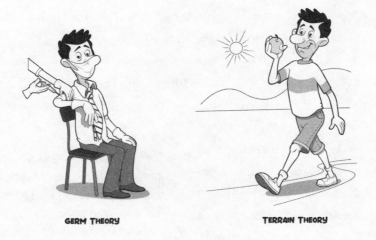

GERM THEORY   TERRAIN THEORY

Pasteur was better connected than Béchamp and his theory became accepted and promoted amongst his peers. The idea that germs make us sick is the basis for much of the conventional medical industry today. Meanwhile Béchamp died in poverty and disdain. We now know that terrain theory is extremely important while germ theory is shortsighted at best. Our insight may have improved but human nature has not changed much, being on full ugly display during the Covid years.

Discord amongst professionals has served greatly to advance knowledge and understanding. Freedom to choose how to address a health issue leads to innovative solutions that can be compared for efficacy. Natural forces of free competition will then ensure the most cost-effective and beneficial solution will be available to individuals. At the turn of the twentieth century there were three main sectors of the medical profession—the eclectics (those that relied mainly on botanicals, also known as herbalists), the homeopaths, and the regular doctors.

The founder of **homeopathy** was Samuel Hahnemann, a German physician. It gets its name from their main doctrinal stance that disease can be cured by compounds that produce the same symptoms when given to a healthy person; the "law of similars." The other main foundation of the approach is that the effects of the compound can be heightened by administering them in minute doses.

The homeopaths dubbed the regular doctors "allopaths" supposedly curing by opposites using high quantities of their often-toxic drugs. Part of the appeal of homeopathy to the masses was that it encouraged a deep relationship between doctor and patient, insisting that symptoms were only the perception of disease and not the disease itself. The reduced dosages also provided a welcome alternative to the pharmacological excesses of conventional physicians.

The eclectics and homeopaths still believed in scientific training and the curriculum of their medical schools was almost indistinguishable

The most commonly known homeopathic treatment today is probably **arnica**, which is a natural herb that looks like a small sunflower and is toxic to the liver if ingested in large amounts. The homeopathic remedy is highly diluted and useful for muscle aches and pains, and especially bruising. You can take it in small tablets that dissolve under the tongue or in roll-on preparations.

from the orthodox schools. While the American Medical Association (AMA) spent years attempting to discredit unorthodox physicians and bar them from membership, commercial pressures led to a temporary truce. In 1903 a new code of ethics was adopted that ignored the kind of medicine doctors actually practiced and the medical schools mostly merged.[5]

Then along came John D. Rockefeller, who had already made his fortune by then at the helm of Standard Oil. He had earned a reputation as a ruthless businessman always focused on the next great venture that would increase profits. Although he had consistently given to charitable causes, he was advised to improve his public image and focus on neglected causes like public health and education.[6] The Rockefeller Medical Foundation was formed with a large infusion of cash given to the AMA. One of the first projects supported was a survey of all the medical schools in the US to assess the quality of the education. The survey was carried out by Abraham Flexnor, a teacher working for the Carnegie Foundation, while his brother Simon Flexnor, a physician, was head of the Rockefeller Institute for Medical Research. The resulting report published in 1910[7] had a lot of positive ideas like requiring a science degree as a prerequisite for medical school, ensuring students received clinical experience in hospitals as part of their training and the use of ongoing research to ensure doctors stayed up to date on current advances. However, the most famous conclusions of the Flexnor report were the ratings given to individual medical schools with the call for the lowest rated to be closed. Given the inherent bias toward the orthodox medical teachings now marketed as "scientific medicine," those focusing on eclectic or homeopathic medicine received the lowest grades and most were forced to close. The Flexnor report is credited with driving the demise of these sectors of the medical profession in favor of the singular approach preferred by the now industry-funded AMA.[8, 9]

The Tide Turns

The twentieth century saw a huge flurry of medical invention going mainstream such as the stethoscope, the microscope, use of X-rays and the electrocardiogram. The patient could clearly see the expertise needed of a trained physician to understand aspects of their body they were unable to interpret. The physician's status started rising.

The surgeons became the real heroes though once antiseptic methods were employed and surgery became a lot safer, almost miraculous in what it could achieve.

Many physicians found that honing their practice to a particular specialty would bring in higher revenues from a broader cross section of customers. The physicians and surgeons relied on referrals though which encouraged getting along with their peers. Consequently, the diversity of thought and ideas seen previously started to diminish; much to our detriment today.

> It's important to ask questions of your doctor as to why they recommend a particular form of treatment. Make sure your doctors are thinking for themselves and are not just going along with the medical consensus to make their lives easier. Ask for the latest studies and what experience the doctor has in treating that condition with the plan they are recommending for you. Does it cure and reverse the condition?

At the same time, all this medical invention needed large capital outlays and this is where big business saw the opportunity in entering the profession. Hospital systems started popping up run by administrators, and doctors sought to work there for the guaranteed salaries they could earn. No longer would clinicians want to give part of their time to the medical schools to educate the next generation. This began the disconnect between scientific discoveries and clinical practice.

The mid-twentieth century also saw the first forms of health insurance introduced.[10] The idea was to spread the cost of diagnosis and medical treatment so they would become affordable to many more people. But to keep premiums low, only certain approved procedures were covered. This design influenced behavior as you were more likely to opt for the treatment that was covered by the plan you had already paid for. Those businesses offering the earliest plans had a vested interest in selling the new commercial treatments they had funded.

It is human nature to be distracted by the latest "shiny object" but newer doesn't always mean better or best. There's no doubt that, for certain illnesses anyway, the progress of medical science has saved lives. But we have done a disservice to ourselves to automatically assume the newer version is optimal for our current needs. While cars with an automatic transmission were embraced as easier to drive, I will always prefer a manual transmission. I have yet to be convinced there is a better alternative to a simple piece of paper and a pencil for flexibility, versatility, clarity, and ease of use.

One "old" discovery that never seems to go out of fashion is hygiene. Simple hygiene does not get the credit it deserves but was revolutionary in preventing many of the illnesses that were common before the mid-twentieth century. Not only handwashing but public sanitation, indoor plumbing, pasteurization of milk products, and refrigeration of food. It's hard to imagine the general living situation of the majority of the population before these inventions became commonplace but abject squalor would not be too strong a description. Malnutrition was common and overcrowding in the cities meant a good night's sleep, something most of us expect to get these days, was hard to come by. You had to work long hours to make ends meet and working conditions were poor.[11]

Bacteriology and its implications for hygiene as well as nutrition were important components of the medical school curriculum in the nineteenth century. However, with all the scientific progress made in the next hundred years, the curriculum got so crowded with all the new diagnostic tools and procedures that these basics were relegated to barely a mention. Obvious malnutrition became less common as wages and conditions improved. Perhaps limiting the study of nutrition in medical school was deemed an acceptable loss as more technical advances took precedence.

The biggest contrast between what was learned in medical school a hundred years ago and today is undoubtedly the weight now given to studying drugs and choosing which drug can cure a diagnosed disease or illness. Understanding this shift is the final piece of the puzzle we need to look at to understand how the medical profession got so one-dimensional as it is today.

The Rise of the Drug Makers

My mum was a pharmacist. She owned a couple of drugstores at either end of the small suburb where we lived. They were the kind of old-fashioned pharmacy you don't see very often nowadays. In addition to picking up your prescription, you could find all sorts of useful household items, over-the-counter remedies and even gifts like fancy soaps and fragrances. Mum knew most of her customers well and she helped them with their health issues over the years. If their doctor had prescribed a drug, she would explain what it did, how it worked and side effects to watch out for. She also treated many common health problems and injuries with over-the-counter products. It was perfectly normal in England to go to your pharmacist first to find health solutions, most of which didn't require a prescription. I found this not to be the case in the US years later when I arrived in 1998 to start my new job in New York. I'd been traveling overseas for a few weeks and had picked up a nasty stomach bug. I went to the nearest chain drugstore I found, asked to speak to the pharmacist, and proceeded to tell her all my symptoms. She looked at me incredulously and stated that I needed to go find a doctor. I called my mum instead!

The simple remedy was plenty of clear chicken broth (which replaces lost electrolytes), and plain easy to digest foods we used to call the BRAT diet. My amazing human body with all its inbuilt intelligence then did the rest. My immune system attacked the bug

BRAT diet for an upset stomach
Bread, Rice, Applesauce and Toast are a good guide for getting through an upset stomach with diarrhea and/ or vomiting.

and eventually restored my body to equilibrium. It was stronger for the fight with no lasting side effects. A doctor's visit would have most likely resulted in a prescription. It may or may not have shortened the course of my discomfort but is more than likely to have unbalanced my body in an unforeseen way.

The pharmaceutical industry is really as old as the medical profession itself. Ancient civilizations across the world documented medicinal preparations made from plants, animals or minerals. You didn't need a medical school degree to use these substances with knowledge passed down through the generations. But purity and consistent efficacy were hard to maintain.

The first compounds to be isolated and purified for medicinal use were mercury and arsenic dating back more than 2,000 years. We now know them to be extremely toxic but up until the end of the nineteenth century and even early twentieth century they were used to cure a variety of ailments including syphilis in products like salvarsan (an arsenic derivative) and calomel (chief ingredient being mercury).

It wasn't until penicillin was able to be made in large quantities in the 1940s that these toxic compounds fell out of favor. Think how recent that is! Penicillin's discovery is credited to bacteriologist Alexander Fleming. Back in 1929 he was studying staphylococcal bacteria in his lab when he noticed mold growing on some of his specimen jars, and the bacteria close to it had died. It took many more years for the significance to be appreciated and still more years to develop the means to grow sufficient quantities for medical use. But penicillin revolutionized the treatment of severe bacterial infections including syphilis and especially for soldiers wounded in World War II. The age of the antibiotic had begun.[12]

However, natural-derived products like penicillin were the exception rather than the rule with the majority of products developed by industrial chemical giants that had grown out of the oil companies. Morris Beale's 1949 book—*The Drug Story: A Factological History of America's $10,000,000,000 Drug Cartel, Its Methods, Operations, Hidden Ownership, Profits and Terrific Impact on the Health of the American People*[15]—recounts how John D. Rockefeller had been impressed with the big meatpacking houses which processed and sold every part of the hog. The book documents various medicinal products derived from raw petroleum, and tells the history of many of today's well-known

Connections to the World Health Organization (WHO)

Beyond the US the Rockefeller Foundation took its special brand of "scientific philanthropy" global with its International Health Board laying the groundwork for the League of Nations Health Organization after World War I. This organization eventually morphed into the WHO with Rockefeller being its principal patron covering most of its operating budget.[13] Interestingly, another capitalist foundation has today taken over Rockefeller's role as principal patron to the WHO. Set up on the ingenious principles introduced by Rockefeller known as "philanthropy for profit" the Bill and Melinda Gates Foundation controversially has an outsized role in today's global health agenda.[14]

pharmaceutical companies, including overseas entanglements with the chemical companies of Hitler's Third Reich. It also describes the reach of the Rockefeller empire to the news media enabling the control of a wide range of advertising assets. The resulting propaganda ensured a growing market for the drugmakers products. It's amazing how relevant this book is seventy years later.[16] Meanwhile Rockefeller himself continued to rely on homeopathy and died at nearly ninety-eight years old![17]

But innovation wasn't all bad with other successes of the early twentieth century beyond antibiotics being the isolation of individual hormones like insulin and understanding their significance in the body. The recognition that certain diseases are a deficiency in a compound secreted by the body enabled cures to be administered once they could be manufactured by pharmaceutical companies. Insulin is secreted by the pancreas and essential to break down glucose for use as energy by cells and manage the amount of glucose circulating in the blood. Without insulin diabetics succumb to uncontrolled blood sugar causing damage to blood vessels, nerves, eyes, and kidneys.

For fifty years the manufacture of insulin was through extraction from pigs and sheep once it was determined their insulin was similar enough to that produced by humans. It took until the 1980s for science to develop the capability to manufacture synthetic human insulin. Similar manufacturing processes were employed to create another critical human secretion known as Epo (erythropoietin) which is an enzyme produced in the kidneys that signals bone marrow to manufacture red blood cells. For the thousands of patients with failing kidneys suffering from anemia this drug, known as Epogen, has been a godsend.

> Today we distinguish between **type 1 diabetes**, which used to be called juvenile or child-onset diabetes and is an inadequate secretion or total absence of insulin. It results from a damaged pancreas or the body attacking the cells of the pancreas as an auto-immune disease. **Type 2 diabetes** is diagnosed when there is poor glucose management resulting from lifestyle choices which is reversible. We'll cover diabetes in Chapter 7.

With these new tools at their disposal doctors were seen as miracle workers now able to save people from infections and severe illnesses that would have previously resulted in death. It didn't matter that for every lifesaving drug there were hundreds that did little for long-term health. The manufacturers of these products grew into large corporations as they reaped the profits. But like all successful companies they had to keep searching for the next great product. In medicine this means looking to cure different bodily afflictions and, as we shall see, inventing some afflictions along the way.

For the doctors in medical school, it means an ever-swelling curriculum of understanding the tools available to them. The pharmaceutical companies make sure their products are top of mind with advertising, scholarships, and consulting fees to professors. In fact, the hallowed Harvard Medical School received the lowest grade by a national group that rates how well medical schools monitor and control drug-industry influence.[18] It noted that 149 professors had financial ties to Pfizer and 130 to Merck. Taking a look at any medical school curriculum[19] you can see plenty of anatomy, biology, chemistry, genetics, and immunology; however, there is an overwhelming emphasis on pharmacology within clinical practice. There is rarely a single mention of nutrition or validated natural methods for managing a body out of balance (as the second half of this chapter will get into). A recent reflection of the impact of the Flexnor report on modern medicine suggests that the pendulum has swung too far, saying "As medical schools clamored for funding from wealthy capitalists to achieve new standards, they lost autonomy and adopted unsaid values that were possibly a danger to humanity."[20]

Pharmaceutical sponsorship of doctors persists beyond medical school with the requirement for doctors to attend Continuing Medical Education (CME) programs. It is estimated that the pharmaceutical industry sponsors 40–60 percent of CME which has long been identified as questionable from an ethical standpoint.[21] Besides the marketing dollars aimed at you, the consumer, the vast majority of the massive marketing budget Big Pharma wields is aimed directly at the doctors with an army of sales representatives at their disposal. By the start of the twenty-first century, doctors have come to rely on these perks such as dinners, sporting events, and even overseas trips and cash. Some get paid consulting fees to speak or write articles supporting the use of a particular drug. After the expense of medical training and the long hours of working with patients it is difficult for even the most ethical doctor to avoid.[22]

If all you have is a hammer, then every patient who walks through your door is a nail.

Drugs Often Do More Harm than Good

While some drugs in use today replace a missing substance that the body itself creates and needs to carry out its processes, the vast majority are compounds that have been observed to act on a symptom or something that is going awry in the body. After testing thousands of chemical compounds, a pharmaceutical company will pick a handful that look promising to test for safety and then efficacy to address the stated need.

Drugs are classified in all sorts of ways such as what disease they address, what action they instill in the body, what their active ingredient is, or how they are manufactured. Perhaps they are derived from a natural substance in nature, perhaps entirely made in a lab. But as consumers our attitude toward them tends to be the same—if I take this it will improve my health. But that is a very dangerous assumption.

For a start, did you know that the majority of drugs don't actually work for most people? This is a commonly known fact in the medical and pharmaceutical industries but one that is not often shared with consumers. As Dr. Allen Roses, a senior executive of GlaxoSmithKline, one of the world's largest pharmaceutical companies, said at a public meeting in 2003: "The vast majority of drugs—more than 90 percent—only work in 30 or 50 percent of the people."[23] While the goal of this meeting was to improve response rates, some of the statistics quoted on therapeutic effects of drugs to treat common ailments included:

- Alzheimer's   1 out of 3 patients (30 percent effective)
- Arthritis   1 out of 2 patients (50 percent effective)
- Autoimmune   1 out of 2 patients (50 percent effective)
- Cancer   1 out of 4 patients (25 percent effective)
- Migraines   1 out of 2 patients (50 percent effective)
- Osteoporosis   1 out of 2 patients (50 percent effective)
- Diabetes   1 out of 2 patients (50 percent effective)

You could hope that you're in the positive group or more typically your doctor will just switch you to another drug with a different profile to see if it does any better. This might be an acceptable path if the substances involved were otherwise benign. But unfortunately that is not the case.

Pharmaceutical drugs are actually the third leading cause of death in the US and Europe.[24] According to one representative study of emergency room visits across the US between 2017 and 2019,[25] there were an estimated six visits for every one thousand people due to medication reactions (in most cases taken as prescribed). Extrapolating these figures suggests that over 2 million people in the US visit a hospital due to adverse drug reactions every year. Common culprits were anticoagulants, diabetes medications, antibiotics, analgesics (pain relievers), and antihistamines. The number of adverse reactions that do not result in a hospital visit are many times higher.

One of the most problematic drugs you may not have considered is acetaminophen, brand name Tylenol in the US and paracetamol or Panadol in other parts of the world. According to a recent study by the US National Institutes of Health, acetaminophen is responsible for 56,000 emergency room visits, 2,600 hospitalizations, and 500 deaths every year due to its toxic effects on the liver. Around half are accidental overdoses from taking multiple medications each having acetaminophen as an ingredient. It is recognized as the number one cause of acute liver failure in the US and the UK. Despite being heavily used for many decades to the tune of billions of doses worldwide every year, there is still no consensus on how acetaminophen actually works. This is a particular concern given its widespread use and clear toxicity to the liver. As we saw from Chapter 1, the liver is involved in so many bodily processes that any negative impact on it will affect your whole body and multiple aspects of your health. In fact, scientists are just starting to amass evidence on the more insidious effects of acetaminophen which can occur gradually over time such as lower fertility rates in men[26] and risks of developmental disorders in babies and toddlers.[27]

Switching to another type of pain reliever such as ibuprofen (Motrin) or naproxen (Aleve) won't improve the situation much either as this whole class of drugs have been shown to elevate cardiovascular risks and cause gastrointestinal problems. The similar drug Vioxx was recalled in 2004 due to the number of excess heart attacks and sudden cardiac deaths it was responsible for with its Big Pharma manufacturer Merck held liable for withholding the safety data.[28]

Many different types of drugs have been found to have anticholinergic effects[29] which means they block the action of the neurotransmitter acetylcholine in the brain. Nerve cells in your brain release acetylcholine to enable signals to be sent to neighboring cells. Interfering with this mechanism can result in a range of symptoms from instability and balance problems to delirium and general cognitive decline. The effects can usually be reversed on stopping the drugs. But the great concern here is the large range of drugs which have been found to have these effects including antidepressants, antihistamines, blood pressure medication, and drugs for incontinence. Studies have shown that taking one or more of these drugs results in an increased risk for dementia and Alzheimer's.[30] In fact, a common treatment for patients diagnosed with Parkinson's disease is an anticholinergic drug to reduce tremors but this may be why patients with Parkinson's are at an increased risk for dementia.

Another little talked about side effect of drugs is the nutrient deficiencies they induce. The best-known example of this is the use of statins to lower cholesterol resulting in a depletion of Coenzyme Q10 which manifests as general aches and pains. But statins[31] also deplete selenium (essential for optimal thyroid health) and vitamin D (critical to immune function and many other processes). Several drugs deplete magnesium (vital in blood pressure and glucose management) including pain medications, blood pressure medications, antacids, and antibiotics. Oral contraceptives and hormone replacement therapy also deplete magnesium, but more concerning is their impact on vitamin B_6, a deficiency of which can cause depression.[32]

Big Pharma would like to keep this information from you or at least let you know they are there to help with another product when the first causes additional health problems. What's more, after years of trying to discredit the vitamin and nutrient sellers they are now getting in on the act by trying to hijack basic supplements to sell at high prices. Vitamin D and omega-3s are most commonly found in prescription form, but now the cheap supplement NAC (N-acetyl-L-Cysteine) is in Big Pharma's crosshairs. NAC became a star for its beneficial effect in preventing and recovering from Covid-19, but its effects are so powerful that Big Pharma is trying to get it banned[33] as a simple supplement so they can sell it at a high price via prescription. In fact, if you did end up in a hospital due to Tylenol toxicity, you're likely to be given NAC in the emergency room as it helps prevent liver damage due to its mechanism of increasing glutathione, your body's chief detoxer.

Speaking of toxins, which we'll get into in Chapter 4, the drugs you're ingesting are not just the pure active ingredient, which, as we've seen, is problematic enough. But in order to make the drugs palatable, circumvent our regular digestive processes, and make them shelf stable, there are many additional chemicals and additives included which create additional challenges for our bodies to deal with.

In many ways we have come full circle from the pre-twentieth century when the medical industry was viewed with suspicion and people relied on their common sense and community to deal with health problems. With the miraculous developments of antibiotics and biologic drugs that could replace human secretions it led to blind trust in physicians and their methods, and eventually the complete abstinence from personal bodily autonomy in knowing what is best for you and your family. I want to help you become a better consumer who is not swayed by the marketing machine telling you what you need. It's important to educate yourself. You need to know what Big Pharma is trying to hide: there are almost always much safer alternatives you can turn to when you have a health problem. Many of them have been known to humans for hundreds of years and now have up-to-date science to understand why and how they work so well.

Alternative or Smart?

Last week, my son Ethan complained of a sore throat as he was getting ready for school. I suggested he eat a teaspoon of the raw organic honey I happened to be pulling out of the cupboard. He came home from school that afternoon incredulous that the honey had worked, and he felt fine. The healing power of honey, a natural antibiotic, has been known for centuries. (Or you may prefer gargling with salt water, another helpful remedy for sore throats.)

Conventional allopathic medical practitioners use terms like disease, standard of care, taken as prescribed . . . but this just serves to put you in a box with people who have similar symptoms or scores on a blood test. The human body is vastly more complex than this system allows for.

Health insurance in the US, UK, and most other countries further propagate this system, relying on specific procedures and drugs approved for documented conditions that are identified through symptoms and blood tests, resulting in an assigned diagnosis. The International Classification of Disease (ICD) is a system maintained by the World Health Organization (WHO) and adopted just about globally assigning unique numerical codes to specific constellations of symptoms being presented. The ICD-10 code for Parkinson's is G20, that for prostate cancer is C61, while diabetes has nearly fifty different codes and subcode depending on all the variations and complications it comes with. The WHO is currently rolling out ICD-11[34] which is meant to further standardize data collection on causes of death and incidence of disease. This might be a boon for the statisticians but doesn't do much for you as an individual.

In the US or UK if you step outside of this system for the most part you are considered to be using "alternative" medicine. This is a deceptive term as, in fact, 80 percent of the world's population does not use allopathic medicine on a regular basis with "Traditional & Complementary Medicine" incorporating a range of alternatives widespread across the globe.[35] The term is part of the marketing machine's playbook to get you thinking you're doing something less than optimal.

The rest of this chapter takes a brief stroll through some broad categories of alternative health modalities to give you a sense of the choices available to you. Most of them will come up again as we get into specific health issues in Part II of this book. What they all have in common is that they recognize the power of the human body to heal itself if treated right and that there are powerful remedies in the natural world intelligently designed by God to work synergistically with us to get a body back in balance.

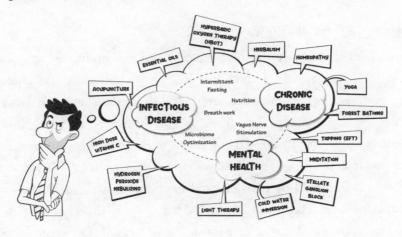

The other key factor about these modalities is that they are tailored to you as an individual. You are unique not only through your genes and more powerfully through your individually microbiome (we cover both of these in Chapter 3), but your lifestyle, likes/dislikes, motivation, thought processes, and culture dictate that your approach to health needs to be customized in a way that only you can discern.

The best part is that ideas from each modality can be mixed and matched—I use or have experimented with just about all of them at one time or another. Plus understanding the alternative options available to us doesn't mean we avoid allopathic medicine altogether. If I get into a car accident, I really hope the ambulance takes me to the nearest hospital where fine doctors will work on me to save life or limb. I'll use modern technology to look inside my arteries periodically to make sure I don't have any buildup of plaque and if I have an unusual pain or lump, I will likely find myself at a specialist to obtain their expert insight. But I will always look to these "alternative" modalities before any drug or surgical procedure so that my amazing body has the chance to do what it was created to do in getting me back in balance and functioning well.

Orthomolecular Medicine

Orthomolecular simply means balancing out the body through correcting nutritional deficiencies. Just like an orthodontist straightens your teeth, an "orthomolecular" approach straightens out or balances your molecular makeup often using supplements. You may not find a practitioner specifically advertising they specialize in this type of medicine but it is probably the most widely used "alternative" because it is generally accepted by conventional medicine as well. That may be because on some level it can be applied using similar methodologies; a blood test can reveal if you have low levels of vitamin D in your blood and your doctor can then recommend you spend more time in the sun or take a vitamin D supplement. However, it's important not to fall into the conventional mindset of "a pill for every ill" even if that pill contains a substance found in nature. Though in some cases it can be that simple.

Big Pharma has been fighting a winning campaign in the past to discredit the supplement industry and paint it as unregulated and untested. In reality pharmaceutical drug trials only need to prove the benefits outweigh the risks accepting known side effects such as incontinence, uncontrollable movements, muscle pain . . . the list can be as long as they like. But if it alleviates the stated symptom better than a placebo it gets approved. They don't have to measure its effectiveness against other older drugs with fewer side effects, only an inert placebo. For dietary supplements there has to be *zero risk* of adverse events. In the US the Food and Drug Administration (FDA) needs to be notified in advance of any new supplement being sold on the open market. They don't have to formally approve it but are aware of it, and if it is found to cause problems in the future, they will step in and take it off the market. The Federal Trade Commission (FTC) on the other hand regulates the claims made for the product. They will step in with fines and even jail time if a manufacturer has been found to make false claims.

This doesn't mean that you can go into your local grocery store and grab any bottle of a given supplement and it will help you. There are a lot of poor products out there particularly those cheaply made in a lab from synthetic materials versus made from whole organic food. Your intelligent body can tell the difference. What it wants is real food created to synergistically provide nutrients to humans in the right proportions. A whole orange for example contains vitamin C but at least 40,000 other cofactors in

Where are all the studies comparing a supplement to a pharmaceutical drug for efficacy? There are some but studies cost money and who is going to fund a study that is likely to show the $30 supplement is way more effective with zero side effects than the $800 drug? You can find plenty of studies[36] on individual efficacy of specific "nutraceuticals" which is a more accepted term amongst conventional doctors and includes individual compounds such as vitamins, minerals, amino acids for example but also products like spirulina, beet powder or medicinal mushrooms in the broader "food-as-medicine" realm.

the orange help you to absorb the vitamin C and create balance in the body.

You can do damage by treating yourself with individual substances and creating more of an unbalance. For example, many people think they are iron deficient, but dosing yourself with iron can be dangerous and lead to poor glucose metabolism and diabetes. The more likely culprit is a copper deficiency. **Copper** is necessary for proper iron metabolism, but copper competes with zinc for absorption. **Zinc** is another critical mineral in the body, a deficiency of which can affect your immune system, thyroid health, and mood to name just three.

During Covid many people started taking Zinc supplements which can then lead to a copper deficiency. This delicate balance managed naturally by the body is why it is always better to get your nutrients from food as God designed. But as we saw earlier, sometimes the playing field is not level if a severe deficiency exists through taking prescription medications or other lifestyle and environmental factors covered in Chapters 3 and 4.

Magnesium is a good example of a potential "quick fix" to what might be ailing you. It is estimated that over half the population in the US are deficient in magnesium. This may be due to the consumption of prescription medications and/or poor diet. Magnesium is required for the activation of vitamin D, protects your arteries from calcification, ensures optimal functioning of all cells but particularly your mitochondria (the energy-generators of your cells). It is required for strong bones and optimal heart and kidney health. A deficiency has been shown to increase your risk of migraines, anxiety, depression, sleep disturbances like restless leg syndrome, osteoporosis, and more. A deficiency won't show up in a simple blood test though as only a fraction circulates in the blood. Supplementing daily with a high-quality absorbable supplement such as 250–500mg of magnesium glycinate can be very beneficial. Supplementing with calcium on the other hand, another critical mineral, can be extremely detrimental to your health.[37]

We will revisit supplementation regularly in Part II with particular recommendations, but for most people a high-quality multivitamin is plain good practice as a start since they are designed with balance and optimum absorption in mind. Don't pay too much attention to the "Recommended Daily Allowance (RDA)" as these guidelines were set many years ago and are mainly minimums for avoiding a deadly outcome like scurvy rather than maintaining optimal health. Everyone in my family takes a daily multivitamin tailored to their particular stage of life even though we eat a very healthy diet. Additional supplements account for specific deficiencies that have built up over the years or address individual requirements. Some people simply need more of certain nutrients than other people. Our supplement regimen is reviewed once or twice a year usually in consultation with a practitioner. See the Resources section to get you started with quality brands.

Herbalism

Remember the eclectics of the nineteenth century who were absorbed into the regular medical profession? While the term "eclectic" generally means utilizing a range of broad ideas, the doctors that practiced eclectic medicine looked for anything that would benefit their patients. They tended to rely on botanical remedies with some nutritional and mineral treatments.

Today there are generally considered to be three main types of herbal medicine:

- Ayurvedic medicine from India
- Traditional Chinese medicine (TCM), and
- Western herbalism that grew out of the eclectic movement.

There are a lot of similarities between these "big three" with around 90 percent agreement on the overall approach to treatment. Some of the herbs used have different names but tend to be of the same species. Which approach you feel most comfortable with is a matter of personal preference and cultural upbringing. The key tenet is that the amazing human body is endowed with bodily functions that can only be unlocked by plants and that our disconnection from nature is one of the biggest causes of disease.

Many herbalists in ancient cultures were women which may have contributed to this modality falling out of favor in Western countries. But if you have the patience to move at the speed of nature, an herbalism approach to health is probably optimal for most people. A body out of balance usually took many years to get there so it can take some persistence to see results. But don't let this make you think their effects are not powerful. Botanicals can be extremely potent and many of them interfere with pharmaceuticals and are thus warned against.[38] Plants are endowed with incredible intelligence and were created to work synergistically with the other organisms on the planet such as us humans.

As an example, one group of herbs is called the adaptogens. They are used to regulate various body systems including metabolism, immune, and hormonal systems, and help you respond to any negative influences or stress. One of the most powerful and best known adaptogens is **ashwagandha**. It has been used for thousands of years for its wide variety of health benefits including chronic pain relief, enhancing sleep quality, hormonal fluctuations and sexual health, supporting healthy adrenal system and thyroid problems, reducing cortisol levels (due to chronic stress), and restoring insulin sensitivity. It also boasts immunomodulating properties which can either stimulate your immune system (in the presence of an infection for example) or suppress it to combat autoimmune problems. Hard to believe a single plant can do all this, right?

I take ashwagandha daily. I buy a large bag of organic ashwagandha root in powdered form and put half a teaspoon of it into a small amount of almond milk. I also drink **tulsi** tea daily with hibiscus. Tulsi, also known as holy basil, is another powerful adaptogen with anti-inflammatory properties. It is antibacterial, antifungal, antiviral and is a known antioxidant.[39] It has also been shown to promote liver health, particularly after damage from pharmaceuticals. Hibiscus is known to lower blood pressure and fight cancer.[40]

Other herbs are used more specifically such as **hawthorn**, which is widely recognized in Europe (even amongst conventional doctors) as a treatment for heart failure.[41] The berries and leaves are made into a tincture and have a potent anti-inflammatory effect on the vascular system.

Some of the most powerful herbs and botanicals you may already have sitting in your kitchen. As we shall see in Chapter 5, there is a fine line between food and medicine. That's why you've likely heard the phrase *food-is-medicine*. It's that connection to nature that is innate in every human being no matter how far we move into concrete jungles we call cities and think we have all the answers through so-called scientific progress.

Garlic is a mighty antimicrobial with anti-inflammatory properties[42] while **turmeric**, **sage**, **paprika**, **rosemary**, and **ginger** have all been shown to have significant anti-inflammatory and protective properties simply using them in culinary amounts.[43] Spices like these were once worth more than gold on trading routes. They are readily available today and can be easily incorporated into our daily cooking. I go through vast quantities of garlic, turmeric, and ginger as well as black pepper (useful in absorption of turmeric) and cinnamon on a weekly basis.

Beyond the culinary spices and other medicinal foods, it's best to get professional help if you're interested in taking an herbal approach to health. While there is plenty of science to back up the efficacy of individual botanicals and a better understanding of the compounds within the plants that are contributing to health improvement, herbalism is more art than science. Practitioners have undergone rigorous professional training with many of them also naturopathic doctors or MDs as well. Obtaining professional help is particularly recommended if you have a specific health condition and wish to avoid allopathic pharmaceuticals to treat it. We will mention a few herbs to treat the conditions covered in Part II and the Resources section has some recommended sources but make sure your practitioner is board certified in herbal medicine or a naturopathic doctor (ND).

An overview of herbal medicine wouldn't be complete without mentioning **essential oils (EOs).** Essential oils are nature in its most concentrated form. They are the extracts of flowers, fruits, bark, leaves, resins or roots of a plant or tree. Just one drop contains a complex network of molecules that work synergistically with your body to deliver a myriad of health benefits. Almost a modality unto itself, I have seen firsthand how simple it is to incorporate EOs into your life and wellness routine. They are invaluable for anyone resolved to avoid chemical products in your home and around your family.

Frankincense and myrrh are mentioned in the Bible, given as gifts to the baby Jesus. It's unlikely these were true EOs as advanced distillation techniques were developed more recently, but using plants in aromatherapy and as salves, ointments, and tinctures goes back to ancient days. Just think how cutting into an orange or lemon makes you feel. That

> Next time you have a headache instead of reaching for the (over-the-counter) pharmaceutical put a drop of pure **Peppermint Essential Oil** on either temple and one at the base of your neck behind your head. Peppermint is one of the most versatile EOs with a range of healing properties.

smell of citrus wakes you up and lifts any black mood you might have been in. **Frankincense** is known as the king of oils for the wide range of healing properties that have been scientifically validated.[44] It is a powerful anti-inflammatory agent, painkiller, and immune booster with the biggest attention given recently to its cancer-fighting properties. Frankincense is one of the more expensive EOs but can be used directly on skin (or a visible tumor) whereas most of the time you will be diluting EOs as a blend in a carrier oil such as almond oil, coconut oil, or my favorite, jojoba oil. We'll be meeting EOs again in Part II. If you're anxious to get started with experimenting just make sure of the quality and source of your EOs. See Resources.

Energy Medicine

Many years ago, before I specialized in health and wellness professionally, a client told me about a practitioner he had seen after being
bedridden for two weeks with a mystery ailment. He described sitting
in a chair holding large electrodes in his hands that were hooked up to
a machine and a computer screen. After a bit of questioning and some
clicks on the computer the practitioner announced he had had a spider
bite that was the source of his problems. A small vial of water was then
placed on a metal platform, also hooked up to the computer. My client
was then asked to drink it. Within ten minutes he started to feel better.
I was completely skeptical but had been suffering from unexplained
digestive problems for a while. My curiosity led me to go check out
what I now know to be Bioresonance Therapy.

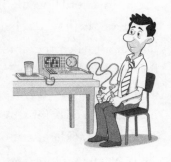

Sure enough, within fifteen minutes
of questioning and some clicks on the
computer, the practitioner stated I had a
parasite. He could tell exactly what type
and infused a similar vial of water with the
correct frequency which I drank. He also
gave me some herbs to take for the next
week or so and I was indeed cured. This is
one form of **Energy Medicine or Bioenergetics** which is based on the
premise that the human body is basically just one big battery generating its own energy field. Ill-health results from an obstructed or imbalanced energy field. Organisms or toxins that are bad for us show up in
the aberrant frequencies that they vibrate in.

In Chapter 1 we looked at the biological parts of the human body,
the cells and interconnectedness of the organs and other parts. In
the previous two sections we touched on the chemistry of the body
at the molecular level and the balance needed between chemical
elements such as essential vitamins and minerals. The missing piece is

understanding a little about the physics of the human body as in fact physics underlies everything in the universe. It's the hardest aspect to understand and manage on your own but I wanted to touch on it for completeness. In fact, the body relies on electrical impulses for countless functions. Disruption to our electrical field is a common contributor to disease. This is why grounding in nature is so helpful as it resets the body's electrical field and provides much needed free electrons we can absorb, to offset the oxidative stress in our body.

The best-known form of energy medicine is probably acupuncture which has its roots in Traditional Chinese Medicine (TCM) and the concept of "qi" (pronounced "chee") which is believed to be the vital energy flowing through the body. According to TCM, qi flows through various meridians throughout the body. **Acupuncture** involves inserting a tiny sterile needle into specific points along these meridians to stimulate the flow of qi and bring balance back to the body. It doesn't hurt at all when the needles are being applied and usually you'll then lie on a comfortable bed with some relaxing music for fifteen minutes or more. Acupuncture is best known for treating chronic pain without medications or combating the side effects of chemotherapy. But it can be used to tackle just about any health problem to great success especially when combined with herbs.

Reiki is a Japanese healing practice based on a similar premise but just using the practitioner's hands to promote healing.

What I referred to as bioresonance therapy or frequency medicine[45] has now developed into a more standardized approach and uses "infoceuticals" which utilize the power of resonance—matching the vibrations of a system, the human body or parts of it—to infuse information into water that can be taken as a tonic. Other therapies that build on the premise of energy medicine include light therapy, sound therapy, and to a certain extent, hydrogen and oxygen therapies. While testimonials and studies abound for the efficacy of these therapies, I find the whole concept of bioenergetics most helpful in understanding why our modern lives full of technology emitting electromagnetic frequencies (EMFs) are so damaging to our health. We will dive into EMFs in Chapter 4.

Functional Medicine

Functional Medicine is now being recognized as a direct contrast to allopathic medicine and is mainly practiced by MDs who started out in the allopathic system but found it lacking. Many of them tell stories of looking for solutions to their own unspecified health challenges and realizing the shortcomings of an allopathic approach. Naturopaths, homeopaths, osteopaths, integrative physicians, and doctors of chiropractic have all been around longer and offer many of the same approaches to holistic "alternative" care. (I've provided a short glossary to help you understand the difference between some of these terms.) While functional medicine incorporates many of these more natural alternatives to drugs and surgery it also embraces the latest research into genetics, epigenetics, the microbiome, and more—we'll get into these aspects in Chapter 3.

Rather than focusing on diagnosing a particular disease and identifying the drugs approved to treat it, functional medicine digs into the root cause of the symptoms or lack of function being displayed. The best way to understand functional medicine is to look at a direct comparison with conventional medicine:

Conventional Medicine	Functional Medicine
Disease centered	Health centered
Diagnosis based on symptoms	Focused on underlying cause of disease
Doctor centered	Patient centered
10-min visits	1-hour+ diagnostic visits

(Continued on next page)

Conventional Medicine	Functional Medicine
Current symptoms and biomarkers	History, lifestyle, and functioning as well
Specialized	Holistic
Standard of care—one size fits all	Personalized biochemical individuality
Early detection of disease	Preventive based approach
High tech	High touch/high tech
Expensive	Cost effective

Functional Medicine[46] is starting to be considered more mainstream with the launch of the first academic research center for functional medicine at the world-renowned Cleveland Clinic in 2014. This is principally due to the efforts of some prominent functional medicine specialists like Dr. Jeffrey Bland and Dr. Mark Hyman. However, the insurance and health plan industry has been slower to catch on, which is surprising given that last bullet in the table—functional medicine is far more cost effective as it focuses on reversing disease and generally avoids expensive pharmaceuticals and surgery aiming to restore the patient to vitality and health such that ongoing care is no longer needed.

If your employer offers it or you can afford it out of pocket, going to a functional medicine doctor is usually a great option, not necessarily because that doctor will have all the answers but because their approach is likely to be highly personalized. A good functional medicine doctor will tailor their treatment plan to your particular health history and environmental exposures, prioritizing natural solutions while also incorporating the best that modern medicine has to offer. These doctors focus on understanding your uniqueness and how your genetics, lifestyle, environment, and behavior intersect to generate health or illness.

Glossary of Key Alternative Modalities	
Acupuncture	Originally part of TCM. Involves inserting a tiny sterile needle into specific points along identified body meridians to stimulate the flow of qi and bring balance back to the body.
Ayurveda	Indian form of herbal medicine.
Chiropractor	A doctor of chiropractic (DC) studies a lot of the same medical specialties such as biology and anatomy but focuses on the spine. Therapeutic adjustments are not just for musculoskeletal problems though, especially now that vagus nerve health is better understood.
Functional Medicine	The newest systematic approach to an individual holistic treatment plan incorporating alternatives and lifestyle factors to get to the root cause of the health problem.
Herbalists	Anyone who practices a form of botanical medicine such as TCM or ayurveda.
Homeopathy	A medical practice based on the premise that a tiny amount of a substance that can cause a symptom when given to a healthy person, can also heal that symptom.
Integrative Medicine	Anyone who integrates different forms of medicine including conventional/allopathic.
Naturopath	A naturopathic doctor (ND) undergoes rigorous medical training and in some cases can prescribe certain medications but their approach focuses on natural healing modalities first such as botanicals, diet, and lifestyle.
Orthomolecular medicine	Focusing on balancing the biochemical and molecular profile of the patient.
Osteopaths	A doctor of osteopathy (DO) undergoes similar medical training and are considered equivalent to MDs in most states but focus on treating illness through the manipulation and massage of bones, joints and muscles.
Traditional Chinese Medicine (TCM)	Chinese form of herbal medicine.

When My Doctor Tells Me Something Different

Whichever route you take or individual therapy you select, it's essential that you take ownership of your own health. No professional, even one that sees you for an hour each week, is inhabiting your body or fully understanding all the nuances of *you*. There are no quick fixes or silver bullets. Health is an ongoing part of life that you need to take responsibility for. Don't worry if that sounds overwhelming from your current vantage point. Once you embrace the basics and figure out what works for you it will become second nature to operate "outside the box."

When you cut your finger, you know you just need to keep it clean and your body will heal the wound. If all the doctors, scientists, and other practitioners the world over pooled their collective knowledge about the human body—how it works and how it breaks down—we still would have barely touched the intricacies of the human organism. The fact is we don't know how most of it works. But it has become clearer than ever that while allopathic medicine is invaluable for acute problems that are immediately life threatening, its shortcomings are vast for anything else.

I find conventional doctors and clinicians generally fall into one of three camps:

1. Those who are open-minded enough to listen to their patients, curious enough to study new developments and brave enough to step outside of the mainstream to improve the health of those in their care or sphere of influence.
2. Those who sense there is something wrong in the way they are practicing but have a family to support and are way too busy helping patients in the day to day to get reeducated so press forward with their conventional tools.

3. Those who are dismissive of any new information and too enam-
ored by the trappings of their profession including status, pride,
and money to be open to a new approach.

I hope those of you already under the care of a conventional physician have experienced the first category. I am blessed to have ben-
efited from wonderful conventional doctors both for myself and
for my children. For the first five years of my older son's life, I did
everything our pediatrician told me to do and never questioned it.
Once I got educated, I forged my own way with various alternative
therapies and used our pediatrician only for annual checkups. She
dutifully recommended immunizations and conventional remedies
but respected my wishes when I wanted to do things differently. It
has been a true partnership for which I am very grateful. I have also
encountered far too many MDs in the second and third categories. If
this is your experience then read on, as we will address how to handle them in light of specific health issues in Part II. The easy answer
would be to find a new doctor, but I recognize that is not always
possible. Sometimes you have to keep meeting with the specialists
to get a complete diagnosis, and many modern tests are helpful to
understand where to focus the healing. But if they aren't willing to
explore a range of treatment options then you are completely within
your rights not to go back to them.

Many of the best healing modalities are completely free and don't
even need a practitioner to be involved. These include things like sleep,
getting outside in nature, sunlight, meditation, mindfulness, exercise/
movement, and upgrading your nutrition. Just because they are free do
not discount their power. We'll be talking about lifestyle practices to
optimize your health in the next chapter.

Points to Remember

1. You know more about your body than any professional, and only you should decide what you do to it.

2. History is littered with doctors disagreeing with each other, and this is how science is driven forward as long as open discussion is permitted.

3. The pharmaceutical industry has grown to such a vast size and wields such power that you cannot trust marketing messages in mainstream media or even what your conventional doctor tells you due to the influence it exerts.

4. The majority of pharmaceutical drugs have efficacy rates well below 50 percent and inflict many side effects on the body including toxicity and nutrient depletions that lead to far more problems than they solve.

5. There are a number of alternatives to conventional medicine that are fully validated for efficacy and safety. They harness the power of nature and the innate healing abilities of the human body in a synergistic way.

CHAPTER 3

Don't Blame Grandpa

23andMe is probably the best-known consumer genetics testing company (named for those twenty-three chromosomes we talked about in Chapter 1). There are many other companies around the world with new start-ups popping up regularly. For various fees from the high end to the fairly reasonable, you can provide a DNA sample usually through your saliva and get reports on your ancestry and what your DNA says about your health risks. But is all the hype around genetic testing justified?

There's a lot of breast cancer in my family. My mum's two sisters died of it at forty-seven and fifty-two. Mum was diagnosed at age fifty, went through standard chemotherapy and radiation, and survived. Over twenty-five years later, she is still going strong playing bridge regularly, growing the most amazing house plants you have ever seen, and enjoying being an important part of her various grandchildren's lives.

My parents tried to talk me into genetic testing in my twenties; they even suggested that I get a prophylactic mastectomy. I ignored this advice and have passed my fiftieth birthday with flying colors! The theme you will keep hearing throughout this book is how the human body has the capacity to heal itself. Simply cutting off the offending part needs to be considered a last resort. However, it's always been in the back of my mind that I have a genetic susceptibility, a potential ticking bomb in my body that could someday explode into cancer. My aunt had come to visit one weekend when I was thirteen after she had gone through extensive chemotherapy. Seeing her pale swollen features barely recognizable as my formidable aunt drove me to quit my budding smoking habit immediately. Over the years I have gradually cleaned up my diet and focused on other lifestyle changes to reduce my risk considerably.

But susceptibility doesn't mean inevitability. As with many new inventions or technological progress we assume the new replaces the old and is always an improvement. In medicine and science this is rarely the case. New discoveries are more often an expansion of our knowledge and frequently lead to more questions than they answer and an increasing sense of "awe" at the phenomenon we call "life."

Twenty years ago it was thought that genetics held the answer to reducing chronic disease. This is why the results of the Human Genome project described in Chapter 1 were announced with such fanfare by the US and UK heads of government. But while that project was an incredible feat of scientific collaboration and development, it has since become evident that the assumption was woefully inadequate. While the expectation was to find at least 100,000 genes, given this is about the number of different enzymes (or proteins) in the human body, in fact they found closer to 22,000 and over 99 percent of them are identical from person to person.

So we have twenty-three pairs of chromosomes in every cell containing a specific instruction set (DNA) but yet we have lots of different types of cells and literally thousands of different enzymes being produced to drive all the chemical reactions to keep us alive and functioning well. What we have learned in fact is that our basic genetic makeup is only a fraction of the story. Gene *expression* is much more relevant which means if they are switched on or off and that is influenced by our **epigenetic factors.**[1]

"Epi" simply means outside of or "on top of" so it's basically your daily experiences we more commonly refer to as lifestyle factors. At the cellular level it's the environment the genes are exposed to that will determine if they are expressed or lie dormant.

This makes sense as chronic disease rates have skyrocketed in a single generation—obesity, heart disease, diabetes, neurological conditions. The gene pool hasn't changed but our environment has, drastically so, over the last fifty years.

But many diseases run in families, I hear you say! Yes, that's true, but this doesn't automatically mean it's due to the genes. Families tend to have similar lifestyles, eat similar foods, and make similar brand choices. When I was first cooking for myself, I followed many of my mother's recipes. As much as I hate to admit it, I have many of the same habits I learned growing up and apply them to my own family. Home cooked meal on the table by 6 p.m., no TV before 5 p.m., play outside in the dirt, read a good book, dessert is for special occasions, candy is not a food group, and if the sun is out, I need to be in it! Growing up in England this last one is critical but now that I live in Southern California you'd think I wouldn't drop everything to get out in the sun but I often do!

Okay, but what about cystic fibrosis and other diseases that can be clearly traced to a single defective gene? They do exist but less than 1 percent of all diseases would fall in this category. Even then, significant progress is being made to show many of these devastating diseases can be reversed when the right environment is applied. We are also finding that specific nutritional deficiencies during pregnancy or early life may trigger the faulty gene expression.

Lessons from China

One of the first books I read once I embarked on my health journey nearly fifteen years ago was *The China Study* by T. Colin Campbell and his son Thomas M. Campbell.[2] *The New York Times* called it the "Grand Prix of Epidemiological Studies." As you read earlier, I am a big Formula One racing fan, so this label resonated with me. It is also full of data and graphical representations that spoke to my inner actuary while explaining complex biochemical processes for the layman. The book has sold over three million copies worldwide and spawned follow up books plus a cookbook (which I also own and still use occasionally). It walks the reader through the groundbreaking study Dr. Campbell led in the 1980s with other researchers from Cornell University, Oxford University, and the Chinese Academy of Preventive Medicine to look at how diet impacts chronic illness like heart disease and cancer.

China is a huge country with stark cultural differences from most Western countries. Family ties are tight. In more rural areas in particular, people tend to stay in the same location their whole lives and continue to eat the same diets that were unique to their region. They also tend to eat a lot more plants, certainly more than modern Western diets. The study compared a wide variety of dietary, lifestyle and disease characteristics of adults (between the ages of 35 and 64, half male, half female) in 130 villages across 65 counties in 24 different provinces. It included personal surveys and blood tests as well as macro-analyses of the produce sold in the local markets and rates of disease in the village.

The Significance of Location
Many studies have shown that people moving to Western countries from a country or area with generally low rates of chronic disease, succumb to the poorer health of their new environment once they adopt the lifestyle of their adopted location.[3]

In all they studied 367 variables including disease mortality rates for 48 different kinds of disease, 109 blood indicators such as vitamin levels and hormonal elements, 36 food constituents including pesticides and heavy metals as well as nutrients, and 60 lifestyle factors from personal questionnaires. What is most useful about this book is that it highlights the difficulties of studying the impact of lifestyle factors on disease in a statistically meaningful way. *The China Study* was the most comprehensive research of its kind and came to rigorous conclusions backed by data points and clearly explained mechanisms of action. Yet it is not even close to telling the whole story of nutrition and chronic illness. But do not let that comment put you off reading this excellent book. The eight principles of food and health it summarizes are worth repeating:

Eight Principles of Food and Health from *The China Study*	
Principle #1	Nutrition represents the combined activities of countless food substances. The whole is greater than the sum of its parts.
Principle #2	Vitamin supplements are not a panacea for good health.
Principle #3	There are virtually no nutrients in animal-based foods that are not better provided by plants.
Principle #4	Genes do not determine disease on their own. Genes function only by being activated, or expressed, and nutrition plays a critical role in determining which genes, good or bad, are expressed.
Principle #5	Nutrition can substantially control the adverse effects of noxious chemicals.
Principle #6	The same nutrition that prevents disease in its early stages (before diagnosis) can also halt or reverse disease in its later stages (after diagnosis).
Principle #7	Nutrition that is truly beneficial for one chronic disease will support health across the board.
Principle #8	Good nutrition creates health in all areas of our existence. All parts are interconnected.

Notice principle #4. The book doesn't mention epigenetics at all but that is basically what it is saying and scientific developments since have greatly backed this up. The only detractors from this truth can be traced back to Big Pharma. If you can find a gene that is responsible for a disease, then it supports their business model to find a chemical that will act on that gene and change something in your body. Just look at the way Big Pharma funded mass media is propagating the myth that genes are the main cause of obesity. Of course they have now got approval for their diabetes drugs to be prescribed for people who are simply overweight. Go seek out some old photographs of your grandparents or great-grandparents, look at historical news clippings or illustrated books of life fifty plus years ago. There were very few overweight people. Genetic makeup cannot change substantially in two to three generations.

Principle #3 may have also caught your eye. Yes, the main conclusion from *The China Study* is that animal protein and dairy in particular is a main driver of disease. Given my susceptibility to breast cancer this book scared me into being vegan for a few years! You can find some valid detractors of *The China Study* who have gone into careful analysis of the raw data and concluded that the correlation between chronic disease and animal protein is not as strong as the book implies. While I agree that removing all animal protein from everyone's diet is not the answer to health, these eight principles do stack up. Just make sure you don't miss the word "virtually" in #3. I explain nutrition in detail in Chapter 5.

Italian Hospitality

From China I now want to take you to a little village in the southern part of Italy called Roseto Valfortore and its namesake Roseto, Pennsylvania, in the eastern part of the US. The author Malcolm Gladwell tells the interesting story of Roseto in the introduction to his book *Outliers: The Story of Success*[4] where he asks the question about a diverse range of people, what makes high achievers different? The high achievers in Roseto seemed to live to a ripe old age with no signs of chronic illness or heart disease in particular. Dr. Stewart

Wolf and a sociologist friend John Bruhn decided to investigate in the 1960s.[5]

The original village of Roseto in Italy is on a craggy hillside organized around a large central square with an archway leading to the local church named Our Lady of Mount Carmine. In the nineteenth century the *paesani* of Rosetto led a hard life working in the marble quarries or cultivating the fields walking up and down the steep hills every day. In 1882 a group of Rosetans set sail for the US looking for a better life and settled near the town of Bangor, Pennsylvania, where they found work in a slate quarry. Word got back to Italy and over the next few years many more Rosetans set sail for the new world. In 1894 alone it is said 1,200 Rosetans applied for a US passport. By the turn of the twentieth century, enough land had been purchased on the hills outside of Bangor and a church had been built, named Our Lady of Mount Carmel. The village was renamed Roseto as almost all the inhabitants originated from there.

Wolf and Bruhn spent four weeks in Roseto in 1961 and carried out rigorous analysis including blood tests and EKGs, food logs and exercise patterns. Most surprisingly the Rosetans had actually adopted a lot of bad US habits such as smoking and cooking with lard instead of olive oil. Very few worked in the quarry anymore; some were overweight. Wolf thought it must be genetics that played a role, so he also analyzed Rosetans who had settled in other parts of the US to see if they enjoyed the same good health. They did not. Nor was it something about the particular location in Pennsylvania. The town of Bangor just down the road had three times the rate of heart disease in those over sixty-five than Roseto. Quoting from Gladwell:

> *What Wolf began to realize was that the secret of Roseto wasn't diet or exercise or genes or location. It had to be Roseto itself. As Bruhn and Wolf walked around the town, they figured out why.*

They looked at how the Rosetans visited one another, stopping to chat in Italian on the street, say, or cooking for one another in their backyards. They learned about the extended family clans that underlay the town's social structure. They saw how many homes had three generations living under one roof, and how much respect grandparents commanded. They went to mass at Our Lady of Mount Carmel and saw the unifying and calming effect of the church. They counted twenty-two separate civic organizations in a town of just under two thousand people. . . . In transplanting the paesani culture of southern Italy to the hills of eastern Pennsylvania, the Rosetans had created a powerful, protective social structure capable of insulating them from the pressures of the modern world.

As the years went by later generations of Rosetans became more Americanized and let go of the tight community bonds. Decades later, a study found their rates of chronic disease matched the surrounding areas. But while none of *The China Study*'s principles have been refuted by the interesting case of Roseto, it is clear the whole story of chronic illness is far more complicated.

Interaction with the World

What I know for certain is that God created this world as a home for us humans and the secret of human flourishing is a better understanding of how He created it all to work together.

God endowed us with five senses: touch, sight, hearing, smell and taste. These are five separate areas of study in the scientific world looking at the impact on health in various ways. I prefer to take a more holistic view that these are the ways God has intended us to interact with the world and as His design is perfect, they must all be important.[6]

We are constantly getting inputs from each one of these senses.

Whether they are positive or negative impacts your health throughout the day and as time goes by. Here's some sample inputs so you get a better idea what I mean:

	Positive	Negative
Touch	• Hugs • Stroking a pet	• Hot stove • Slap in the face
Sight	• A sunset • Smiles	• Car accident • Porn
Hearing	• Birds singing • Laughing	• Shouting • Police sirens
Smell	• Citrus • Flowers	• Dry-cleaning • Rotting flesh
Taste	• Apples • Mushrooms	• Sugar • Pesticides

Hang on, I hear you say, why is sugar in the negative column and perhaps eating a mushroom would not be considered a positive experience? These are positive or negative effects on your health not your immediate pleasure centers of your brain. Ingesting cocaine will excite your pleasure centers, but I bet you would be a little horrified to see that anywhere but in the negative list.

This is a tiny sample to get you thinking about all the ways your body interacts with this world. Hopefully you can think of many more in each row. Now think back to the day you were born. You don't remember? Unsurprising. But let me use myself as an example. I am aged fifty-two. This means on my birthday this year I have been alive for 52 x 365.25 days =18,993. (We actuaries use 365.25 as the multiplier to account for leap years). That is 18,993 x 24 hours = 455, 832. Sure, I probably spent about a third of these hours asleep in bed not doing much interacting at all, but stick with me here. It's 455,832 x 60 minutes = 27,349, 920 (as in over 27 million minutes). Multiply once more by 60 and we deduce I have been alive 1,640,995,200 or 1.64 billion seconds.

Now if you think about all the possible positive and negative influences you have experienced over the billion or so seconds you have been alive, you are starting to get an understanding of how complicated it is to really understand all of the epigenetic or lifestyle factors that generate or impact good health. Well-designed studies have their uses, but they must be taken within a broader context and never look only at the headlines and assume the latest study discounts all that have gone before.

I like to think of our bodies as a bucket where we're taking in good stuff, wholesome food with plenty of nutrients, smells from nature like flowers and trees, hearing the birds singing and the laughter of children, seeing the smiles from a friend or even a stranger, getting regular hugs or a hand squeeze from a loved one. These good influences build up our reserves and make us strong, so that the bad influences such as toxins (whether they are chemical, physical, relational, or emotional) do not overwhelm our reserves, which is where illness sets in.

Quite often it is one factor that sets off a major illness and triggers the bucket to overflow. The body gets so out of balance that it can't immediately right itself. This might be a virus you picked up along the

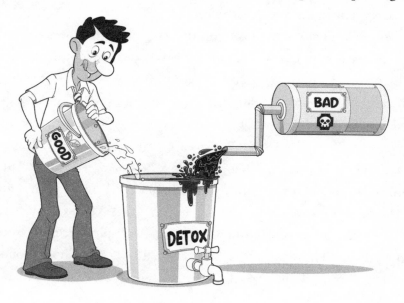

way: one that didn't seem to affect your friend or family member too bad but you are having a hard time getting over and feeling like yourself again. There is a lot of talk about "Long Covid" these days, but the truth is many viruses like influenza (flu) or even the common cold can trigger people into chronic illness. It's not the virus acting alone but a combination of all the other experiences the body has encountered in the days, weeks, months, and years before.

It might not be a pathogen that physically entered your body as the trigger but a relational or emotional trigger. Divorce or other major upheaval can greatly affect your whole body. We'll talk about trauma in Chapter 8 and how your body might have fully healed on the outside or it's been years since the events that so greatly affected you. But studies have shown that trauma makes permanent changes in your brain and the interconnectedness of your whole body can manifest as a physical or mental illness. Remember how the human eyeball doesn't work without its connection to the brain and that it's actually your brain that does the seeing? So, what enters your eyes through the sense of sight, even if none of your other senses are involved, affects your brain and, through the vagus nerve, every organ in your body.

The quality of our nourishment via taste is probably the single biggest impact on our health which is why I have dedicated a whole chapter to it: Chapter 5. To make sure you have a good sense of all the toxins you are being exposed to on a daily basis, we cover that in the next chapter. But before we leave the subject of genes altogether, I want to mention a set of genes that seems to have more of an impact on your health than your 22,000 human genes. It is the way you interact most intimately with the rest of the natural world that God created. It's called your **microbiome**.

Microscopic Bugs

Your microbiome is simply all the bacteria, fungi, viruses, and other microorganisms that live in and on you. Remember in Chapter 1 as we discussed the amazingness of the human body? I explained that you actually have more cells in your body that belong to microscopic organisms than human cells. This is why the germ theory of disease—propagated since the turn of the twentieth century and continuing in much of mainstream medicine today—is so inaccurate. While we've identified plenty of pathogenic bugs over the years (those that cause illness) there are many thousands more that are not only beneficial to our bodies but essential to their healthy functioning.

The bugs that have been identified and studied have been shown to be involved in a huge range of bodily processes such as immunity, metabolism, hormone regulation, and neurological function. At least 80 percent of these bugs hang out in your gut, that is your digestive tract that runs from your mouth all the way through to your stomach, your small and large intestine, your colon, and out your butt. It is essentially one long tube that is open to the environment anytime you open your mouth. This is why what you put in your mouth is so critical to your health. But not

Microbiota or Gut Flora

You'll often see the reference to flora that tends to be used interchangeably these days with microbiota (the technical term for the organisms) or microbiome (technically the genetic material they contain). Flora is Latin for flower and is usually used to describe the plant environment in a particular area. However, I like to use the term gut flora as it conjures up the garden inside your body that can get overgrown with weeds (pathogenic microbes) if you eat too much sugar for example or wiped out altogether with drugs or pesticides. You need to feed it well with healthy nutrients and fiber from plants.

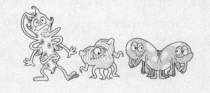

just your health, it's actually the health and diversity of your microbiome that is key.

Many diagnosed diseases are now being tied to a depleted or unbalanced microbiome.[7] A single course of antibiotics is enough to wipe out up to one-third of your flora and it is not easily restored. Serial antibiotics for ailments like acne, ear infections, or recurring urinary-tract infections are particularly detrimental to overall health. Many non-antibiotic drugs also adversely affect your gut flora. In one study[8] almost one in four (24 percent) of one thousand drugs tested were detrimental to at least one of forty gut bacteria strains. The relationship is bidirectional though such is the synergy with our microscopic friends. So that if you are placed on a drug, your microbiome affects your response to it, a fact that has not gone unnoticed by Big Pharma who are investing heavily in microbiome research to turn it to their advantage with so called "drugs from bugs."[9]

The study of the microbiome is one of the hottest specialties in medicine right now, but it is still in its relative infancy. In fact, it's estimated that we have no idea what 95 percent of the microorganisms that make up the microbiome do.[10] We do know that a fraction of 1 percent is likely to be pathogenic and even then it's the balance and the diversity of all the different organisms that seems to lead to health versus illness.

Given the number of different types of microbes found in healthy humans it is estimated that the microbial genome is collectively at least two hundred times the size of the human genome.

The malleability of your microbiome is tremendously complex and not yet well understood. What we do know is that it builds from birth and is impacted greatly by what type of birth you had and whether or not you were breast-fed as to how much flora you accumulated from your mother. From there your own personal experiences will influence its development in terms of what you eat, your social interactions (how many other microbiomes you interact with), how much time you spend in nature, and what insults you encounter like antibiotics, pesticides, or preservatives in food for example. All of the interaction with the world we discussed in the last section, affects your microbiome.

Your microbiome can be manipulated over weeks or months if your circumstances or lifestyle change. There is no "silver bullet" though and even the promise of precision medicine is unlikely to find instant cures for a body out of balance. It is the highly complex interaction of both your human genome with the diversity of your microbial genome, your environment, and your personal lifestyle day by day that makes the difference.

Getting in the Blue Zone

Yesterday, out of nowhere, I developed a really sore neck as well as an ache deep in my left hip socket. I immediately tried to figure out what I must have done that day to cause my pain so I could figure out the best remedy. I realized I had spent all day writing in my home office without the benefit of my anti-EMF device to protect me from the damage of all the electronics in that room (more on EMFs in the next chapter). I'd also gotten into a rather intense two-hour discussion after dinner with my sixteen-year-old son Max on the evidence for God. (He's spent his entire life in weekly church but currently thinks God is make-believe. He has some good arguments, but he is aggressive in his stance and demands my recollection on the spot of very specific information which can raise my blood pressure.) I had also done a workout that morning with some free weights and perhaps my form was off. I had been distracted and forgot to drink much water, relying on one or two cups of herbal tea all day, so perhaps I was dehydrated. I have been trying out a new probiotic (experimenting with my microbiome!) and I had spent a good portion of my writing time poring over some notes and research. Thinking it would be good not to sit down all day I was standing peering down at this information on my desk much lower down. Maybe my pain is due to one of these triggers or maybe it's a combination of some or all of them. The important point is that I don't just reach for some Advil or Aleve (ibuprofen or naproxen) but I'm trying to figure out the cause so I can remedy it and take steps to avoid further pain in the future.

I hope you are appreciating by now that there is never a single cause of our illness or pain but it's also not just bad luck due to the genes you were handed at birth. Similarly, there is no single prescription for a long life. This brings me to the last population study I want to share with you. I have been fascinated by the concept of Blue Zones™ since I first read Dan Buettner's book over a decade ago.[11] *Blue Zones: 9 Lessons for Living Longer from the People Who've Lived the Longest* is a great read. Local culture (and gene pool) is taken out of the equation in looking at the similarities between the communities in five very different parts of the world with the largest proportion of centenarians (reaching the ripe old age of 100).

Before we get in the blue zone, I want to take a moment to talk about longevity and life expectancy. As an actuary I can get a bit hung up on life expectancy numbers particularly when you look at statistics that show life expectancy in the US has actually been dropping since 2014[12] whereas other countries have been improving. The US life expectancy rate climbed steadily for the seventy years prior, reaching a maximum of 78.9 years. However, the latest statistics from the US National Center for Health Statistics indicate an age of 76.4 years for someone born in 2021, a reduction of 0.6 years since 2020.[13] The focus and blame has been put on the pandemic in the write-up referred to in the notes. However, life expectancy in the US was falling well before Covid-19 came on the scene and, as we shall see in Chapter 6, blaming one germ is diverting attention from the underlying factors discussed in this book.

I've provided a table with the life expectancy of a few other countries for comparison.[14] This is all 2019 data as the latest worldwide statistics available. Notice I've also included a statistic called "Healthy Life Expectancy." This is defined as "the average number of years a person can expect to live in full health by taking into account years lived in less than full health due to

Country	Life Expectancy (years)	Healthy Life Expectancy
Australia	83.0	70.9
Canada	82.2	71.3
China	77.4	68.5
Costa Rica	80.8	70.0
Greece	81.1	70.9
Israel	82.6	72.4
Italy	83.0	71.9
Japan	84.3	74.1
Singapore	83.2	73.6
Switzerland	83.4	72.5
UK	81.4	70.1
US	78.5	66.1

disease and/or injury." While the calculations for this second statistic are a little more squishy, it highlights the fact that it's not just about living longer but about compressing the time between disability or infirmity and your ultimate demise. We'll come back to this important point again in Chapter 9.

What is life expectancy anyway? It sounds simple enough but I want you to understand it is just another data point statisticians use for comparisons and doesn't itself provide any indication of your expected lifespan. Let me give you an example. Suppose we have a family where Mom died at age ninety, Dad at age ninety-five, but of their two children, one died in a bicycle accident at age five and the other died of cancer at age sixty-two. The average age at death for this family is (90+95+5+62)/4=63. Does that seem representative to you for the expected lifespan[15] of any of their relatives? I'd love to study how Mom and Dad lived compared to the one who died of cancer.

That is exactly what Dan Buettner did with a team of demographers from National Geographic once they identified the first Blue Zone—an area with a higher proportion of centenarians than anywhere else in the world. I love how Buettner describes the details of the lives and cultures of each of the locations studied.[16] He quotes very few data points but instead paints a picture of the day-to-day experiences of the inhabitants: how they spend their time, how they interact with other humans, what they eat, and their recognition of something greater than themselves in the world. It makes you long to go visit these wonderful people. The five locations studied are:

- **Sardinia, Italy**—the mountainous highlands of this island to the west of mainland Italy with the world's highest concentration of male centenarians.
- **Okinawa, Japan**—an island south of the mainland, with the longest-living female population in the world.
- **Loma Linda, California**—high concentration of Seventh-Day Adventists where health is built into their faith disciplines. Live ten years longer on average than the rest of the US.
- **Nicoya Pennisula, Costa Rica**—second-highest concentration of male centenarians.
- **Ikaria, Greece**—Aegean island between Turkey and Greece with one of the world's lowest rates of middle-age mortality and lowest rates of dementia. Ikaria is not covered in the book, but you can read about it on the website.

Even if you can't afford to visit them you can still create a blue zone in your little corner of the world. These centenarians are some of the poorest people on the planet. They don't have access to all the latest expensive health technology, pharmaceuticals, or convenience tools. They live traditional lives full of faith and community.

Nine Lessons for Living Longer from *The Blue Zones*	
Move	Move Naturally
Eat Wisely	80% Rule
	Plant Slant
	Wine at 5
Right Outlook	Purpose
	Down Shift
Connect	Right Tribe
	Loved Ones First
	Belong

While each location has its own unique recipe for longevity, Buettner teased out nine common ingredients that he calls the Power Nine: lessons for living longer. These are further grouped into four categories as can be seen from the table. Two of these we have discussed already, Eat Wisely (per *The China Study* and to be covered more in Chapter 5) and Connect (as highlighted in the Roseto study and covered more in Chapter 9). Before we leave this chapter, I want to touch on Movement and Outlook.

Your Body Needs to Move

I have a desk job. I can sometimes spend twelve hours a day at my desk. This is seriously detrimental to my health if I don't take steps to counterbalance it (pun intended!). Studies abound on the risks of inactivity on our health. One study a decade ago calculated the impact on chronic disease and associated deaths worldwide due specifically to inactivity.[17] Given the numbers were similar to deaths from smoking we started to see headlines comparing sitting to smoking cigarettes. This is impactful given the well-accepted understanding of what cigarettes do to your health. I have this headline in mind almost every day I am deskbound.

We are only starting to understand all the different mechanisms involved though. When you move you are engaging your musculoskeletal (MSK) system. This includes your skeleton—your bones of course, and your muscles which need to contract to create movement. But it also includes ligaments, tendons, joints, and a wonderful substance called fascia that connects everything together with your nerves and organs. Your fascia can actually cause more discomfort than the better-known elements as it has a sort of memory of past insults which can lead to a "weakness" like I have in my neck. After an impact injury some years ago which took over a year to heal I can have a lesser "relapse" if I don't take care of my MSK system. For me this means an ergonomic setup for my desk and office chair, 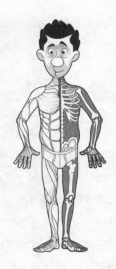 getting up regularly to go for a walk or refill my water, daily stretches, strenuous hiking twice a week with my husband and more high-impact exercise or sports when I can fit it in.

But movement doesn't only impact your MSK system. There are many other mechanisms at play. One obvious one is that you use up less fuel when you're sitting around compared to activity. Notice I don't refer to fewer calories burned, as that is oversimplification. There is a complex effect on your overall metabolism which is heavily influenced by your microbiome. Getting back to our bugs, the effect of exercise on the microbiome is particularly fascinating. It seems that there is a bidirectional relationship such that exercise encourages the growth of healthy bacteria in your gut which produce metabolites called short-chain fatty acids (SCFAs), which are critical to digestion, insulin sensitivity, and mood regulation. But the microbes also stimulate your nervous system to promote the desire to exercise more. Cool right? This is why it is so hard to start an exercise routine but once you form the habit you crave it.[18]

Another mechanism at play in movement is exercising your heart which is basically one big muscle pumping blood all around your body into every nook and cranny. We talk about cardiovascular exercise but basically anything that makes you huff and puff is exercising your heart. Going up and down stairs counts. Being sedentary can result in poor circulation which in turn depletes not only oxygenated blood and nutrients getting around your body but all the chemical processes keeping each part healthy become compromised.

While your circulatory system relies on a pump—your heart—the lymphatic system has no pump. The lymphatic system is basically the waste disposal department of your body: working closely with the circulatory system it's responsible for cleaning the cellular environment, enabling the absorption of fats, and most critically producing and transporting antibodies to fight infection. Without a pump, it relies on the contraction of muscles and joints to keep things moving. A sluggish or stagnant lymph system is a recipe for disease.

Those of you who have a manual job in a factory or on a farm are ahead of the game here. If you live in a blue zone and spend a lot of your day walking to the shops, to your social gatherings or to tend to your sheep or customers, again a check mark. But if you're like me and are stuck behind a desk much of the time, you need to take matters into your own hands. We'll come back to movement throughout Part II and especially in Chapter 9 on aging well.[19]

Rest Is Part of Life

My younger son is an Eagle Scout. It took a lot of years of camping and other outdoor activities to reach that rank. I was very involved and loved every minute of it. Mostly because a lot of our campouts were in the far-off wilderness, often with no cell service, no showers, sometimes no toilets and only the wonders of nature to focus on. After a day of hiking, rock climbing, caving, or just teaching survival skills, we'd eat around a fire and often be tucked up in our sleeping bags not long after dark. I slept SO well on those trips even though

I was basically sleeping on the ground and usually a little chilly. My mind totally shut off from the business of my executive job, chores around the house, and other commitments. Even though camping can be strenuous physically, it forces you to be in the moment and move at the speed of nature. In fact totally at the mercy of nature. You don't control anything when you're out in the elements as we found out a few weeks ago caught in a fierce lightning storm while camping on Pisgah Crater, a very remote piece of volcanic rock in the middle of nowhere, California. But I feel fully restored and refreshed when I return home from these trips.

The human body was designed for hard work followed by periods of rest. There are numerous places in the Bible that direct us on this point starting with the story of creation in the book of Genesis. In the second chapter, there is an explanation of God resting on the seventh day, but we also find the instruction in the law of Moses and in Jesus's teachings.[20] The centenarians in Buettner's blue zones all have structured periods of rest and reflection. Plus, at the end of every day they unwind and let their routines be dictated by the rhythm of the sun going down. I bet our blue zones friends sleep as deeply at night as I sleep in my tent.

I find the majority of commentary on sleep in media and health information tends to focus on a lack of sleep as a symptom of something out of whack in the body. This is entirely true. If you are attempting to sleep a solid seven or eight hours a night and having difficulties, unless there's obvious external influences like a crying baby or noisy neighbors, it's likely a sign of an imbalance in the body. We'll address these as we get into the health issues in Part II. The bigger problem is that sleep is not better recognized as critical to our good health and longevity.

Business executives and young people nowadays seem to wear a shortage of sleep as a badge of honor. I wonder if they would change their tune if it were more commonly understood what sleep is and what it does for our body. Matthew Walker, in his internationally acclaimed book *Why We Sleep* refers to sleep as "really quite magi-cal" and explains of years of sleep research: "We had learned a subtle, but important lesson: sleep was far more intelligent than we had once imagined."[21] While I share Walker's fascination for sleep as well as some of his life story (he went to the University of Nottingham in England and now resides in the US), I am blessed to have an under-standing that God created the mechanism of sleep whereas Walker clumsily tries to use evolution as a way to explain what doesn't make sense. Having to spend one-third of our daily allotted hours uncon-scious seems counterintuitive to the survival of a species, but that is exactly how God has designed it.

Healthy sleep involves cycling through REM and non-REM sleep throughout the night. REM sleep is named for the rapid eye move-ments involved in an otherwise completely motionless (purposefully paralyzed) body. Each sleep cycle lasts about ninety minutes but the design of our sleep process is particularly curious as the ratio of REM to NREM sleep in each cycle changes throughout the night. The first part of the night is heavily weighted toward deep "slow-wave" NREM sleep. This is the brain's repair mechanism when neurons are pruned and memories consolidated. Not only your memories of the report you read or skill you learned the day before, but your immune system's memories of pathogens it has encountered, enabling you to better fight infections in the future. The body also uses "slow-wave" sleep to flush out toxins and recycle cellular waste (a process known as autophagy).

The second half of the night is more heavily weighted toward REM sleep, also known as dream-sleep. Interestingly your brain waves ramp up during REM sleep to levels sometimes even in excess of brain activ-ity when you are awake. In this phase your brain is processing emotions and motivations. If slow-wave sleep provides reflection, dream-sleep is focused on integration; interconnecting all the various experiences of life to build an ever more accurate model of how it all works. It's quite incredible how on entering REM sleep every muscle in your body, other than those you use to breathe, are completely disabled to ensure you can't act out the activities in your dream.

Impact on Teenagers
Teenagers naturally have a circadian rhythm that puts them in bed later but we insist on waking them up early to attend school. This creates a shortage of REM sleep which would be concentrated in the later parts of their sleep period. The impact is particularly damaging to their emotional health.

Both types of sleep are equally important to our healthy functioning for different reasons. A shortage of good-quality sleep has been shown to weaken your immune system, increase your risk of cancer, disrupt your blood sugar management, increase your likelihood of cardiovascular disease, and contribute negatively to any psychiatric disorder like depression, anxiety and increase your risk of dementia and Alzheimer's. Focusing on getting good-quality sleep is one of those free solutions that is simply a no-brainer for the currently healthy and those struggling with a health issue.

Sleep has always been a priority in my life with a strict 10 p.m. bedtime or earlier if my global job demanded a 5 a.m. conference call for example. Full disclaimer: those calls were taken in my pajamas with the alarm set just one minute earlier. The arrival of video calls in recent years didn't alter this scenario, as some of my colleagues can attest.

In Part II we'll look at some strategies if you are struggling to get a good seven to eight hours sleep at least six days a week.

A Word on Faith

As we wrap up this chapter, I did want to point out what is probably obvious to some of you but every one of the Blue Zones™ lifestyles highlighted faith. All the healthy centenarians participated in some sort of religious community. Other studies have supported this observation showing that in general people who have a commitment to one of the traditional religions such that they attend religious services regularly have a longer life expectancy, lower rates of cardio-vascular disease, lower rates of depression and anxiety, and generally stronger immune systems. Maybe it is because people of faith tend to follow most of the other healthful practices such as being socially connected, having a strong sense of purpose, treating their bodies well so as not to engage in harmful behaviors like smoking, taking illegal substances, or drinking and driving. They tend to be more physically active through service opportunities and are encouraged to have daily periods of self-reflection and meditation or prayer.

It seems that science is only just catching up with what has been documented for two thousand years. For those interested in exploring faith further I go into some detail in Appendix C but for now I will just address the myth that science and faith are somehow incompatible. If you dig a little into the origins of various scientific disciplines you will find that strong Christians led the way. In fact the oldest universities operating today, and three of the most prestigious, are the Universities of Paris, Bologna, and Oxford that were all founded on Christian principals. These then gave rise to several other well-known universities in Europe also founded on Christian principles including Cambridge and St Andrews. Sadly, while Harvard and Yale in the US were founded on Christian principles, they have clearly moved far away from them in recent years. Those who believed in God understood their world to be the product of a singular, orderly, rational mind, and they were driven to better understand God through the natural world He created. They were motivated by their desire to worship God through studying His universe and these universities were just the place to do that.

Scientific discovery exploded after Jesus arrived, with the vast majority of scientific breakthroughs being led by Christians across a wide variety of disciplines such as astronomy, mathematics, geography, medicine, chemistry, geology, botany, paleontology, and zoology to name just a few. You might think these faith-based discoveries slowed after Darwin came on the scene with his theory of evolution that provided an alternative explanation to God. But Christians have dominated even the post-Darwin period of scientific discoveries, and this continues to this day across the widest possible list of scientific disciplines.

Of course it's a little harder to identify who believes in God these days as it's a badge that tends to be kept hidden. However, at the 100th anniversary of the Nobel Prize, statistics were gathered on religious affiliations and it was found that 65 percent of all winners had identified as Christians. The next biggest group were Jews at 21 percent, then atheists/agnostics at 7 percent and other religions or movements at 3 percent or lower.[22]

So if you already belong to a religious community, get more involved. If you don't, then, if for no other reason than your health, I recommend you keep an open mind and give it a go!

Points to Remember

1. Your genetic makeup has only a tiny impact on your health. Susceptibility to disease can be overcome with healthy behaviors.
2. The genetics (diversity) of your microbiome and lifestyle factors (epigenetics) have the strongest impact on your health.
3. It is all the millions of interactions of your body with this world, positive or negative, across days, months, and years that dictate whether it is kept in balance or falls into illness.
4. Staying active provides a range of health benefits beyond your musculoskeletal system.
5. Quality sleep of seven to eight hours a night is critical for maintaining good health.
6. Faith in God has been scientifically proven to be good for your health.

CHAPTER 4

A Toxic Planet

What comes to mind when you hear the word toxin? A noxious chemical oozing out of the back of a factory? A nerve agent used in war? My old print edition of the Oxford English Dictionary defines a toxin as a "poison produced by a living organism, especially one formed in the body and stimulating the production of antibodies."[1] We find a lot of naturally occurring toxins in nature, such as ricin, which is produced by the castor plant and is a by-product when you process the beans to make castor oil. Ricin has been used as a biological weapon. The bacteria *Clostridium botulinum* creates the toxin botulinum which causes the illness botulism if you eat food tainted with it. Botulism symptoms of muscle paralysis, which can include the muscles you use to breathe, have been exploited by Big Pharma to create the drug Botox used to treat various medical and cosmetic conditions. Death cap mushrooms are the most toxic to humans, producing the toxin cyclopeptide, which ravages the liver if ingested. Tetrodotoxin is found in various marine animals, most famously the puffer fish or blowfish consumed in Japan as sushi. It acts by blocking the sodium channels in the body, resulting in cardiac, neurological, and stomach problems, and can be fatal.

But in today's language toxin or something that is toxic to you has a much broader definition. It includes anything that is harmful to the body in any way and that's the context we're going to use in this book.[2] The damage inflicted from toxins under this broader definition may be just as vicious as the examples above but as they act slowly and some-

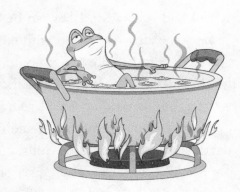

times imperceptibly, we are prone to ignoring them. We are like the frog who is sitting in a pot of cold water as we slowly apply the heat. He will die once the water boils rather than jump out as he doesn't feel the immediate damage all at once.

I bet you have a hard time being told what not to do. Believe me, I prefer to focus on healthy additions to your life rather than recommendations on what to take away. But it's important to give you the whole truth about interacting with this world and the place and time God has put you into it. Often this means not completely taking things away, but adjusting the details, which I'll explain as we go.

When Dan Buettner conducted his longevity research in the early 2000s, most of the people he interviewed were born at the turn of the twentieth century. This was before dangerous and unnatural chemicals introduced into our lives really took off. Buettner's nine principles of longevity are all positives: recommendations to add to your life rather than pitfalls to watch out for. It is always difficult to prove a negative (that taking something away is good for you). Plus, the more Buettner's centenarians nourished themselves with good principles, the better equipped their bodies were to deal with any negatives. As the toxic load has increased in recent decades this balance is harder to maintain.

Remember the camping trips I took with my younger son the Eagle Scout? While I do find camping in the wilderness incredibly restful and restorative, I have to be honest that I'm always ready to come home after two nights with no running water or other modern amenities. I'm happily dirty (my microbiome appreciates the boost) but life takes an extra effort out there to keep the bugs out of your sleeping bag, wrestle a tent collapsing in a storm, cook the food on an open fire with no refrigeration, and manage temperature extremes of daytime heat and nighttime chills.

Modern conveniences are part of the human condition. We can recognize a number of human failings we used to call the seven deadly sins in our embrace of the trappings of modern life such as sloth or laziness—we'd prefer to spend less time cleaning or cooking. Gluttony drives our desires for fast food and ultra-processed ready-to-go food as well as constant entertainment and instant satisfaction of our desires. The greed of big industry to drive profits through making more products cheaper and marketing messages telling us we need what they are selling. Pride in our appearance and our envy at wanting to follow the crowd to embrace the latest products. God frowns on these qualities because He knows they are detrimental to us when pleasure and enjoyment can be easily found in contentment and optimism. As we learned from our study of the healthcare industry in Chapter 2, newer doesn't necessarily mean better.

Of course there is a safety aspect to some modern conveniences such as antilock brakes, air-conditioning, and fireproof building insulation. But the incessant adherence to germ theory has driven the herbicide, pesticide and disinfectant craze beyond measure which is particularly misguided. Not only do the risks outweigh the benefits but the perceived benefits were based on faulty science to begin with as we'll get into in Chapter 6.

You may think that there are plenty of controls in place to protect us from harm but in one example a government subcommittee was convened in 2010 to look at the public harm from chemicals in the environment.[3] It found that of eighty thousand chemicals we are exposed to in everyday products only two hundred of them had even been tested by the Environmental Protection Agency. There is a total lack of regulation and the studies that do make it to mass media are often controlled by the very industry pushing their dangerous products.[4] This means that reducing your exposure to toxins, just like all aspects of your health, is a personal responsibility.

There are many ways to categorize toxins such as the class of chemical or element they fall under (e.g. solvents, pesticides) or the system in the body most affected (e.g. endocrine disruptors) but to make it easiest for you to apply to your own lifestyle and figure out how to reduce your exposure, we're going to look at the most common areas of our lives where we encounter toxins. While we'll only be touching on a fraction of the toxins we are exposed to, I hope it will open your eyes to the many bad influences getting into your own bucket. Hence making it more important than ever to increase the good influences in our overall interaction with the world.

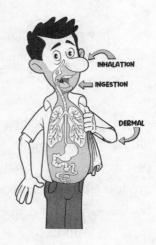

The three major routes of exposure to toxins are through ingestion (our mouths, stomachs, intestines), through inhalation (our lungs, respiratory tract) and dermal (through our skin). But thinking about our five senses we'll also touch on negatives we take in through our eyes and ears toward the end of the chapter. So fasten your seatbelt and let's see why we need to jump out of the boiling pot.

Avoidable Consumption

Arguably this should be the easiest way to control the toxins you are exposed to given the influence you have over the orifice known as your mouth. But in my experience it is one of the likeliest culprits given the power of the food and agriculture industries (we'll collectively refer to as Big Food) and the impact of convenience over nourishment.

We're going to focus on real food in Chapter 5, so here I'm going to limit the commentary to the "food-like-substances" many of us put in our mouths regularly. Packaged foods that we buy at the grocery store or eat on the run as "fast food" contain a dizzying array of food additives including flavor enhancers, coloring, emulsifiers, preservatives, artificial sweeteners, thickeners, and bulking agents. Not to mention the residues of pesticides, herbicides, and antibiotics that have been used in creating the base ingredients as cheaply as possible. Many of these are presumed safe only because each one individually makes up a small percentage of the total food product. But remember our bucket—if you're consuming these food-like-substances that have very little nutritional value to help your body run its detoxification systems you're getting out of balance at double speed.

> **Ultra-Processed Foods**
> All forms of cooking tend to involve processing food such as curing, drying, fermenting, smoking; all of which are healthy ways to prepare food. If it comes in a package made by Big Food though for maximum profit it is more likely to be full of toxins with very little nutritional value and engineered to be hyper-palatable (i.e. addictive). We call these products ultra-processed food. A study in the *British Medical Journal* in 2019 showed consuming large amounts of UPFs resulted in a 62 percent increase in mortality over the fifteen year study period.[5] Other studies link UPFs to specific diseases.[6]

Let's start with **Emulsifiers and Gums**. These help to improve the texture and consistency of processed food. Carrageenan is one of the worst offenders, common in dairy products in particular but also found in a wide variety of other packaged foods such as dairy-alternatives, deli-meats, and even coconut water. It is derived from seaweed and hence Big Food claims it is natural and safe; there is much push-back on those of us who claim it causes health problems. But it's been linked to digestive tract ailments in scientific studies[7] and anecdotally when conscientiously eliminated from diets symptoms tend to improve.[8] Xanthan gum is derived from fermented corn using industrial processes and tends to lurk in gluten-free baked goods. You may also come across guar gum which has similar properties but is more often used in cold foods. Guar is derived from a legume, the guar bean, but again don't think this makes it good for your body. The gums have been associated with digestive ailments and autoimmune disease.[9]

Glutamate in all its many forms is the most common flavor enhancer used throughout the packaged food industry but also in restaurants. It is similarly derived from a natural product, usually seaweed. While natural glutamate is a major amino acid used by the body as a neurotransmitter, too much of

> **Hiding in plain sight—the many names of Glutamate**
> - MSG—monosodium glutamate
> - Glutamic acid
> - Yeast extract
> - Soy protein isolate
> . . . and many more

it, and the synthetic form in particular, has been strongly associated with neurological diseases such as Alzheimer's, Parkinson's, and Huntington's.[10] I find I get a headache when unwillingly exposed to MSG. If you have to eat that takeout food, studies have shown that natural spices like garlic and curcumin and the nutrient quercetin can be protective against the cell damage.[11]

Nitrates and nitrites are the next "innocent"-sounding additives endemic in our food, particularly in processed meats such as bacon, hot dogs, and salami to enhance the color and to preserve and flavor the meat. Nitrates are found in natural forms in many healthy foods like beets and leafy greens. However, when included as a food additive and subject to high heat in the processing, they get broken down first into nitrites and then combine with the amines in the protein to form nitrosamines which are carcinogenic. One study of half a million Americans estimated about half the increase in mortality they found with the consumption of processed meats could be attributed to nitrites.[12]

While we're on the subject of meat, the unwarranted campaign against meat (explained in Chapter 5) has led to an explosion of fake meats on offer. These food-like substances contain far more harmful ingredients which your body doesn't recognize as food. If it's not identified as "friend" by your body then it must be a "foe" and attacked as an invader, which creates inflammation. When inflammation is chronic and ongoing it leads to illness.

Vegetable and seed oils were also developed in response to reductionist science claiming saturated fat found in meat and butter is bad for you. We'll get into the benefits of healthy natural fats in Chapter 5 but the resulting reliance on cheap highly processed fats has contributed more to chronic disease than possibly even sugar. They have only existed in the last hundred years or so with the invention of the hydrogenation process by Procter & Gamble to convert surplus unused cotton seeds into synthetic cottonseed oil sold under the brand name Crisco. Margarine was invented shortly afterwards followed by a range of highly processed oils such as canola, sunflower, safflower, corn, and soy. You might have heard that trans fats are the main contributor to poor health and steps have been taken to ban them but don't be fooled that removing one processing method has solved the problem.

Did you know it takes ninety-eight ears of corn to make five tablespoons of corn oil, which is the amount you're typically consuming in a plate of tortilla chips? Or that it takes 2,800 sunflower seeds to make five tablespoons of sunflower oil, a typical amount in a bag of potato chips? Not only is the amount ingested highly unnatural, but these oils are almost entirely a type of omega-6 fat called linoleic acid (LA) which the body needs in only minute amounts. LA is unstable, easily oxidized to create free radicals in the body, causing chronic inflammation and leading to mitochondrial disfunction, immune system impairment, damage to the cells lining your blood vessels, and cognitive impairment to name a few.[13] There are other documented health risks and studies highlighting the overall increase in mortality from consuming these processed oils. It's been calculated that for every one teaspoon of these oils you consume your risk of death increases by as much as smoking two cigarettes.[14]

Sugar and sweeteners have become such a problem partly because fifty years ago we were brainwashed into thinking fat is bad for us so we replaced our eggs cooked in butter for breakfast with low-fat flavored yogurt which has about as much sugar as a can of Coke. Low-fat products abounded swapping out the fat for sugar in its various forms. Sugar is not a food group. It is more than just empty calories though; it causes heart disease, diabetes, cancer, and fatty liver disease for a start.[15] Part of the challenge is that it is more addictive than cocaine, meaning that while I hate to preach total abstinence, in the case of refined sugar found in most packaged products, this tends to be the best approach.[16] If you have a sweet tooth grab an apple or home baked goods made with coconut oil which are naturally sweet and do not have the same damaging effect. High-fructose corn syrup has made it into just about everything these days from baked goods to salad dressings, ketchup, breakfast cereals, and other ready-made foods and ice cream, but it's not the only perpetrator of your ill-health.. Added sugar is hidden in all sorts of ingredients such as anything with the suffix "-ose" like fructose, dextrose, sucrose, or with the word "cane" or "syrup" such as rice syrup and agave syrup (which might sound healthier but is pure fructose and processed with toxic chemicals).

Similar to the history of processed fats Big Food thought they had a great marketing campaign with artificial sweeteners such as saccharin (Sweet 'N Low), aspartame (NutraSweet, Equal), and sucralose (Splenda) but these chemical additives are even worse for you. Studies have shown they are carcinogenic, and a recent study of sucralose showed it was genotoxic which means it damages DNA when metabolized.[17] It is a huge mistake to consume diet sodas thinking you are taking in fewer calories when in reality these artificial sweeteners wreak havoc on your gut microbes, destroy beneficial bacteria, and end up causing glucose intolerance which leads to diabetes.[18] They have also been linked to neurological effects such as seizures.[19]

While it might be a particularly tough lifestyle change, the good news is that cutting out sugar improves your health rapidly even without any other interventions.

About a year after Covid-19 came on the scene, I was watching an online health conference and heard a talk by eminent research scientist Stephanie Seneff from the Massachusetts Institute of Technology (MIT). The presentation focused on **Glyphosate** and its role in bad Covid outcomes, but the implications were far wider. You may not have heard of the chemical glyphosate but maybe you have heard of one of its most common manifestations, the weed killer Roundup? The pervasiveness of this herbicide in our food and environment together with the dramatic and myriad ways it affects our health drove me to research more. Happily, Seneff was about to release her now award-winning book *Toxic Legacy: How the Weedkiller Glyphosate is Destroying Our Health and the Environment,*[20] which I highly recommend.

Industrial players that create and utilize glyphosate try to tell us it is safe for humans because it utilizes a metabolic pathway in plant cells that human cells don't possess known as the shikimate pathway. This enables it to be so effective at killing weeds. The big problem though is that our gut microbes do have a shikimate pathway which is central to their metabolism enabling the synthesis of amino acids we rely on. It's these beneficial microbes that are most damaged by glyphosate causing pathogenic ones to thrive in our guts instead.

The effect on the shikimate pathway is not the only concern with glyphosate as it has a number of mechanisms detrimental to human health such that Seneff refers to its toxicity as "unique and diabolical." It is generally recognized that glyphosate causes cancer particularly in workers exposed on farms or in gardens but the wide

Implications for GMOs

One of the main drawbacks of Genetically Modified Organisms, found in packaged food and amongst conventional fruits and vegetables in the grocery store, is that they have been bred to withstand the spraying of glyphosate to kill the weeds and pests while maintaining the food crop. So called "Roundup Ready" corn and soy in particular are now ubiquitous in the food supply particularly UPFs. But any GMO produce tends to have more residue from harmful chemicals like glyphosate and are best avoided.

range of health problems Seneff explains includes fertility, hormone disruption, autoimmune diseases, and mental health problems. The effect on the liver is particularly concerning given the importance of the liver to our overall health compounded by all the other chemical toxins our livers are having to deal with each and every day.

I've focused on glyphosate here because of its unique and complex action in our bodies but also because of its pervasiveness in our food and environment. In addition to being sprayed on crops it is used as a drying agent on grains like wheat and barley making them easier to harvest. This could be contributing to the rise in celiac disease and non-celiac gluten sensitivity. The best way to protect yourself is to avoid ultra-processed foods that rely on glyphosate-treated crops but also avoid conventional fresh produce and buy only organic that may not be completely chemical-free (the organic label has some workarounds) but should have vastly lower quantities of herbicides and pesticides.

Beyond glyphosate the other major culprits are **Atrazine**, known
to cause extreme hormone disruption even at low levels, and **Paraquat**,
which is particularly linked to Parkinson's disease.[21] Atrazine is another
herbicide used on crops, especially corn, but also in gardens and on
golf-courses. It has been shown to induce testosterone to be converted
to estrogen resulting in a range of problems such as sexual disfunction
as well as cancers of the breast and prostate.[22] It has been implicated in
contributing to the rise of gender dysphoria.

Breakfast, lunch, and dinner are obviously the biggest concern but
for completeness I want to include those recreational ingestions such as
cigarettes, alcohol, and caffeine in the thought process of your overall toxic load. Now you may be surprised I'm grouping these together
but hear me out. I promise I am not a puritanical killjoy. These have all
been part of my lifestyle in the past but their long-term health consequences are just not worth the temporary pleasure.

I probably don't have to try too hard to convince you that cigarettes are bad for health. It's not the nicotine per se naturally occurring in tobacco plants (although it is highly addictive and raises
blood pressure putting a strain on the cardiovascular system), but
the recipe of chemicals included in the products we consume and the
damage done to the lungs through inhaling irritating substances.
Smoking cigarettes is quite simply playing Russian roulette with
your life.

Alcohol may be a bit harder to sell you on its toxicity given it's
usually derived from fermentation of grapes or other produce and
organic wines are touted for their antioxidant properties. Indeed one
of Dan Buettner's Power Nine principles from the Blue Zones is "Wine
at 5" (though it has to be said one of the five Blue Zones, Loma Linda
California, abstains from alcohol altogether). A recent review of the last
forty years of research has called into question whether alcohol has any
healthful benefits at all.[23] Other studies have concluded that alcohol

consumption accounts for a "considerable proportion" of cancer incidence and mortality across the US.[24] Alcohol is metabolized in the
liver into toxic by-products such as formaldehyde, with women more
prone than men to the effects. So while the occasional glass of wine on
special occasions is to be enjoyed, the amount of alcohol you consume
in a particular week should definitely be on your negative bucket list.

As if that isn't upsetting enough, I'm now going to go after
caffeine. I am British, remember. The craving for a good strong cup
of tea particularly midafternoon and preferably with a chocolate
digestive biscuit (American readers can think cookie!) is burned into
my soul. My husband is a huge coffee drinker. When I met him, the
need for coffee as soon as he awoke and regularly throughout the day
impacted our schedule more than I would have liked. He has cut down
immensely but afternoon coffee is an occasional treat we like to enjoy
together (though I usually regret even a decaffeinated version at this
point as decaf doesn't mean non-caf with up to 10 percent of caffeine
still remaining).

Caffeine is "the most widely used (and abused) psychoactive stimulant in the world."[25] It works by taking over the adenosine receptors
in your brain. Adenosine is the chemical that builds up in your brain
the longer you have been awake and tells you when it's time to sleep. If
caffeine has taken over the receptor sites, the adenosine is still building
up but you don't feel the effects, so your brain doesn't know to begin
its sleep routine. This is why you might get a caffeine crash, as once you
have degraded the caffeine (another job for your liver) suddenly all that
built-up adenosine registers. Caffeine has an average half-life of five to
seven hours though it depends on your genetics and age (your body
gets less efficient at processing it as you age). But in general, if you've
had a cup of coffee at 4 p.m., by 9 p.m. at the earliest you've still got
half the caffeine circulating. So you are not going to benefit from a full
measure of adenosine sending you into a natural restful sleep for many

more hours. Trying to combat caffeine with alcohol is a terrible idea as alcohol is a sedative that makes you unconscious which is not the same as sleep. Alcohol has been specifically shown to suppress REM sleep, which is partly why it is so damaging to unborn babies.

Beyond the sleep impact caffeine can escalate psychiatric problems like depression or anxiety, increases your blood pressure, and can trigger cardiac irregularities. It is a diuretic, so it can induce dehydration and is linked to headaches in those who consume it due to its effect on the blood vessels in the brain. Whether the antioxidants found in the coffee bean outweigh the negative effects on your body only you can decide, however the synthetic caffeine used in Big Food products has no redeeming qualities.[26] Coffee and tea have some, but I prefer a handful of blueberries on most days.

Lastly, as you'll recall from Chapter 2, medications need to be put into the negative category of what is going into your bucket. Even if they resolve a particular symptom you are suffering from, they are metabolized by your liver and should be treated as toxins for the adverse effects they have on the overall balance in your body. And that's just looking at the active ingredients without even considering the inactive additives and fillers to make them palatable and shelf-stable.

Putting on Your Body

Moving from ingestion to absorption. Did you know that your skin is actually the largest organ in your body in terms of overall size and weight? It is also one of the most complicated. We are still learning all the functions of healthy skin but those we do know include working as a barrier to protect against water loss, physical and chemical injury, and bugs. It helps regulate our temperature and protects us against UV radiation from the sun. It gives us our sense of touch. It enables the synthesis of vitamin D when sunlight falls on it. However, for all its protective properties, skin is remarkably absorbent. We call this *dermal permeability*. Big Pharma studies this phenomenon to find new ways of delivering drugs for convenience or to avoid the digestive tract. You've probably heard of nicotine patches to help quit smoking or hormone patches to manage the symptoms of menopause or for contraceptive action. It's why essential oils are powerful remedies immediately absorbed by the skin acting without interference from other bodily processes.

Given the knowledge of dermal permeability and the significant surface area of our skin compared to any other part of our body why are we so careless with what comes into contact with it?

Starting with **cosmetics**, the list of harmful ingredients is endless such as benzene (strongly linked to leukemia), triclosan (an antimicrobial that damages your microbiome), parabens, formaldehyde, phthalates (also used in plastics and discussed more below), and hundreds of other industrial chemicals. Fragrances are a particular problem as you are inhaling the chemicals as well as absorbing through your skin. Whereas historically botanicals such as essential oils and naturally occurring compounds were used to add pleasant aromas, in the twentieth century it was found to be far cheaper to manufacture synthetic forms of fragrance from chemicals that have since been found to be endocrine disrupters. This means they upset the balance of hormones in your body with wide ranging health impacts such as on fertility, on puberty and on metabolism for example. If you see the word "fragrance" as an ingredient that can mean a range of synthetic chemicals. Some manufacturers will put "natural fragrance" on the label to throw you off but while this may exclude the worst offenders it still involves a harsh industrial process with a range of chemicals. For example, Lilial can be included under natural fragrance in the US to add floral aromas to the substance but has recently been banned in the EU as carcinogenic and mutagenic (causing cancers and reproductive problems).[27]

Deodorant is a particular problem due to the common addition of **Aluminum** as an antiperspirant. The human body has no use for aluminum, a known neurotoxin that builds up in tissues over time. But as a stable metal with a range of helpful properties it has become all too common in our environment not only in personal care products but in cookware and in pharmaceuticals. To make matters worse aluminum binds to glyphosate with the combination finding it easier to cross the blood-brain barrier enhancing its toxicity.[28]

While we're on the subject it's worth a special callout for the whole category of **heavy metals** which wreak havoc on our bodies in insidious ways. These include lead, arsenic, cadmium, and mercury. The list of negative health impacts is vast including gastrointestinal and kidney dysfunction, nervous system disorders, skin lesions, vascular damage, immune system dysfunc-

> **Combating Heavy Metals**
> While medical chelation may be necessary in severe cases, supplementing with natural zeolites daily can help to detox the body from heavy metals. Zeolites work by attracting and trapping heavy metals from your cells to enable them to be eliminated. See Resources for recommendations.

tion, birth defects, and cancer, with the simultaneous exposure to two or more of them likely having cumulative effects.[29] The neurotoxic effects of mercury are said to be one thousand times greater than lead. They get into our bodies in a variety of ways from beauty products, medications, dental fillings, vehicle exhausts, household products, the fish we eat, and even the water we drink. Given their ability to accumulate in the body and wide-ranging effects it is worth a special effort to avoid this category of toxins.

Aluminum is just one of a range of nasty chemicals that show up in **sunscreen**, which is another hot spot I want to call out particularly living in Southern California where people tend to slather on thick layers of sunscreen multiple times a day. Why is it that skin cancer rates have gone up the last fifty years in line with the increase in use of sunscreen? We are encouraged to go for higher and higher levels of protection, SPF 50 or even 65 but the chemicals get even nastier to achieve that level of "sun protection factor." Going back to where we started in Chapter 1, the sun is vital to human existence.[30] Why are we trying to block it?

Indeed it can be damaging to your skin to stay in the midday sun until you burn but putting toxic chemicals on your skin is not the answer. There are nutrients that can boost your skin's natural sun protection such as astaxanthin (found in aquatic animals like salmon, shrimp, and lobster and responsible for the pink pigment of flamingoes), lycopene, beta carotene, and vitamins D and E, i.e., through a healthy diet. I decided to try an astaxanthin supplement on this summer's family vacation and found 12mg a day to work well for even the two fair-skinned members of my family. The vegetable and seed oils I denigrated earlier have been linked to higher levels of melanoma (a type of skin cancer)[31] and I have heard anecdotal stories of people who used to burn easily in the sun having less of a problem once they cut out these oils. If you simply must be out at the beach all day in the height of summer, there are a few less harmful products available (see Resources). Better yet, come in for a siesta (nap) during the hottest part of the day, a great concept practiced by many cultures living in sunnier places.

What about your clothes? I've found that a typical bottle of laundry detergent doesn't even contain a list of ingredients. This highlights the attitude that only small amounts of any one ingredient are being used so it's not enough to worry about. In the case of detergent, it's diluted with water and your clothes are only loosely on your body. But this is not accounting for the accumulation of microscopic amounts of all sorts of harmful chemicals throughout the day. **Dry-cleaning** raises the alert level further. Trichloroethylene (TCE) is widely used to dry-clean clothes (as well as decaffeinating coffee, degreasing metal parts, and processing vegetable oils) and has been associated with a 500 percent increased risk for Parkinson's disease not only in those who work with it but in those exposed as hobbyists using it as a solvent.[32]

Fortunately, I only have a handful of dry-clean-only clothes these days and I leave them in our garage without the plastic wrap for a couple of days to air out afterward. I've never been into wearing makeup, reserving that ritual for weddings and other major evening events once or twice a year. Some of you may push back in horror at the thought of not wearing makeup, but if you treat your skin well, avoiding harsh chemicals and letting it get some morning sun and plenty of nourishment, you won't be in such a hurry to hide it.

For my own wedding I also decided to treat myself to a manicure at a nail salon. What a den of toxic soup those are. I will never return.

Being prone to eczema I am extremely careful with what I put on my skin in terms of moisturizer or sun care, finding even brands like Neutrogena to be problematic. I include some recommended brands in the Resources section.

Hair care is a particular challenge for me as I have exceptionally thick hair that is starting to grey. While I don't mind the salt and pepper look, those grey hairs are very unruly! For years I had used a leave-in conditioner but after studying the ingredients one day I decided I'd be better off without it. My hair started falling out in clumps once I stopped using it. I was really worried. This went on for weeks before it stabilized and thankfully thickened right up again. This incident highlights that products we use to improve texture like dry hair or fine lines and wrinkles are actually weakening the underlying cells and creating damage. Conversely if you nourish your body as we'll get into in the next chapter, you'll find you won't need these artificial products that are contributing to ill-health.

Around the House

While the products in closest contact with your body are obviously the worst offenders there is an even wider variety of chemicals around your house.

Starting with all those **plastics**. Cheap to produce, these petro-chemical-based products are relatively unstable when you expose them to heat or cold, breaking down into particles we call microplastics, which have been found to damage our immune systems and disrupt our hormones.[33] Found in just about every room in your house including the food containers you put in the microwave, the plastic wrappings your food comes in, the toys your children play with, and the pens you chew on. You might have heard of BPA (bisphenol A) a substance added to plastics to increase strength which has been linked with cancer and autoimmunity.[34] While manufacturers now tout products as BPA-free, do not think this excludes them from being harmful. Many of the substitute chemicals are just as bad.[35]

From food storage to food preparation introduces a different category of harmful substances. In **pots and pans** the biggest danger is a group of chemicals collectively called "forever chemicals" because they are so slow to break down in the environment and in our bodies. The best known is a substance called Teflon you might have heard of used in non-stick pans brought to prominence in the documentary *The Devil We Know*. But this is only one of around nine thousand chemicals including per- and poly-fluoroalkyl substances (PFAS), also PFOA, and PFOS. The list of documented health problems is long but includes high blood pressure, infertility, birth defects, cancers, and liver problems. If you've gone to the trouble of avoiding chemicals in the food itself, upgrading your cookware is the next step. I prefer solid ceramic cookware, but cast iron is also more inert though a little more onerous to take care of. Also watch out for that roll of aluminum foil you might be using to put underneath the items you're roasting or grilling.

Moving out of the kitchen you can also find toxic products in your **furniture**, your mattresses and even your carpets. Have you ever noticed that "new" smell around these products in the store? Or that "new car smell" in the showroom? These smells are known as Volatile Organic Compounds (VOCs) that off-gas known carcinogens. Exposures increase with heat, so think about all that healthy sleep you're aiming for, up to one-third of your life is spent in bed where there is heat from your body and increased carbon dioxide from your breath. These conditions have been shown to enhance the detrimental effects of these toxins.[36] Organic mattresses do exist. For other products it's best to allow them to air out like my dry-cleaning and ensure plenty of ventilation for the first few weeks in your house.

We like our homes to be clean, sometimes too clean. The dizzying array of **household cleaners** we use can be a big source of toxicity. All those cleaners, wipes, and sprays we use on every surface have chemicals linked to immune suppression, endocrine disruption, and cancer.[37] Natural products such as baking soda, vinegar, and botanicals can work just as well. (See Resources for commercial brands if you don't want to make your own.)

The last toxin I want to bring up in our homes is actually naturally occurring. **Mold** is more often associated with easily identifiable food gone bad but can be a problem in our homes and in particular the mycotoxins they emit as part of their metabolites. Mold requires moisture to grow but in damp or high humidity environments, mold species can live on dirt, dust, paint, paper, insulation, and just about any building material. Mycotoxins are tiny molecules that can get into our cells absorbed through the gut, skin, or lungs and carried to just about any part of our body. They cause inflammation and interfere with our immune response, disrupt hormones, and inhibit our ability to absorb nutrients. Mold can directly cause illnesses such as upper respiratory infections that don't seem to go away, and be the source of muscle weakness, tremors, fatigue, and brain fog to name a few. However, the insidious nature of molds (of which there are thousands of species) more often affect the ability of the body to fight secondary infections such as Lyme disease and Epstein-Barr or contribute to autoimmunity. Once you have ingested mold, it has the ability to take up residence in the warm wet places in our body and must be eliminated before other health problems can be addressed.

So keep your eye out for any obvious mold growing on your walls, corners of the ceiling, in your dishwasher or washing machine, and on any furniture. Make sure to fix a leaky roof, broken pipe, or overflowing toilet right away and thoroughly dry out and vent the area.

The Dark Side of Technology

Years ago, I was reviewing the emerging health "wearables" market to see which products had the best offering to help our clients' employees monitor and improve their health. These are gadgets that attach to your body in some way and measure how many steps you are taking throughout the day with the more sophisticated now measuring the quality of your sleep, pulse rate, blood pressure and even blood sugar and hormone levels. At the height of my review, I was wearing three or four of these gadgets at once. One of them attached to my shoe, another on each wrist and one just looked like a ring on my index finger. However, after only a few days I began to experience all sorts of aches and pains, and I became quite incapacitated until I realized it was the gadgets themselves. They all used various forms of wireless technology to "talk to" my cell phone and record all the data. This began my investigation into the dangers of **EMFs** or electromagnetic frequencies.

Some people are more sensitive than others as with everything we are discussing in this book and outlined in Chapter 3. But EMFs are detrimental to the human body whether you can feel it directly or not.

In Chapter 2 we briefly touched on bioresonance therapy which works because of the electrical nature of our bodies. An EKG is an electrocardiogram which measures the electrical conduction of our heart tissue to see if it is healthy. An EEG, electroencephalogram, assesses the electrical activity in the brain. EMFs interfere with our own electrical processes.

Anything electronic emits EMFs. You might have been told to avoid standing in front of a microwave when it is running. But damage from EMFs is dose dependent; the longer you are exposed, the more damage is done. So you need to start by looking at the electronics you spend the most time with. Our cell phones are the biggest problem, but also your laptop, desktop, wireless router in your house, and yes even those wearables you've chosen for convenience (Apple Watch anyone?) or to help improve your health.

The industry and a lot of mainstream health institutions continue with the narrative that there is no clear link between EMF exposure and health. But there are now hundreds of independent scientists around the world who say the opposite.[38] In their view the thousands of peer-reviewed studies on EMFs completed in the last two decades clearly demonstrate that our current exposure to 2G/3G/4G Wi-Fi and Bluetooth radiation is linked to a myriad of health problems. Beyond the brain cancers caused by cellphone radiation[39] EMFs have been shown to degrade your mitochondria and make your blood-brain barrier more permeable exacerbating the effects of other toxins you might be exposed to. EMFs have been linked to other neurological effects such as depression, anxiety, dementia, and autism. They have been linked to cardiac irregularities, reduction in sperm quality for men carrying their phone in their pants pocket and breast cancer in women carrying their phone in their bra.[40] The effects on children are far worse since their heads absorb twice the radiation of adults.[41] The risks of 5G cell phones are likely to be far worse.[42]

There was a small chink in the industry's armor this year when the French government outlawed sales of the iPhone 12 due to its failing European radiation standards. The story was quickly quashed, but the red flag has raised the alert for many people.[43]

While I'd love to live on an organic farm far away from technology, that is not reality for me, and likely not for you. So I use a variety of strategies to protect myself such as:

- I avoid carrying my cell phone on my body and keep it at least three feet away as much as possible. If I am out and about, I use a shoulder bag that has built-in protection.
- If I'm taking a phone call, I use the speakerphone. If I'm in a public place, I'll use special headphones that do not carry the electric current to my ear.
- All the computers in our house are wired (rather than using Wi-Fi) and I use a wired keyboard and mouse with my desktop. We minimize the use of Bluetooth and connected technologies.
- The Wi-Fi is shut off when we go to bed. There are no electronics in the bedrooms. All phones are left downstairs overnight.
- I use various devices to offset the damaging radiation including a cylinder that sits right beside me on my desk emitting calming electrons. My laptop has a protection device on the underside, and I have various plug-ins around the house. See the Resources section for recommended products.

As with all the toxins we've talked about, nourishing your body as we'll get into in Chapter 5 fortifies your body and can help protect it from the worst damage. Spices like cinnamon, turmeric, ginger, and rosemary have been shown to help, as has magnesium.

Of course there is more to technology than just the EMFs it emits.

The use of technology, especially as a replacement for in-person activities, exerts a negative effect on our mental health, as we'll pick up again in Chapters 8 and 9. For now we'll wrap up this chapter with a broader look at the way we spend our leisure time that has the potential for negative impacts to our bodies and our overall health.

Entertainment and Relationships

I have been careful not to mention "stress" itself as a toxin although many health advocates will put stress in that category. But it is more complicated than that as stress can sometimes be a good thing. When you work out in a gym you are putting stress on your muscles, which strengthens them. I tend to do my best work when I am under a deadline. When your body fights an infection, you are putting stress on your immune system but like your muscles, it is ultimately strengthening it. Problems arise when the stress is ongoing and pervasive without giving the body a chance to return to baseline.

When we watch, read, or listen to the news headlines it creates emotional stress in our body. Hearing about a car accident or break-in three towns away from you provides no benefit. While we need to be good citizens and stay up to date on major issues in our country, and vote when given the opportunity, it is only a negative input to our body to constantly follow and internalize all the shenanigans of our government. I spent many years staying up to date on news around the world, particularly anything that could have an impact on my multinational clients or their employees. But during the Covid years it became particularly apparent that most news has a negative bias and only serves to generate fear. The weaponization of social issues is also presented in such a negative light it acts as a toxin we need to rid our bodies of. As I have conveyed throughout this book, every one of us is a unique creation carefully designed to love other human beings in your own sphere of influence. I now purposefully limit my exposure to news and focus on facts that are useful in deepening my knowledge without all the associated commentary.

Beyond news there are other negative influences entering our bodies through our eyes and ears. Anytime you choose to watch a violent movie or listen to a podcast with an angry personality you are chipping away at the positive balance in your body. When you track through social media to see what others are up to it more often generates a feeling of envy or missing out than anything positive. Negative emotions cause biochemical changes in our bodies and contribute to overall ill-health, as we'll explore in Chapter 8.

Are there any negative people in your life? If it's a spouse or family member we might not be able to do much other than create some boundaries and healthy routines to offset those encounters. But if it's a friend or a manager at work then taking action to rid yourself of this negative influence may be critical to your good health. Chapter 8 will look at emotional and mental health and its role in your physical health.

Whew! That's a lot of toxins. A rather negative chapter, but it's important for you to know the extent of the problem. Toxins are everywhere! Unless you can pick up and move to a pristine desert island or a yacht sailing around the world (my preference!), they are impossible to avoid. The best approach is to aim to minimize the amounts of toxins you are subjecting your body to, as achievable within your own lifestyle, while nourishing it well to keep your detoxing systems in optimal working condition. We'll go there next.

Points to Remember

1. Anything that is not a positive influence on your body is a negative weight on its balance and should be treated as a toxin.

2. Newer doesn't necessarily mean better. Many modern conveniences negatively affect our health. If it didn't exist a hundred years ago, look at it suspiciously.

3. The appearance of government controls to protect us from harm are heavily influenced by the industries being regulated. Protection is a personal responsibility.

4. You are exposed to toxins most critically through what you put in your mouth in the form of processed foods as well as recreationally through smoking, alcohol, and caffeine.

5. Your skin is the largest organ in the body and readily absorbs anything you put on it as well as any toxins it interacts with around your home.

6. The technology you use as well as entertainment and personal relationships can negatively impact your health.

CHAPTER 5

A Body Needs Nourishment

A nice way of putting it would be to say I'm a foodie, but the truth is I am obsessed with food. When I take my family on vacation, I plan the major meals and research the restaurants where we will eat before scheduling any other activities. One of my daily priorities is to feed myself and my family good wholesome food. It hasn't always been this way though.

Food is the single most important influencer of your health and longevity. What you put *in* and *on* your body matters. The good news is that however far offtrack you are from good health, optimal nourishment can turn the situation on its head and protect you even when you struggle to change other factors. Food really *is* medicine.

The Nostalgia Factor

Many of our food preferences are rooted in our culture and upbringing. I grew up in a traditional Jewish household. Mum cooked dinner almost every night even though she worked full-time as a pharmacist for many years with her own business to run. My father was the head of our household and demanded a two- or three-course dinner on the table by 6:30 p.m. every evening. There was usually homemade soup;

mushroom or watercress soup were favorites, followed by from-scratch cooked main courses with meat/fish, vegetables, and a starch (potatoes, rice, or pasta). Dessert was often fruit unless it was a special occasion, which in a Jewish household was a regular occurrence.

Dinners were family affairs; everyone was expected to be present no matter how much homework we had or activities outside the home. Every Jewish festival brought extended family and even bigger meals. Friday nights were particularly special as we had a shabbat dinner. Shabbat marks the beginning of the day of rest for Jews. We enjoyed chopped liver on challah bread, chicken soup, roast chicken or lamb, roast potatoes, and vegetables of all kinds. Desserts of pies and crumbles often followed.

The foundation of this way of eating was firmly imprinted on my brain. While I veered heavily off course once I went to university, I found myself drawn back to those foundational principles when I started a family of my own. I'm lucky that I grew up with healthy eating habits and home-cooked meals being such an important part of my upbringing. My two brothers and I were taught to cook from a young age. But it's never too late to learn.

Most Americans today do not regularly eat dinner as a family. In a recent poll covered by *Newsweek*, the average person estimates they only eat three dinners a week with loved ones.[1] The other four days are typically grab-what-you-can affairs consisting of convenience foods. When I first met my husband at the go-kart track, food was just a necessary inconvenience to him, a frustration almost. Like an empty car, he had to stop life to fuel up so he could keep going. He was living alone and didn't cook. Meals were generally fast food devoid of nutrients and ingested on the run, at his desk, or in front of the TV. This is not a healthy way to eat, as his annual blood tests would display. Almost prediabetic and at risk for prostate cancer, my not-yet husband was seeing a doctor who proposed medication and biopsies. We got married and he moved into my house where I made meals every night which we ate together as a family. I suggested he give me three months to turn his numbers around before following the doctor's plan. It worked! Now eight years into our marriage, at nearly sixty years old, he is super healthy and on no medication.

My desire for you, if not to turn you into a complete foodie, is to give you an appreciation for how food and other living elements can nourish your body to promote vibrant health and heal just about any health condition.

Eating Badly

University was one big party for me. I lived on Pot Noodles (essentially British ramen with processed soy and artificial flavorings—just add boiling water and stir!), pizza, and peanut butter sandwiches. The balance of my calories was from beer and alcohol. In my first year, I got seriously addicted to Diet Coke, downing upward of six cans a day from the vending machine. My twenties weren't much better. I ate fast food multiple times a week: Kentucky Fried Chicken, McDonalds, Taco Bell.

My favorite foods were bread, cake, and cereal with dairy of all kinds, the creamier the better. One spring I got physically addicted to hamantasch, one of those Jewish delicacies, that I miss to this day. The festival of Purim (the origin of which is told in the Old Testament book of Esther) is celebrated with these pastries that literally translate as "Haman's Ears." Haman was the villain in the saga. They are traditionally made from sweet bread filled with a paste made from almonds and poppy seeds (remember poppy seeds are used to make opiate drugs!) They are available from Jewish bakeries for about two weeks around Purim. I was eating six to eight of them a day (they are about the size of your hand and one or two inches thick) and nothing else! This went on for several days and almost required an intervention. Cheesecake, crème brûlée, and my absolute favorite—sticky toffee pudding and custard—are at the top of my list of favorite foods.

The end of the line for me was when I got pregnant with my older son Ethan and proceeded to put on seventy-five pounds. I read the pregnancy books and dutifully avoided raw fish and perhaps made some attempt to eat a little better. But I followed the principle that, as I was eating for two, I could eat as much as I wanted. I could easily put away a whole baguette with copious amounts of fancy cheese, and a store-bought chocolate cake would barely last twenty-four hours. My younger son Max followed less than two years later, so I hadn't lost all the weight I had put on with the first and food cravings continued to drive my existence.

Being overweight was an entirely new experience now in my mid-thirties with two small boys. I didn't like how I looked or felt and decided to do something about it. Enter a low-carb diet recommended by friends and complete elimination of breads, cereals, and cake. I ate a lot of sliced turkey and string cheese. I lost most of the weight, but I now know it wasn't a healthy way to do it.

It was only after Ethan was diagnosed with Asperger's and ADHD that I began to research causes and treatments, nearly all of which involved avoiding foods that were detrimental to him and supplementing with nutrients he was deficient in.

It was during this critical period in our family's health journey that I read *The China Study* and promptly became vegan! We had already cut dairy out of our lives, which was tough enough, as well as gluten, so now we explored the world of plant-based protein sources. I had become a single parent during these years and my boys will tell you I was militant when it came to what they could eat and the lengths I would go to make sure they had healthy food every day, no matter what activities we were juggling.

In recent years, meat, poultry, and especially fish have made it back on our table with my growing sons (who are both now gym rats with high protein requirements) fortified through their stepdad's influence as head of our household. While my husband will happily eat my vegetable curry or another plant-based meal a couple of times a week, he prefers a little meat and poultry, so we have found a balance.

You are unique, as is every person in your household. Plus, your nutritional needs today may not be your needs two years from now. But there are certain principles that will help you figure out the best way to nourish your body. These won't change. You will need to tweak the details for you over time. I'm going to show you the difference.

The Placebo Parsnip

Part of the problem in making food choices is that the research is so confusing. I've had a doctor tell me there is no research that definitively proves eating more vegetables can reduce your risk of various diseases. But doctors are taught to only trust in randomized, double-blind placebo-controlled studies as we discussed in Chapter 2. This would require two groups of people fed very controlled diets (one the diet being tested and the other the placebo) without knowing exactly which they were eating (the concept of "double-blind") and then followed for years. It would be almost impossible, not least because it's rather difficult to disguise a parsnip or a carrot so that you don't know if you're eating one or not!

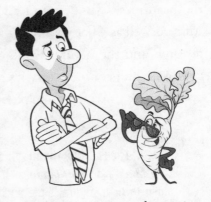

Nutrition research, therefore, relies on large group studies using questionnaires of what people are eating through food-recall surveys. If I asked you to list everything you've eaten in the last week, how much would you remember? I expect it would be rather subjective too. If you knew the survey was about nutrition, you're likely to over-report the healthier items and under-report the ice cream and fast food.

Nutrition science also tends to focus on individual dietary components such as fats, carbohydrates, and proteins, or even individual vitamins or minerals. This approach might be appropriate to study the effects of a medication, typically a single molecule designed to target a specific bodily process, but it's not helpful to evaluate how to nourish our bodies. God has provided a wonderful variety of other living organisms on this planet each designed with a complex recipe of hundreds of different nutrients that work synergistically with each other and with our human bodies to provide fuel and medicine. It's when we step away from this natural worldview that problems arise.

Finally, you have to consider who is funding the research. It's the Big Food companies that have the most to lose if we stop buying their packaged, processed, convenience products. As with pharmaceutical research covered in Chapter 2, there is much bias in many of the nutritional headlines that you read.[2]

I have continued to research and study the data, looking beyond the headlines to understand all the factors that have gone into the study as well as what we already know from other studies, from health research and the natural world as I've presented. While it can seem confusing and contradictory it's really quite simple.

Here are the three principles to remember:

The Healthy Human Simple Principles for Nutrition

1. *God-Made Not Man-Made*—Make sure you are eating whole foods as close to their natural state and with as few man-made ingredients as possible.
2. *When and How You Eat*—Be mindful of how and when you eat. Respect food as something intelligently designed to nourish and sustain you.
3. *Address Special Needs*—One man's medicine is another man's poison. Understand your body and what it needs at different times of your life. Adjust accordingly.

Principle #1: God-Made not Man-Made

Let me make it clear that all food groups are generally good to eat as long as they are as close to their natural state as possible. So if your gym buddy is pushing you to avoid grains entirely, your lactose-intolerant mom tells you dairy is the devil or eggs will raise your cholesterol, or your spouse is rejecting the fruit salad you lovingly made due to its sugar content, just smile sweetly. They're wrong. There is no science to back up their claims.

How do I know this? Because God has made it clear in his written word, the Bible. Indeed, the Bible has a lot to teach us about food! For example, Genesis 1:28–30 indicates that, initially, God gave Adam & Eve all the plants for food, and the animals separately would also live on plants (not each other). And then in Genesis 9:1–3 God gives Noah and his sons all the animals for food as well. What changed? The Flood. Genesis chapters 6 to 8 tell the story of when God reset everything on the Earth due to the corruption, finding

And God said to them, "Be fruitful and multiply and fill the earth and subdue it, and have dominion over the fish of the sea and over the birds of the heavens and over every living thing that moves on the earth." And God said, "Behold, I have given you every plant yielding seed that is on the face of all the earth, and every tree with seed in its fruit. You shall have them for food. And to every beast of the earth and to every bird of the heavens and to everything that creeps on the earth, everything that has the breath of life, I have given every green plant for food." And it was so. (Genesis 1: 28–30, ESV)

And God blessed Noah and his sons and said to them, "Be fruitful and multiply and fill the earth. The fear of you and the dread of you shall be upon every beast of the earth and upon every bird of the heavens, upon everything that creeps on the ground and all the fish of the sea. Into your hand they are delivered. Every moving thing that lives shall be food for you. And as I gave you the green plants, I give you everything. (Genesis 9:1–3, ESV)

only Noah and his family worth saving. While plants were originally designed as our sole source of food, once corruption and fear
entered the world, we were expected to also eat animals. But animals
throughout the Bible and other sources of history were an accompa-
niment, a treat, not a staple daily food, and certainly not the main
feature of every meal.

While science backs up the Bible's teachings about food, our
modern approach to eating can unnecessarily complicate matters.

In the simplest terms what we eat can be broken down into **plants**
and **animals**.

Carbohydrates, fats, and proteins are the macronutrients we need
to live and all three can be found in both plants and animals. Vitamins
and minerals are then known as the micronutrients that we still need,
but in much smaller amounts than the macronutrients if measuring
by weight.

The more plants you eat throughout the day, the better your body
will be nourished. With plants, you're not just feeding and nourishing
your human cells; you are also feeding your microbiome. The beneficial
microbes that live inside your body thrive on plant matter, particularly
fiber that is only found in plants. Those hardworking microbes inside
you regulate hundreds of bodily processes. They need plant matter to
thrive, and the more variety the better.[3]

Plants contain hundreds of different phytonutrients. ("Phyto"
quite simply means from plants.) They are sometimes called phyto-
chemicals. These phytonutrients include carotenoids such as lutein
(known to promote eye health), beta carotene, and lycopene which
tend to give vegetables their bright colors particularly red/yellows. Also
flavonoids (such as anthocyanins found in blue/purple foods like blueberries and purple potatoes known to promote vascular and neurological health), coumarins, indoles, isoflavones, lignans, organosulfurs (the
best known being sulforaphane found in broccoli and other cruciferous

vegetables known for its cancer-fighting properties), and plant sterols (best known for their effect on reducing absorption of bad cholesterol).

There are hundreds, if not thousands, of different chemicals and nutrients in different plants. But it is the synergistic effect of these hundreds of phytonutrients working together that creates optimal health.

If you want to improve your health, it is time to learn to love the huge variety of plants God has created to nourish us. If a salad to you is iceberg lettuce and tomato, or "eat your vegetables" brings up child-hood trauma of being forced to eat boiled Brussels sprouts or over-cooked green beans, then we have some work to do. Plants have been intelligently designed to be our main source of food. Plus Hippocrates was entirely correct when he said "Food is medicine." This is what he's talking about. But here's the interesting part—plants are delicious! The varieties and flavors are incredible. Once you start experimenting with real plants prepared properly you will marvel at what you've been missing.

Eating a lot of man-made processed food can dull your taste buds. Just wait until they wake up! Plants should make up the majority of our intake, and the more variety the better to maximize the different types of nutrients we are ingesting.

Some plants are best cooked while others are better eaten raw. You need a combination of cooked and raw for optimal health. Appendix A provides some food hacks and recipes to get you started on your food adventure.

Vegetables

Let's start with the **leafy greens and cruciferous vegetables**. Leafy greens can help to protect against cellular damage and support the body's detoxification from all those toxins we covered in Chapter 4. Greens tend to be fairly delicate and lose their nutritional value when heated so eating them raw is good. If you're going to cook them, make sure it's with low heat for a short amount of time.

Leafy greens are easy to add to any meal, breakfast smoothie, fresh juice, omelet, soup, salad, or pasta sauce.

Cruciferous vegetables are the edible versions of the Brassica family of plants. They all contain plenty of soluble and insoluble fiber, vitamins, potassium, selenium, and many phytonutrients, including sulfur-containing compounds that are known to fight cancer.

Cabbage, cauliflower, Brussels sprouts, broccoli or its little sister broccolini can each make a great side dish all by themselves. Try roasting any one of these with some olive oil and spices. Cauliflower is also a useful addition to any soup to make it taste creamier. Bok choy is awesome in a main meal stir-fry. Arugula is a great alternative to lettuce in any salad, and its peppery taste makes it a natural with eggs.

Bulbs, or a subset of which are called **Allicins**, are known for their antimicrobial, antitumor, antiarthritic, anticoagulant, cardioprotective, antioxidant, and anticancer properties. Pretty amazing! Allicins include onions, garlic, leeks, scallions, and shallots. These are plants that you probably already eat due to their flavor-enhancing qualities. I recommend you eat them at every meal.

Leafy Greens
- Cilantro
- Collard Greens
- Dandelion Greens
- Kale
- Mustard Greens
- Parsley
- Spinach
- Swiss Chard
- Watercress

Cruciferous Vegetables
- Arugula (rocket)
- Bok Choy
- Broccoli
- Broccolini
- Brussels Sprouts
- Cabbage
- Cauliflower
- Radish

Bulbs/Allicins
- Chives
- Garlic
- Leeks
- Onions
- Scallions
- Shallots

Roots and Tubers are a diverse set of vegetables that grow underground. Tubers include cassava, yams, and sweet potatoes and are staple foods in many parts of the world including two of the blue zones, Japan and Costa Rica. The humble white potato is also part of this family. I don't recommend eating white potatoes, given their high starch content and as they tend to be enjoyed as fries cooked in toxic oil or mashed without their skins, which removes their beneficial fiber. They are not that bad eaten with the skin on such as baked, but you probably don't need encouragement to eat more of them.

Sweet potatoes, on the other hand, come in a number of colors including orange, purple and white. All are chock full of nutrients and incredibly tasty. One of my own staple meals is sweet potato hash, which is quick to make and a nutritious powerhouse. Check out the recipe in Appendix A.

Ginger and turmeric have powerful anti-inflammatory actions in the body[4] and can be bought fresh though only tiny amounts are needed to season whatever dish you are adding them to. They can also be bought in a dry powdered form to keep on your spice rack and used as an herbal seasoning. I buy mine in individual frozen one-serve pods, so I always have it fresh on hand.

Roots and Tubers
- Beets
- Carrots (various colors)
- Cassava
- Ginger
- Jicama
- Parsnips
- Sweet potatoes (various colors)
- Turmeric
- Turnips
- Yams

Stems and Fruit Vegetables

Next comes a miscellaneous collection of super healthy vegetables that you should eat regularly. (Can you spot which are technically fruits?)

- Asparagus is a curiously unique vegetable if you're going to try and grow it at home. The spears sprout directly from the ground before any stems or flowers appear and the roots persist in the soil for many years. It is an excellent source of nutrition, particularly folate (for healthy pregnancies) and various vitamins and minerals. Lightly sauté with some lemon juice or chop into a stir-fry or hash.

Stems and Fruit Veg
- Acorn Squash
- Asparagus
- Avocados
- Bamboo shoots
- Bell Peppers
- Butternut Squash
- Celery
- Cucumber
- Eggplant
- Olives
- Plantains
- Spaghettis Squash
- Tomatoes
- Zucchini

- Avocados should be a daily staple for their healthy fat content. Beyond guacamole they lend thickness and creaminess to smoothies and substance to salads, and they are a versatile topping and garnish to just about anything.
- Bamboo shoots are often enjoyed in Asian stir-fry.
- Celery is a great snack especially loading it up with hummus or tahini dip. Although many people flavor their soups with celery, I am not a big fan of it cooked.
- The humble cucumber is surprisingly nutritious. Include it in your salads and with dips.
- Olives, like avocados, are highly nutritious with a high healthy fat content. They make a great snack right out of the jar or add to salads.
- Plantains are one of my favorite "vegetables" (a cousin of the banana, they are technically a fruit). They cannot be eaten raw and are best cooked when really ripe and the skins have started to turn black. Awesome in stir-fries, my sweet potato hash, or with scrambled eggs. A little more difficult to peel than a banana, slice them up and they can be boiled or cooked in a

little healthy fat such as coconut oil for a stir-fry or grass-fed butter to then add eggs for an amazing scramble.

- Zucchini, also known as courgette or baby marrow in some countries, is another underestimated and nutritious vegetable. Full of fiber, antioxidants, and nutrients.

Water and Sea Vegetables

There is a whole class of vegetables that do not grow on farms. Chlorella and spirulina are freshwater algae. You'll usually find them as a powder to add to smoothies or as part of a "Super Greens" supplement to mix with water for a quick fix of detoxifying power. Spirulina has been called "the most power-ful superfood on the planet" due to its par-ticularly impressive nutrient profile. Just one

Water and Sea Vegetables
- Chlorella
- Dulse
- Kombu
- Nori
- Spirulina
- Wakame

tablespoon of powder contains 4g of protein. Known health benefits include reducing bad cholesterol, reducing inflammation, lowering blood pressure, increasing blood flow and oxygen uptake by your mus-cles, and potentially fighting cancer.[5]

Sea vegetables, generally known as seaweed, contain nutrients hard to find elsewhere such as iodine, which is critical to good thyroid function, and manganese. Nori is available nowadays dried to eat as a snack. It makes a wonderful substitute for potato chips!

* * *

That wraps up our vegetable tour! Ideally you should be eating vegeta-bles with every meal and at least one item from each list every day. A good exercise would be to see how many different types of vegetables you are getting through in a week. That might seem daunting but it's a good goal to set, to expand the types of vegetables you are eating. It is not uncommon for me to look back over my day and I've eaten over ten different types of vegetables, and we haven't even got to the rest of the plant family yet!

Mushrooms

Mushrooms are a category all to themselves as they are not strictly a vegetable even though we eat them as such. In fact, many scientists would say a mushroom is neither a plant nor an animal. This unique and rather mysterious organism has been appreciated by nearly all cultures around the world for thousands of years. In fact, it's often treated more as a medicine in the herbalism realm than a food to be enjoyed at the family dinner table. But that's the wonder of God's creation.

Some of you are turning up your noses and equating mushrooms to those detrimental fungi like mold that can cause serious health problems. But just like the universe of bacteria there are bad guys but also very good guys. Don't forget the discovery of the penicillium fungus, which is the core ingredient of the lifesaving drug we call penicillin. The natural world calls for balance.

Mushrooms
- Baby Bella
- Chaga
- Chanterelle
- Cordyceps
- Cremini
- Lions Mane
- Maitake
- Oyster
- Portobello
- Porcini
- Reishi
- Shiitake
- Turkey Tail

Edible mushrooms have incredible health properties. Some species in particular are considered modulators or adaptogens. This means they have the ability to boost bodily processes that might be out of balance, including supporting your immune system and nervous system. Mushrooms are also an excellent source of vitamin D. Other known health properties of mushrooms include reduced inflammation, immune system boosting, neurological protection, and regulation of blood sugar.[6] The cancer-fighting properties of mushrooms are where a lot of the latest research is focused though. This has led to a plethora of supplements being available.[7] But the best idea is just to incorporate actual mushrooms into your diet!

While it's preferable for all your food to be organic it's particularly important to buy organic mushrooms as they are especially absorbent of contaminants in the soil or air. Mushrooms are also easy and fun to grow on your own! See Resources.

Fruits

Are you eating the right types of fruit and enough variety to optimize your health? Orange juice or apple juice at breakfast does not count as a serving of fruit. A whole orange or an apple is a different story. Once you separate the juice from the fiber you are ingesting an unnaturally large amount of fructose. It takes a number of oranges or apples to create a glass of juice which your liver will have a hard time metabolizing all at once, creating a spike in your blood sugar leading to insulin resistance and weight gain. However, the whole fruit comes in a neat package with fiber that slows down the fructose absorption and feeds your friendly gut bacteria at the same time.

As we discussed in Chapter 4, fructose has been highjacked by the processed food industry and you'll often find high-fructose corn syrup or similar derivative on those packets which is very detrimental to your body. Run away from

Fruit
- Acai
- Apple
- Apricot
- Banana
- Blackberries
- Blueberries
- Cherry
- Cranberry
- Fig
- Grape
- Grapefruit
- Guava
- Lemon
- Lime
- Kiwi
- Mango
- Melon
- Nectarine
- Oranges
- Papaya
- Passion fruit
- Peach
- Pear
- Pineapple
- Plum
- Pluot
- Pomegranate
- Raisin
- Raspberries
- Strawberry
- Tangerines

those products! But natural whole fruit in reasonable amounts is essential nourishment to your body due to all the nutrients and antioxidants that come in the package.

I'm sure you've heard the saying *"An apple a day keeps the doctor away."* A simple apple has been found to have hundreds of different nutrients that work together to nourish our body. I reach for an apple daily as a fallback snack or a sweet and crunchy addition to a salad.

All fruits are good and should be enjoyed daily in moderation, preferably whole and fresh. Those lowest in sugar and highest in their identified health properties are the berries. Blueberries, for example, have been shown to reduce inflammation, improve immune response, and help manage blood sugar.[8, 9] I make sure to have a big handful everyday! Raspberries, strawberries, and blackberries are similar powerhouses.

Nuts and Seeds

It's interesting how we think about nuts and seeds these days, perhaps as an unhealthy snack food. If you go looking for nuts and seeds in a regular grocery store, you'll probably find them in the snack aisle with the potato chips and other junk fare. This treatment stems from decades of bad nutritional advice that high-fat foods are bad for us.

In fact, nuts are close to a miracle food. That's because nuts are actually the seed or embryo that grows into a whole new plant. They are therefore chock full of monounsaturated, saturated, and omega-3 fats to provide the energy necessary to grow into that new plant. The myth that fat is bad for us is so pervasive and wrong that we're going to dig into it a bit more in a separate section below.

Nuts
- Almonds
- Brazil
- Cashews
- Coconut
- Hazelnuts
- Macadamia
- Pecans
- Pistachios
- Walnuts

Seeds
- Chia
- Flax
- Hemp
- Pumpkin
- Sesame
- Sunflower

In addition to healthy fats, nuts contain plenty of fiber, certain antioxidants, minerals like zinc and magnesium, and amino acids. They have been shown to lower cholesterol, stabilize blood sugar, and reduce the risk of diabetes, improve bone health, thyroid function and digestive health, support detoxification, improve vascular health and blood flow, and reduce the risk of cancer. Like I said—miracle food!

You can incorporate a variety of nuts and seeds daily as:

- On-the-go snacks
- Toppings for salads
- Additions to smoothies
- A substitute flour in baked goods

Nut butters can be a useful way to get your daily fix, and a yummy addition to a fruit snack, but be discerning about what kind you buy and how much you eat. Make sure there are no added sugars or preservatives. Tahini is made from ground sesame seeds and is delicious as a savory dip or as a salad dressing with a bit of lemon juice.

The other caution with nuts and seeds is that nature gave them mechanisms to protect themselves from predators. These "antinutrients" can make nuts hard to digest particularly in larger amounts. Some people are more sensitive than others but if possible try and soak your nuts overnight and then warm in a low oven or dehydrator to dry out. Or purchase sprouted versions which are ready to germinate (grow) thus deactivating the antinutrients.

Notice I don't mention peanuts in this discussion. That's because peanuts, by growing in a pod, are actually legumes!

Beans and Legumes

Beans and legumes are a staple food across the world. They tend to be easy to grow and are the most common home-grown food plant after the tomato. This makes them a cheap source of protein, fiber, and nutrients.

What categorizes these foods as legumes is the pods they grow in. Some are eaten without the pod, and some include the pod in what we eat. Runner beans (often called simply green beans), snap peas (called mange tout in some countries), and snow peas tend to be eaten more like vegetables. Green peas also.

Hummus is a staple in Mediterranean countries and is becoming more popular across the world. It is most often found

Beans and Legumes
- Black beans
- Broad beans
- Garbanzo beans
- Green peas
- Kidney beans
- Lentils
- Peanuts
- Pinto beans
- Runner beans
- Snap peas
- Snow peas
- Soybeans

with pita bread and falafel, both made with chickpeas (a.k.a. garbanzo beans). It can also be made with lentils and is a delicious dip for veggies of all kinds.

Soy can be misunderstood. Soybeans are healthy in certain forms. Edamame—the whole beans in their pods—are a great snack. The fermented versions, one of which is tempeh that you can use as a meat substitute in just about any ground beef recipe, is a good option. Miso is a fermented paste made from soy which has a great nutritional profile overall and is a good base for soups or stew flavoring. But avoid any of the highly processed or GMO soy products as mentioned in Chapter 4.

Grains

So remember how I used to be a complete carbo-addict living on bread, pizza, and cereal? Grains have become such a problem in our modern diet that many nutritionists and functional medicine doctors suggest avoiding them altogether. I mostly avoid grains myself these days. It is not the type of plant that is necessarily a problem. God created these grasses of which grains are the seeds and technically they are fit to eat with bread appearing all over the Bible. It's the amount of genetic modification they have undergone over the last hundred years and the advanced processing they tend to endure before they get to our table in the twenty-first century that turns them into a problem. Remember our principle here—God Made, not Man-made. There has just been too much human interference in today's staple grains that seem to be causing problems for us.

Wheat is by far the most eaten grain in Western countries today, mostly in the form of bread, pizza crust, cookies, pasta, and breakfast cereals. We covered in Chapter 4 the problems of glyphosate which is sprayed on wheat crops at the time of harvesting and other chemicals used in big agriculture. So what if you focus on organic versions?

Even though whole wheat has fiber in its bran (the outer layer) and some helpful nutrients (all available in other plant sources), when wheat is processed into flour it's basically metabolized as sugar in your body. It's going to spike your blood sugar and leave you craving more.

Grains
- Amaranth
- Barley
- Buckwheat
- Corn
- Millet
- Oats
- Quinoa
- Rice
- Rye
- Teff
- Wheat

Then there's the problem of *gluten*, a particular protein in wheat and a few other grains like rye and barley. You might have heard of gluten sensitivity and a more severe form known as celiac disease, either of which can manifest with a range of symptoms we'll get into in Chapter 7. Both have been on the rise in the last fifty years.[10] As Big Food has bred types of wheat with higher gluten content and our love affair with convenience foods has grown, gluten has become much more of a problem. I recommend avoiding it altogether.

You might have heard of "ancient grains" which are simply grains that haven't been genetically altered and industrialized like wheat and corn. Amaranth, buckwheat (no relation of wheat), quinoa, and teff are examples. These can be nutritious additions to your meals. Quinoa cooked as a side dish either on its own or made into a salad is a great option as it's a complete protein, contains a full range of amino acids, unusual for a plant, and also contains some good fiber for digestion.

Oats can be a decent option as long as they are not contaminated with gluten or pesticides and have not been processed to death. If you're making oatmeal for breakfast start from a package of whole oats, cook them slowly and add some healthy fats like nuts. A few blueberries will add sweetness if needed. Instant oatmeal is a man-made food-like substance that you should avoid.

What about rice? Another staple in many parts of the world. Various varieties of unrefined brown, red, purple, or black rice are great options. The more colored the better. Just be mindful of the lack of fiber in refined white rice, which is just treated as sugar by your body and is often devoid of any nutrients. There is an issue with rice taking up arsenic in the soil often from the run-off of chemical fertilizers so buy organic and always rinse well before cooking. Probably best not to eat it every day for this reason unless you are really sure it's clean.

We should probably mention pasta and noodles here as a few of you have a cold sweat going lest I have anything negative to say against these universal comfort foods. Pasta and noodles made from buckwheat (soba noodles), brown rice, or any ancient grains can be made into a healthy meal with the addition of healthy fats and vegetables. If you're following my three principles for nourishment carefully you won't go wrong.

The same goes for bread. Still one of my favorite foods. Stick to wholesome breads made from nuts and seeds with no additives.

Beyond Plants

Hopefully you are so motivated with the variety and appeal of plants right now that you have forgotten there's a whole other category of food I lumped together as "animals" (covering meat/poultry/fish). In my experience people are in two camps—you either love to eat animals and think meat is synonymous with protein, or you are convinced animals are bad for you, bad for your body, or bad for the environment to cultivate for food. You have to dig deeper to find the truth.

Animal foods have unique nutrient profiles that our bodies are designed to utilize but it's the quantity and the quality that can get us in trouble.

Back in Chapter 3 we took a look at *The China Study*, which laid out clear evidence that high amounts of animal proteins promote cancer and other diseases. The *Blue Zones* research indicated that animal-based foods tended to be weekly treats rather than staples in the longest-living communities. Let's see if we can unpack the details.

Meat and Poultry

Organic grass-fed beef is extremely nutritious containing many nutrients including vitamin B_{12} that is almost impossible to obtain from plant foods. It contains all the essential amino acids your body needs in one package and various minerals and antioxidants as well as a range of healthy fats. Organic chicken contains the same amount of monounsaturated fat as olive oil as well as palmitoleic acid, which is antimicrobial and fights infection. (A hearty bowl of chicken soup known as Jewish penicillin is not a myth!)

Meat and Poultry
- Beef
- Bison
- Chicken
- Duck
- Eggs
- Elk
- Goose
- Kangaroo
- Lamb
- Turkey
- Veal

Conventionally raised and factory-farmed beef and chicken is a whole different story. The nutritional profile is completely altered. It bears no resemblance to what nature created and is practically a different food. The animals are fed a diet of typically GMO soy, corn, or other cheap grains, live in stressed-out conditions which requires them to be pumped full of antibiotics and hormones to limit the diseases they are susceptible to in such conditions, and which also makes them fatter. (Don't miss that point—antibiotics and hormones make them gain weight; us too.) There are very few rules in place on what can be included in conventional livestock feed with a long list of unnatural items you would never want in the food supply such as re-cycled excrement, plastics, toxic chemicals, and all sorts of sugar products including candy.[11]

While it is true that organic grass-fed meat is up to 50 percent more expensive than conventional, the saying holds—*would you rather pay the farmer or the pharmacy?* It is worth the investment in your health now to buy food that will nourish you and not add to the negative flow into your bucket. See the Resources section for where to shop for lower-priced healthy meat. But also note that you don't need as much meat as you might be used to. We definitely don't need a 12-ounce steak! 4–6 ounces of meat or poultry is a healthy portion size. Your plate should be three-quarters plants with any meat almost as a side dish.

I've included eggs in this section as they are essentially baby chickens. Eggs have got a bad reputation the last fifty years with fearmongering about cholesterol levels which has been completely debunked.[12] Eggs from organic pasture-raised chickens are a health food and should be enjoyed particularly for breakfast where the protein and fat content will keep you feeling full and alert well into the day. But make sure you know where your eggs are coming from as "free-range" or "cage-free" just means they weren't imprisoned all their lives and says nothing about their feed or whether they got to forage outside. And don't mess around with those cartons of egg-whites you can buy at the store. The yolk is the most nutritious part of the egg, all the nutrients needed to create new life, and a whole egg comes in that neat little package preserving the nutrients until you are ready to eat it.

Lastly, on the subject of cholesterol, you might have also heard that liver and other organ meats are bad for you. Nonsense. Liver contains a wide variety of vitamins including folate and vitamin C, minerals, and other substances like coenzyme Q10 that we need for good health. Score again for my Jewish upbringing as I regularly crave chopped liver or search out liver pate when eating out.

In general, meat and poultry are an important part of a healthy diet but as a side dish, not the main event. Quality is much more important than quantity. If budget is an issue, I'd recommend saving for a quality piece of meat once or twice a week instead of inferior toxic meat at every meal.

Dairy

Dairy foods are problematic for a lot of people. Yet the government insists that milk is good for you, pushing parents to give it to their kids and set a good example by drinking it themselves. This is one of the worst dietary recommendations imposed on us. Digging a little further you can find the vast influence of the dairy industry behind it. On the one side you've got the propo-

Dairy
- Butter
- Cheese
- Cream
- Ice cream
- Milk
- Yogurt

nents of the "calcium for strong bones" crowd but in actual fact the highest rates of osteoporosis (lower bone density) is found in those who drink the most milk.[13] On the other side you've got the "low-fat milk is best" crowd whining about the saturated fat in milk, which is not the problem. But in combination you've got terrible advice. So let's get real.

The connection between dairy foods and cancer rates was shown to be strong in *The China Study*. Studies continue to indicate drinking milk raises your risk especially of breast cancer and prostate cancer.[14] The exact mechanism is not yet clear though and it may be more due to the modern-day mass production of milk involving pasteurization (killing all the healthful bacteria) and the unhealthy conventional cows it comes from. The reason I am including dairy in this chapter on nourishment is that while we don't need dairy for strong bones (there are far better plant-sources of calcium and it turns out your vitamin D level is more important) it can be a healthy source of fat, vitamins, and probiotics to boost your microbiome.

Given the toxic effects of modern vegetable and seed oils (discussed in Chapter 4), organic grass-fed butter is a great option especially for cooking. Studies have clearly shown no link between eating butter and cardiovascular disease, and that butter is even protective against diabetes.[15] Clarified butter or ghee may be even better for cooking at high temperatures or for those who have an identified allergy to dairy.

I do miss cheese but occasional treats of fresh organic Parmesan or goat cheese work well for me. You might even do fine with other locally sourced organic cheeses from grass-fed cows or try sheep cheeses like feta. Just make sure to avoid any processed cheese that is full of additives.

The Benefits of Goat Milk

Part of the reason goat milk is more digestible is that it only contains A2 casein, a milk protein. Whereas modern cows have been bred to have high levels of A1 casein which is highly inflammatory and responsible for most of the stomach upset many people experience. A1 casein forms casomorphins in the body which act on the brain similar to morphine-like peptides with negative consequences for brain, behavior and ability to detoxify.[16] When my son was first diagnosed with an autism spectrum disorder he was entirely addicted to milk, and it took some painful weeks to wean him off it. A1 casein is also implicated in autoimmunity and diabetes while A2 casein doesn't seem to have the same effect.[17]

Yogurt is a misunderstood food that has lost its way due to hype. Most of it comes from conventional cows and is full of added sugar and preservatives but if they add some probiotics they can convince you it's healthy. However naturally probiotic dairy like unsweetened yogurt or kefir from grass-fed cows is healthy for most people. Sheep's yogurt has a higher protein content, but I prefer unsweetened goat milk yogurt, which is delightfully creamy and easier to digest.

Coconut milk, cream, and ice cream can be a great alternative as well as some other nut milks, but watch for those man-made additives.

Fish and Seafood

Seafood is one of the best dietary sources of protein and it's hard to have a healthy diet without fish and seafood at least three times a week. It's packed with nutrients like iodine, selenium, and vitamins but the biggest health benefits come from the two types of omega-3 fatty acids, DHA, and EPA, that we get from seafood and nowhere else. You might argue that certain plant foods have omega-3s like walnuts and flaxseeds but this is ALA that the body has to convert into DHA and EPA with some inefficiency.

The many health benefits have been shown to reduce cardiovascular risks, as well as lower the incidence of cancer, type 2 diabetes, rheumatoid arthritis, and other autoimmune diseases.[18] Consumption of fish has even been shown to lower the risk for depression.[19] Fish is brain food. Our brains are more than half fat, with children and even developing fetuses requiring the omega-3 fats found in fish. But as you're likely getting the hang of at this point, quality is more important than quantity.

Fish/Seafood
- Anchovies
- Herring
- Mackerel
- Mussels
- Oysters
- Salmon
- Sardines
- Scallops
- Shrimp

The type of seafood you eat as well as where it comes from is important. Size matters. In this case the smaller the better. The larger fish at the top of the food chain like tuna and swordfish have extremely high levels of mercury due to water pollution. Stick to wild-caught salmon from clean waters like Alaska, mackerel, anchovies, sardines, and herring. Remember SMASH for short. Fresh or canned is fine but avoid farmed fish. With few exceptions farmed fish are given manufactured feed consisting of corn, wheat, soy, and vegetable oils and contain other pollutants much like factory-farmed meat. If you're shuddering at the thought of sardines or anchovies, then let me recommend canned mackerel from a reputable brand. Mackerel is less fishy than their cousins and I eat it several times a week. If you must have canned tuna, there are some safer brands now available. See Resources for recommendations.

Shrimp has lower levels of omega-3s but other useful nutrients like zinc similar to the other seafoods listed, all healthy protein sources if good quality.

Healthy Fats

While we've concluded our survey of plants and animals that nourish us, it's worth a separate look at fat as probably the most misunderstood part of our human diet. Myths continue to propagate on whether or not fat is good for us and what types. We covered the great toxicity of manufactured vegetable oils in Chapter 4. Here I just want to reiterate that the macronutrient we call fat is a very important part of the nourishment our body needs. Some vitamins and minerals are fat-soluble. This means we only absorb them if they are eaten at the same time as we are digesting fat. You should therefore make sure you are getting plenty of healthy fats each day.

You should eat fat with every meal. Learn the healthy fats listed rather than fret about the marketing machine telling you saturated fat is bad for you or you should limit your fat/cholesterol intake. Science has acknowledged that these were some of the worst recommendations in history and have undoubtedly contributed to the rise in chronic disease.[20] Remember the God-Made principle and include fats that are as much in their natural state as possible and that existed a hundred years ago.

Healthy Fats
- Avocados
- Beef/chicken fat
- Extra-virgin olive oil
- Ghee
- Grass-fed butter
- Coconut oil
- Nuts and seeds
- Olives
- Tahini (sesame seed paste)

I've talked quite a bit about protein and fats in these sections. I haven't mentioned the word carbohydrate as it generates too much confusion. I prefer you focus on getting a good amount of protein and fats and then just load up with plants! Simple as that. No calorie counting, no turning your plate into a pie chart with percentages, no keeping track of grams of this or that. I love numbers, as we've established, but I don't want to have to do a math problem every time I sit down to eat. I just want to focus on enjoying the food in front of me.

Hydration

Water is magical. It is the only substance that can shift its form from a solid, liquid, or gas without any extreme force applied. Most substances when they form a solid become more dense but when water freezes it becomes less dense, enabling solid water (ice) to float. Our bodies are 70 to 80 percent water. Every plant and animal we have discussed above is 70 to 80 percent water. The planet itself is over 70 percent water. Don't you think God is trying to tell us how important water is? It flows all around us and is essential to our existence.

At the most basic level water helps regulate our body temperature through respiration and perspiration, it flushes waste and toxins from the body, it carries oxygen to cells, it helps break down food into nutrients we can use, it insulates the spinal cord, brain, and organs, and lubricates our joints. It facilitates the electrical activity throughout our body enabling every cell to function properly. I didn't leave liquid nourishment for last to imply it's less important than food. If you do nothing else after reading this book, I hope you assess the amount of clean fresh water you are drinking daily. This single act can transform your health without making any other changes.[21]

The simplicity of water may be the secret behind its potency. Water has an intelligence that is difficult to grasp. I mentioned alternative health modalities of homeopathy and bioresonance back in Chapter 2. Both of these depend on the intelligence of water to heal us. It is one of the best conductors of electricity, which helps explain why dehydration compromises just about all our functions.[22]

Whatever else you are drinking containing water be it herbal teas, homemade lemonade, soup for dinner . . . do not fall into the trap of including them in your daily needs for pure water. Carry a water bottle around with you, and keep track of how often you fill it up. It can take some effort to get to an adequate daily level but it's a habit that will pay huge dividends.

> **How Much Water Do I Need?**
> A broad approximation of eight 8-oz glasses a day is a good start.
>
> If you take your weight in pounds, you need one-half to two-thirds of it in ounces. So if you weigh 150lbs you need 75–100oz a day.

Make sure you are drinking clean water though. Tap water is usually contaminated with toxins including deliberate additions of chlorine and fluoride in municipal systems which can negatively impact our health especially our thyroid.[23] A water filtration system is probably your best approach (see Resources for recommendations). Bottled water is an alternative, but do your research. Many brands of bottled water are just marketing hype and come straight from a tap.

Food Labels

The marketing hype of bottled water leads me to an important sidebar. Even before you learn to cook healthier you need to learn to read food labels. Most health claims on food packaging are just the marketing machine trying to get your attention. Don't fall for stickers like "low-fat," "diet," "zero trans fat," "gluten-free," or "whole-grain." If it's in a package you need to treat it with suspicion and investigate more closely. Read the ingredients. Chapter 4 covers the worst offenders to watch out for. If you are new to cooking and baking or heavily pressed for time and can't avoid premade products, then try and buy local or investigate the brands now available that try to stick to natural ingredients. The Resources section has examples of brands and websites to help including how to eat well on a tight budget.

As we wrap up the discussion of Principle #1 (God Made not Man-Made) I want to reassure you that we are not aiming for perfection. Depending on the state of your own bucket (from good health to poor) you are likely to camp somewhere on a continuum between the

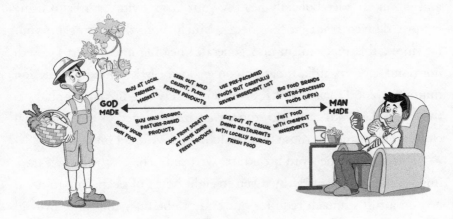

two extremes as shown in the illustration. If you can move yourself a little more to the left with each passing week you are going to be reducing the bad stuff going into your bucket and increasing the good. See Appendix A: Food Hacks to get You Started.

Principle #2: When and How to Eat

I'm a foodie, remember? Food is one of my big enjoyments in life. Once I was eating well my body no longer craved bad and unhealthy foods. I craved apples or an avocado. You can't imagine the enjoyment I get from a fresh salad with some canned mackerel or a bowl of goat milk yogurt with some nuts and blueberries. A big treat is finding the time to bake my famous turmeric seed loaf to enjoy with some herbal tea. I reasoned if all my food options were healthy I could eat whatever I wanted whenever I wanted. I grazed all day long. My global job had me at my desk early in the morning and often back there late at night. I ate mindlessly, often sitting right at my desk. This is not how God intends us to eat.

We have two primary energy systems. One is activated when we eat. Our blood sugar goes up and we use glucose for energy as we go about our day creating metabolites that generate free-radicals and inflammation. When you don't eat for a period of time your blood sugar drops and if you are metabolically healthy your body switches over to using ketones derived from fat for energy. Much more than using up your fat stores, this mechanism also generates healing and repair. Growth hormone goes up, inflammation comes down. Mitochondria function improves, blood sugar stabilizes, and autophagy is ignited. Autophagy is the renewal of your cells with those that are damaged or dysfunctional cleared out including those that could have developed into tumors.

Think about the word breakfast. We need to break the fast we have imposed during our healthy seven to eight hours of sleep. But going to bed on a full stomach requires our body to be busy digesting instead of working on all the processes designed to occur when we sleep. To optimize the sleep process we need to finish eating at least three hours before we start our sleep routine. When we wake up, we shouldn't start eating right away. Instead take advantage of the optimum brain function running on ketones. Even before you worry about *what* to eat, I recommend you make sure you are leaving a minimum of twelve hours fasting overnight. This is a baseline for everyone. We'll get into the benefits of longer fasting in Chapter 7 to see how it can address various health issues as an extremely powerful (and free!) health intervention.

So you haven't eaten in a while and now you're going to load up on your wonderfully nourishing proteins, healthy fats and lots of plants. Don't cram it down in between phone calls. Take time out of your day to sit down at a table and marvel at the colors and textures before you. A little prayer goes a long way to show appreciation for the food. Make sure to chew carefully; digestion starts in your mouth with a good mix of saliva. Avoid drinking a large glass of 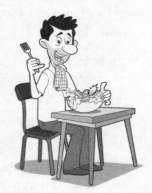 iced water just before you eat as that dilutes your digestive juices and slows everything down. Many cultures start a main meal with a raw salad as that contains the live enzymes needed to break down food. I'm also a fan of the large breakfast (for me it's around 10 a.m.), substantial lunch and light dinner routine. Above all acknowledge that the meal is designed to nourish and not just provide fuel.

Principle #3: Addressing Special Needs

My food journey has been an adventure. From ultra-processed foods at university, to crash diets after pregnancy, veganism to food sensitivities to a general awareness of how food affects different symptoms. As we are all entirely unique our nutritional needs are distinct and one prescribed diet is not going to be right for everyone all the time. You must learn to make the connection between what you eat and how you feel. This simple skill is all you really need to fulfill this last principle.

The trap you don't want to fall into is to think: What is the minimum I can do that will improve my health? I want to keep eating cheeseburgers and fries but if I add some blueberries to my processed cereal will that reduce my risk of cancer or heart disease or whatever my genetics say I'm predisposed to? That's just not how it works. It's why I've not called this chapter "what to eat or not eat." It's about nourishment; having respect for the amazing body God has given you and His provision to sustain it with plants and animals.

But there are some special needs that you'd be wise to consider eating a certain way if only for a short period to heal your body. If you have severe acne, eczema, or digestive issues you might find that eliminating dairy altogether provides relief. I personally avoid all grains except for the occasional serving of quinoa or wild rice. This is due to the extra effort to digest grains and their propensity to elevate inflammation. Gluten is a problem for so many people and might be causing you problems without you even being aware. Eliminate it fully for an entire month (or more) before you pass judgment. I'll talk more about gluten in Chapter 7.

We'll be getting into solutions for specific health issues in Part II of the book, but I've provided a short glossary of some common diets for reference. I know it is sometimes easier to follow a set program in order to take out the guesswork and get into better habits. There are many excellent books written on these diets, and I encourage you to try whatever sounds most helpful and will fit with your lifestyle and the health issues you are facing. I've provided some basic food hacks and recipes to get you going in the meantime in Appendix A.

Whether or not you choose to follow a prescribed diet my three principles still hold. If one approach doesn't work for you try not to fall back into old ways of eating. Make some tweaks, experiment, be in tune with what works or not but keep pressing forward.

Most people know that eating good food is healthy for them. But I find that most don't understand the true scope of food's power to prevent, treat, and even reverse disease. We'll see this again and again in Part II.

Points to Remember

1. Food is not an inconvenience. It should be appreciated for the nourishment it provides us. Our food selections have more impact on our health than any other aspect of our life.
2. It is never too late to change our food habits and certainly never too late to learn to cook.
3. Much nutrition science is highly flawed, so avoid the headlines and concentrate on the three principles:
   i   God-Made, Not Man-Made
   ii   When and How You Eat
   iii Address Special Needs
4. Eat a wide variety of plants at every meal. Experiment with those you are not familiar with.
5. Meat, fish, and eggs are healthy but quality is more important than quantity.
6. Eat healthy fats and protein at every meal and then load up with plants.
7. Plenty of clean fresh water daily is critical for good health. Increasing your water consumption can heal many ailments before any other interventions.
8. Make sure to leave at least a twelve-hour fasting window overnight to give your body the chance to switch into repair mode.

Some Prescribed Diets	
Anti-inflammatory	Typically prescribed for autoimmune conditions. It eliminates sugar, gluten, dairy, grains, and legumes. Restrictive but very effective for serious conditions and for those wishing to avoid medications.
Blood Types	Often dismissed as a fad, the science is quite interesting. It indicates the foods you should avoid or enjoy based on whether your blood type is A, B, AB, or O. This blood categorization is based on the antigens found on the surface of your red blood cells. Lectins are a type of protein molecule found in plants and animals. The problem is that they are shaped like certain antibodies causing them to react with our blood type antigens. Read more at deadamo.com.
Low FODMAP	The acronym refers to fermentable oligosaccharides, disaccharides, monosaccharides, and polyols, which are short-chain carbohydrates that the small intestine may have difficulty absorbing. Some people experience digestive distress after eating them particularly those with Irritable Bowel Syndrome (IBS) or SIBO (small intestine bacterial overgrowth). There is some crossover with the anti-inflammatory diet, but it can be more restrictive.
Keto	Originally developed to treat epilepsy, it focuses on high fat, moderate protein, and ultra-low carbohydrates forcing your body into ketosis, the second energy mechanism discussed under Principle #2. Can be useful for certain severe conditions like MS, schizophrenia, and to improve insulin resistance in metabolically unhealthy individuals (though fasting can have the same effect).
Mediterranean	Named for the diets of countries around the Mediterranean, I appreciate this way of eating growing up Jewish with regular trips to Israel. It emphasizes cooking with whole foods, lots of plants, healthy fats like olive oil and some animal foods. You may simply love the recipes. There are lots of versions and it's less prescriptive than most.
Nutritarian	Popularized by Dr. Joel Fuhrman it focuses on maximizing the nutrients in each bite. Heavily plant-biased it pushes G-BOMBS which stands for greens, beans, onions, mushrooms, berries, and seeds. Very low in animal foods.
Paleo	The idea is to eat like our ancestors did before agriculture came along a few thousand years ago. This means no sugar, no grains, no dairy, no beans or legumes. Focusing on nonindustrial meats, whole vegetables, nuts, and seeds. While restrictive this can be a healthy option for people as long as it's not used as an excuse to load up on meat and not incorporate enough plants.

Some Prescribed Diets	
Pegan	This term has been coined by Dr. Mark Hyman as somewhere between Paleo and Vegan. It's probably closest to how I eat. Mostly plants, low-glycemic fruits other than occasional treats, lots of healthy fats, limited dairy (I stick to goats), meats as a side dish, low-mercury fish, no gluten, other grains very sparingly, beans/legumes only sparingly. Highlights avoiding toxins and junk to focus on organic, wild-caught, and pasture raised.
Vegan	Removing all animal foods and focusing on plants. The healthier version is referred to as the plant-based diet to make clear that processed fake meats should also be avoided. Can be helpful temporarily to detox and if currently fighting cancer. But is generally low in important omega-3 fatty acids and certain minerals, takes a lot of effort to get enough protein with the range of essential amino acids, and will require a vitamin B_{12} supplement as it only comes from animal foods.
Vegetarian	Similar to vegan but includes eggs and dairy. Can be healthy but too much conventional dairy is often a problem.
Wise Traditions	Focused on the work of Dr. Weston A. Price who studied the diets of ancient cultures around the world. Focuses heavily on animal foods and saturated fat with an emphasis on proper preparation techniques to avoid problems. Many similarities with Paleo. Read more at westonaprice.org.

PART II
IMPLICATIONS

The doctor of the future will give no medication, but will interest his patients in the care of the human frame, diet and the cause and prevention of disease.

—Thomas Edison

CHAPTER 6

It's Flu Season Again

In Part I, I laid the foundations to human health and some basic principles to understand. Now in Part II, I look at health issues or conditions you might be facing so you can see how all illness is essentially connected and how to apply the principles to specific health situations. Do you expect to get a cold or the flu every year once the weather turns colder? If you have children in your house, do you worry they will bring home some sniffles or worse from school? I can tell you right now it doesn't have to be this way.

The last time I was really sick was in 2012. My boys were seven and five. I was a newly single mom juggling an executive job and the special needs of a not-yet-recovered Aspergers/ADHD kid. It started as your typical virus; congestion, headache, fatigue but after a week it was getting worse and had moved into my chest causing difficulty breathing. I had to actually take some time off work. I was miserable. I did end up seeing a doctor who prescribed some antibiotics (the last I have ever taken) and eventually I came out of it, but it was a good few weeks before I was fully well, and my digestion has never been the same since. Interestingly I was so offended that a virus (and then opportunistic bacteria) had got the better of me I did some research to discover the root cause. In addition to the immense stress I was under, I had become fully vegan (thanks to *The China Study*!) and was eating large amounts of nuts. Nuts are very high in arginine, an amino acid. It turns out viruses love arginine and need it to multiply. Too much arginine in the body disrupts the balance of another amino acid called lysine as they share an absorption pathway. I started taking a lysine supplement which I take to this day. I'm also aware if I feel a sniffle coming on I'll stop eating nuts for a few days.

Dominance over Microbes

Antibiotics are a blessing and a curse. As we saw in Chapter 2, they revolutionized the treatment of bacterial infections like syphilis, saved many soldiers wounded in battle, and turned the former butchers of the surgical wards into heroes. They also contributed to the tide turning in favor of doctors being consulted for basic illnesses given the training needed to understand and administer these new industrially prepared products.

Since penicillin became available in the 1940s there are now many different types of antibiotics. One of the more common versions of penicillin you've probably heard of is amoxicillin/Amoxil used to treat bronchitis, tonsilitis, ear infections, and even pneumonia. A few other classes of antibiotic are:

- Tetracyclines, e.g. Vibramycin I was treated with several times in my childhood for frequent sinus infections;
- Cephalosporins, e.g. Keflex, used for strep throat, urinary tract infections (UTIs), and meningitis;
- Fluoroquinolones, e.g. ciprofoxacin/Cipro, which came to prominence during the US anthrax attacks in 2001 but has since become the poster child for unsafe antibiotics as we'll get into;

- Macrolides, e.g. azithromycin/Zithromax, used for skin infections, pertussis (whooping cough) and forms of pneumonia;
- Sulfonamides, e.g. Bactrim and Septra, used for UTIs and ear infections which have become less effective in recent years due to widespread resistance;
- Glycopeptides, such as Vancomycin used heavily in hospitals to treat MRSA (methicillin-resistant staphylococcus aureus) and *C. difficile*–associated diarrhea—see below).

There are more classes and many different products in each class making a lot of competition for Big Pharma to deal with. Each class has a different structure or mechanism of action targeting different types of bacteria. But the paradox is that the more an antibiotic is used in the population, the quicker bacteria can mutate and adapt around it. This is why over the decades the number of infections that are no longer treatable with oral antibiotics is rising. This means Big Pharma needs to constantly invent new antibiotics but the market is small (i.e. unprofitable) for new (more expensive) versions due to the crowded space.[1] Plus hospitals are required to maintain antimicrobial stewardship programs that optimize antibiotic use (and often limit the newer more expensive ones) given their overuse is what causes the resistance in the first place.[2]

Remember the discussion of germ theory vs. terrain theory in Chapter 2? Penicillin was brought to market long before we understood the importance of the microbiome to overall health. When you take any of these antibiotics they might be targeting a particular bug but end up indiscriminately killing many more bugs including the good guys, leading to worse problems. One example of this phenomenon is a bacteria called *Clostridium difficile* or *C. diff* for short. It causes severe diarrhea and colitis (inflammation of the colon) and can lead to death if not controlled. It often shows up in hospital or nursing home settings and after rounds of antibiotics have already been used to combat other infections. While considered a last resort the standard of care for *C. diff* includes a **fecal microbiota transplant (FMT)**. This is basically someone else's poop inserted directly into the patient's colon during a colonoscopy procedure thereby repopulating a heathy diverse microflora which can then control the *C. diff*.[3]

While the effect on our microbiome and growing bacterial resistance to our man-made arsenal are bad enough, there is an even more sinister side of antibiotics. A recent report[4] found that antibiotic use is linked to inflammatory bowel disease, obesity, and even colorectal cancer. Antibiotic use in children is also linked to asthma, allergies, and airway illnesses. Vancomycin, the first line of defense against *C. diff*. and the most often prescribed antibiotic in hospital settings, is associated with kidney failure.[5] This has been known for years but particularly came to light during Covid-19 hospitalizations where doctors were adding antibiotics to the arsenal they were throwing at this viral infection. News reports began to appear that Covid-19 seemed to be affecting the kidneys.[6] The interesting sidebar here is that when your kidneys are failing you cannot excrete fluid from the body, and it can build up in your lungs causing a pneumonia-like condition. Just one of the revealing facts of the poor Covid response.

Other antibiotics are known to cause delirium, confusion, and hallucinations but their effects often go unnoticed particularly when used in older patients.[7] There is an FDA warning for causing "disabling and potentially permanent side effects" from fluoroquinolones related to tendons, muscles, joints, and the central nervous system that were so serious they "should be reserved for use in patients . . . who have no alternative treatment options."[8] Not everyone heeds these warnings as Former Secretary of State Hillary Clinton was reported to be taking Levaquin for pneumonia when she had difficulty walking at a

ceremony in 2016. Not long after this the term "floxed" began showing up in social media.

Infections are not always due to bacteria, of course. The broader
antimicrobial armory includes antivirals, antifungals, and antiparasit-
ics. We'll only touch on them briefly but I want to step away from
the action for a moment and ponder the bigger picture of man's war
against germs when it is so clear that God's design is for humans to
live in harmony with microbes. The discussion on bacteria reminds
me of one of the clearest pieces of evidence in science that God intelligently created the world and everything in it at a single point in time.
Do you remember my explanation of the human eyeball as being
an example of irreducible complexity? It couldn't have evolved as it
needs every complicated piece to operate. Well let me introduce you
to *Helicobacter pylori*, *H. pylori* for short. It's a bug that exists in your
stomach and many people have no problem with it at all. But it is
thought to contribute to stomach ulcers probably when there is a shortage of good bacteria to keep it in check. *H. pylori* is a type of bacteria
that uses a flagellum to swim along. This one-cellular organism rotates
its filaments in a whiplike fashion using this motor-assembly.

It's difficult to see from these crude illustrations but there are over
forty separate teeny-tiny parts that make the flagellum motor work.
The similarities to our carefully designed rotary engines are striking.

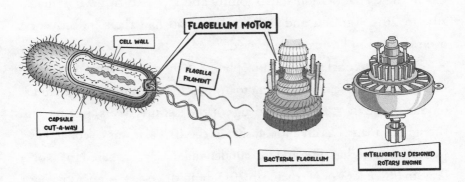

Random mutations, even when assisted by natural selection couldn't possibly achieve this task.[9]

Back to our commentary on anti-microbials. Not to be outdone by the antibiotics, let's take a moment to consider the current darling of the media, the antiviral, **Tamiflu** (generic name oseltamivir). It also has a cousin, Relenza (generic name zanamivir), which is an inhaled form with a similar mechanism. You'd think from the massive marketing campaigns starting in 2005 when the world was introduced to so called bird flu (H5N1) and in 2009 with the latest swine flu (H1N1),[10] that Tamiflu was highly effective against these viruses with minimal side effects. Especially since the US and UK government rushed to stockpile supplies contributing nicely to the bottom line of Swiss pharmaceutical giant Roche, the maker of Tamiflu, earning over $3 billion from it in 2009 alone.[11]

In fact the effectiveness and safety of both Tamiflu and Relenza has been challenged in the scientific literature for more than a decade.[12] With "no clear evidence that oseltamivir reduces the likelihood of hospitalization, pneumonia, or the combined outcome of pneumonia, otitis media [inflammation of the inner ear], and sinusitis" and reporting "that renal disorders, high blood sugar, psychiatric disorders, and heart rhythm disturbances may be related to Tamiflu use." It has been linked to allergic reactions, skin rashes, worsening of diabetes, and even suicide.[13] As the *British Medical Journal* and the nonprofit Cochrane Collaboration stated jointly and reported by *Nature* magazine in 2014 Tamiflu and Relenza have had had their "effectiveness overplayed, and harms underplayed."[14]

Before you conclude that I am opposed to the whole idea of man-made medicines (and an embarrassment to my pharmacist mum!) let's just touch on one of the most important drugs of the last fifty years, **ivermectin**. Brought to market as an antiparasitic in the 1980s, it was celebrated as a wonder drug at that time and its founder and developer shared the Nobel Prize in Physiology or Medicine in 2015 for its discovery. A microbiologist in Japan named Satoshi Omura grew up on a farm and was convinced that the secret to a healthy productive life lay in the nature all around us. While searching for new antimicrobials he discovered a completely new type of bacteria in the soil a few hours south of Tokyo, Japan. On studying the organism, it was found to produce a very active compound dubbed avermectin, which was highly effective against worms and other parasites. It was approved for animal use in 1981 while human studies continued. In Africa, the parasitic worm known as *Onchocerca volvulus* caused river blindness, with over seventeen million people infected across thirty-five countries. The socioeconomic burden was huge with some countries counting half their population over aged forty blind due to the condition. In 1987 it was finally approved for human use under the brand name Mectizan. River blindness was finally under control, with the WHO now moving to total elimination with over one hundred million people treated in a single year.[15]

The safety profile of ivermectin is unmatched with over four billion doses administered in its first thirty years, demonstrating it to be far safer than (for example) acetaminophen (Tylenol/paracetamol).[16] Studies found unique properties of the compound including antiviral and anti-inflammatory effects showing efficacy against a wide range of parasitic as well as viral diseases such as influenza, Zika, dengue, tuberculosis, malaria, HIV, and even cancer. So, yes, I was happy to take ivermectin myself when I finally succumbed to Covid-19 in June 2022.

The Miraculous Immune System

One of the interesting facts about the organism that gave us ivermectin is that it has not been found anywhere else in the world other than the original location in Japan. I like to think God had a hand in a nature-lover like Mr. Omura discovering it. To help you really understand the significance of this discovery as well as the next section on natural remedies against infectious agents, I need to build a little bit more on where we started in Chapter 1 with the miracle of the human body. Specifically the incredible marvel that constitutes our perfectly designed immune system.

As you can see by the illustration, what we call our immune system actually involves a complex network of molecules, cells, tissues and organs, each with a specific role in protecting the body through an intricate orchestra of processes.

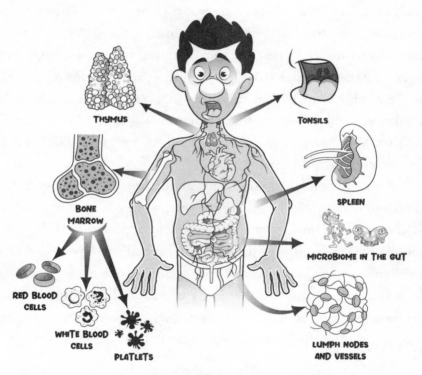

Starting at the top, the **tonsils** function as both gatekeepers and messengers. They are the first line of defense when germs enter our bodies through the air we breathe and the food we eat. They are actually lymphatic tissue rich in different types of immune cells directly engaged in fighting pathogens. But they also send signals to other parts of the network to bring in different kinds of troops. During these battles they often become swollen and red which is a buildup of lymph fluid and increased blood flow. Modern medicine is still performing 500,000 tonsillectomies a year in the US[17] while studies show children who had their tonsils and/or adenoids removed before the age of nine were at significant increased risk for a broad range of diseases as they grew older.[18]

The **thymus** is a little-known organ at the top of the chest most active in the first two years of a child's life as it is responsible for "training" T-cells, the most powerful adaptive immune cells in the body. (They are called T-cells because of their relationship to the thymus.) It begins to shrink after puberty but it continues to play a vital role as it is also part of the endocrine system making those messenger-like substances we call hormones to help regulate ongoing immunity.

You may think of your bones as those structures that are holding up your body but in fact the **bone marrow** is the heart of your immune system. The soft jelly-like structure inside of your bones is where an amazing array of blood cells are created. Without getting into the technical details of all the specialized roles, it includes neutrophils, basophils, eosinophils, mast cells, macrophages, and dendritic cells as well as lymphocytes—the T cells, B cells and natural killer (NK) cells that you may have heard of as the key warriors of the immune system. But each of these cells have incredibly unique jobs and all are important for optimal health.

The **spleen** is a fist-sized organ that sits under your rib cage beside your stomach. It has a number of critical functions in the body including recycling red blood cells. But it also filters the blood to remove pathogens that made it through the lymphatic system and is the main factory where antibodies are created. When you are fighting a serious infection, your spleen can grow significantly in size.

We've covered the importance of the gut and your **microbiome** in Chapter 3. But while we're on the subject of blood and blood cells I wanted to mention the fascinating studies that are now showing how neutrophils (a type of white blood cell) and gut microbes talk to each other and how your microbes help generate new white blood cells when levels are low.[19] Like I've said before—scientists haven't even scratched the surface of how the human body works or its interaction with the rest of nature.

This brings us to the lymph nodes and vessels of the **lymphatic system**. This is the "immune network manager" in which a clear fluid called lymph circulates while eliminating waste, toxins and foreign particles including viruses. It also helps clear fat from the body. The central hubs filtering the fluid are called lymph nodes, and there are about eight hundred of them in your body. It works closely with the cardiovascular system circulating blood but while the heart is busy pumping blood, the lymphatic system has no active pumping mechanism and relies on movement to function. This includes breathing and intestinal activity but it's one of the reasons active physical movement is so critical to good health. Long periods of inactivity are detrimental to your lymphatic system.

Got all that? I'm not going to test you on the details, but I just wanted to give you the smallest sense that our immune system is vastly more complex than the medical establishment would have you think. Consuming a product that has a single mechanism of action pales in comparison to the multitude of processes going on inside your body in response to an infection. We are far better served to nourish and support the body's natural processes so that the orchestra can play in tune.

Remedies That Nourish and Support

If you nourish your body as discussed in Chapter 5, reduce your exposure to toxins as discussed in Chapter 4 and incorporate other positive lifestyle features discussed in Chapter 3 like strong social connections, regular exercise, and uncompromising sleep you will no longer think of the year as having "a flu season." But I do want to provide a bit of commentary on what to do if your current state of health makes you more susceptible to infection or life got in the way of an optimum life-style and a germ seems to be overpowering the natural defenses God endowed you with. Just don't fall into the conventional medicine mind-set that one of these is the silver bullet to your situation. My intention is to open your eyes to the possibilities and give you some tools to figure out what will work for you and your family in any given situation.

The **Open-Air Factor (OAF)** is a real thing! The term first appeared in the 1960s and 1970s when various studies in microbiology established the powerful germicidal properties of outdoor air especially in rural settings (i.e., free of pollution).[20] But the remedy goes back centuries before this with one advocate of the "open-air method" documented as Dr. John Coakley Lettsom (1744–1815) who used the sea air and sunshine to heal children with tuberculosis in Kent, England. The first institution considered a tuberculosis sanitorium was run by Dr. George Bodington (1799–1882) near Birmingham, England, using fresh air, gentle exercise outside, and a nutritious diet.[21] In addition to its healing properties for an individual, it has also been established that outdoor air reduces transmission and infection. Clearly this fact is not appreciated by our modern "high-tech" hospital designers with their enclosed spaces probably contributing more to disease spread than the open-air or highly venti-lated hospitals of the old days.

Ditch the Masks!

The OAF is one reason to understand why covering your face even in the presence of microbes is a really terrible idea. The other reasons stem from the fact that viruses are teeny tiny; magnitudes smaller than say an oxygen molecule and also most bacteria. So if you are breathing through that cloth or chemical-infused disposable mask you are likely to be breathing in plenty of bacteria and there is zero protection against viral particles. Medical masks that surgeons wear are to protect the patient's open cavity from bodily fluids. Outside of a surgical setting they are really only good for generating fear.[22]

OAF is not fully understood, but it is likely a synergistic blend of features that results in a "secret sauce." Sunlight is certainly part of the story as ultraviolet light is known to inactivate viruses in its own right. Plus of course the sunlight would have boosted patients' vitamin D levels. But there is more to it as demonstrated by experiments carried out at night.[23] Outdoor air is high in ozone, another known germicidal agent (with a range of therapeutic applications such as chronically infected tonsils[24]) but even this is insufficient to explain the wonderful properties of fresh air.

Remember my friend's elderly relatives in Oakland who were scared to go outside during Covid? It was a demonstrably terrible public health measure to encourage people to stay indoors. But it does seem to have generated renewed interest in this once commonsense remedy and calls for improved ventilation in schools, homes, offices, and larger buildings.[25] So open your windows (put on more clothes if necessary!) and get outside as much as possible.

It's worth revisiting **Vitamin D** that we touched on in Chapter 1 under Nourished by Our Sun. While not germicidal itself, vitamin D acts more like a hormone in the body, binding to many types of cells with vitamin D receptors and thus activating over one thousand different genes including those responsible for immune health.[26] In other words, it keeps all the pieces of your miraculous immune system working optimally. It has been well established that low levels of vitamin D were a major risk factor for contracting Covid-19, being hospitalized with it, and having worse outcomes.[27] A simple blood test can measure your vitamin D levels but conventional doctors will typically tell you that 25ng/ml is good and that you shouldn't supplement more than 600–800IU per day. However, functional medicine doctors will argue that levels of 40–60ng/ml are better and that most people who are not getting daily sun should be supplementing with 5,000IU per day, even up to 10,000IU per day if levels are very low. Studies are clear that the upper limit for safe vitamin D consumption is far higher than previously assumed.[28] Even though I live in Southern California and get outside every day I take a vitamin D supplement about half the year. I take one that also has an optimal amount of vitamin K2 in it as well, as supplementing vitamin D without vitamin K2 can lead to the over-absorption of calcium (affecting cardiovascular health). A magnesium deficiency could also affect the absorption of vitamin D and calcium as mentioned under Orthomolecular Medicine in Chapter 2.

Vitamin C is one of the most misunderstood and underutilized nutrients on the planet. Part of the problem is it being classed as a vitamin rather than its medical name ascorbic acid, a powerful anti-oxidant.[29] The other problem is that only tiny doses of the nutrient are typically recommended, just enough to avoid scurvy, the fatal disease that sets in when a complete deficiency of vitamin C has gone on for months. While your multivitamin probably has some vitamin C in it, the "Recommended Dietary Allowance (RDA)" is typically in the range of 50–100mg whereas a therapeutic dose of vitamin C needs to be several-hundred times this or more.

Vitamin C has been documented in the scientific literature to cure polio, measles, mumps, chicken pox, shingles, viral pneumonia, pertussis (whooping cough), influenza, Chikungunya, Zika, and Ebola, to name just a few.[30] Part of the issue is that viral infections rapidly consume any vitamin C in the body, thereby effectively inducing scurvy in the patient. The resulting bleeding complications seen in some of these diseases are what lead to poor outcomes. The body needs a constant supply of vitamin C to maintain vascular strength and integrity. The dosages involved though are a minimum of 1,000–2,000mg (1–2 grams) three times a day for mild disease and something like 50,000mg (50g) infused intravenously (IV vitamin C or IVC) for severe illness. There is really no upper limit of vitamin C particularly when administered intravenously. When taken orally you might find a bowel-flushing effect which is nothing to worry about and part of the process. In fact experts will suggest you keep taking vitamin C until you are experiencing two loose bowel movements a day and continue that dosage until the infection is cleared.

Most doctors continue to ignore the healing power of vitamin C despite a huge body of evidence dating back to the 1930s and every decade since. For example, one of the leading causes of death in hospitals worldwide is sepsis (also known as septicemia or septic shock) which is essentially when your body is overwhelmed by an infection leading to multiple organ failure and death if not properly treated. In 2017 Dr. Paul Marik and others published a paper detailing the success in a small clinical trial of their protocol using IVC, thiamine (vitamin B_1) and the steroid hydrocortisone.[31] While the hospital where Dr. Marik works has made the protocol standard of care for sepsis patients, most other hospitals are reluctant to try this safe and cheap therapy.

The pandemic brought renewed interest in vitamin C with several countries embracing it as a therapy in addition to whatever else was being used.[32] But there is unlikely to be a marketing campaign on the benefits of vitamin C anytime soon as it is a cheap nutrient that doesn't

Types of Vitamin C

Natural vitamin C from plenty of fruits and vegetables should be a priority. Oranges, lemons, kiwi, papaya, strawberries, broccoli, parsley, sweet peppers, and kale are good options.

To supplement, sodium ascorbate is your best option for regular use. It can be bought cheaply in a bulk powdered form and has a neutral PH (whereas pure ascorbic acid can be acidic on the stomach).

Liposome encapsulated vitamin C is more expensive but highly absorbent. It comes in packets and can be useful for babies (just rub on the gums) and when dealing with illness.

Calcium ascorbate (such as Ester-C) is not recommended long term due to the high intake of calcium.

need a doctor to administer (at least orally). Hopefully you will now keep some at the ready.

Hydrogen peroxide (HP) nebulization is another powerful tool particularly for respiratory viruses and infections of the mouth, teeth, or gut. While you may have heard of HP as a strong disinfectant used on open wounds and to clean countertops, here's a few properties of HP you may not be aware of[33]—it is a naturally occurring molecule (H_2O_2) present everywhere in the body; it is continually being produced inside and outside cells and naturally detectable in the exhaled breath of healthy people and in urine. Intriguingly, production is increased in the presence of an infection or inflammation. It is basically a naturally generated antibiotic while being completely nontoxic, breaking down into water and oxygen once it has completed its pathogen-killing task.

Nebulization, also known as inhalation therapy, converts a liquid into a fine mist that can be inhaled and has been used for thousands of years.[34] You might have some reservations about inhaling a substance used to clean wounds or that stings you sharply when you do so. But I assure you it is completely safe and incredibly effective when nebulized. I first started using it to help eliminate my own Covid-19 symptoms in June 2022 but have gone back to it here and there multiple times due to its amazing properties to not only kill pathogens on contact but to oxygenate the blood (essential for all healing) and to help restore a healthy gut microbiome.

It's best to purchase food grade HP at 3 percent concentration to avoid any additives. This can be nebulized directly but some people find it irritating to the nasal passages at this concentration. So in that case simply dilute with pharmaceutical-grade saline. I use a 50/50 ratio which causes no discomfort. For example, I'll put 5ml of HP and 5ml of saline into my nebulizer. When dealing with an infection you'll want to nebulize for about ten minutes at a time, three times a day. If you've been on a plane with someone coughing in the next seat, you might want to nebulize for five minutes when you get home to nip any potential threat in the bud. HP can be particularly useful after dental work or to address any chronic infections in the mouth. We'll look at the connection between underlying infections (that may go undetected) and chronic disease in Chapter 7.

While HP is highly effective on its own, it is turbocharged in the presence of adequate doses of vitamin C which becomes a catalyst to its pathogen-killing power in a process known as the Fenton reaction. For more detail on the amazing properties of HP and vitamin C as well as other modalities considered bio-oxidative therapies like ozone, ultraviolet blood irradiation, and hyperbaric oxygen therapy (HBOT) I'd highly recommend the short book *Rapid Virus Recovery* by Dr. Thomas Levy.

Zinc and **quercetin** came to prominence during the Covid years for their antiviral properties. Zinc impairs viral replication and quercetin is known as a zinc ionophore—helps it to be absorbed into the cells where the virus is trying to replicate.[35] (Ivermectin and hydroxychloroquine are also zinc ionophores.) Zinc is critical for many functions in the body, but deficiencies are common especially in those who don't eat meat or legumes. Supplementing with 10–25mg a day of zinc can be helpful but beware of inducing a copper deficiency as mentioned in Chapter 2. I take quercetin daily for its many properties including helping me absorb more zinc from the food I eat. I'll only supplement with zinc if a virus takes hold.

Another invaluable tool in my toolbox is **grapefruit seed extract**, also sold as Citricidal. It is known to be effective against a wide range of bacteria, viral strains, and fungi but I use it mostly for parasites.[36] I love sushi, and so do my kids. It's not particularly healthy given the high mercury content of tuna and amount of nutrient-free white rice usually involved but it's a family favorite for a treat or special occasion.

I found in recent years though that my stomach was often upset afterward, perhaps not dealing adequately with the parasites that are typically found in raw fish. Citicidal was my answer! It's extremely potent so just three drops in a glass of water is all it takes. I use it after any sushi meal whether my stomach is upset or not, and then for any other suspected tummy bug.

Several **Essential Oils** are known for their antimicrobial action such as lemongrass, oregano, tea tree, thyme, clove, eucalyptus, and peppermint. EOs work synergistically such that their efficacy is amplified when they are blended together in specific quantities. Each oil can be effective against an organism on their own but often you have multiple symptoms including inflammation and pain so the blends can address the various manifestations.

There are many other foods, herbs, and spices with antimicrobial properties such as garlic and cinnamon. Just incorporating them into your recipes is the best way to take advantage of their benefits with the added bonus of flavor enhancement.

The last remedy I wanted to mention for now has also been known since ancient times and that is **silver**. Colloidal silver is a liquid suspension of microscopic silver particles and is considered a homeopathic antimicrobial agent. It can be easily purchased often as a spray and is far cheaper than you might expect as only tiny amounts of silver are needed. It is gaining renewed interest in conventional medicine due to the emergence of antimicrobial resistance[37] but has always been available to the discerning patient for at-home use.

Lessons from History

The common theme running through the last few pages is that remedies that have been known for well over a century are still valid today without the expense and side effects of modern pharmaceuticals. It's not difficult to understand why they are no longer embraced within the context of the rising fortunes of the medical profession as covered in Chapter 2. But there remain two myths that must be addressed head-on for a full picture. The first myth is that modern pharmaceuticals and vaccines in particular were responsible for wiping out deadly infectious diseases of old. The second myth is that these products, first widely introduced in the 1940s, have been carefully studied for safety and efficacy. Anyone willing to delve into the history books even a little can see through these myths, and I challenge you to do so as the implications are vast.

In the spirit of "a picture tells a thousand words," I'm going to start out by showing you two graphs. The first shows the reduction in infectious disease mortality in the US between 1900 and 1996. The second focuses only on children under the age of four over the same period. As can be clearly seen the numbers had fallen dramatically before any vaccines were introduced and before antibiotics were widely available in the 1940s.[38] The reasons for this (covered in Chapter 2) include public sanitation, personal hygiene, refrigeration of food, and better nutrition.

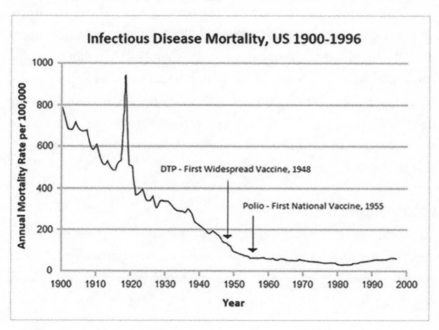

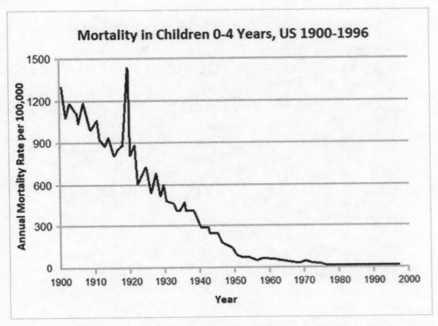

Data from JAMA article Trends in Infectious Disease Mortality in the US During the 20th Century (1999).

If we drill down into a single disease, say **measles**, the data is even more striking. The next graphs show the deaths due to measles in both the US and England during the twentieth century. In the nineteenth century, measles was definitely an illness to be feared with epidemics sometimes claiming 20 percent of children who caught it (one in five). But it was well known that it was the complications such as susceptibility to other infections like tuberculosis that were the problem rather than the measles itself. As nutrition improved the death rate plummeted. By the time the vaccine was introduced in the US in 1963, deaths had fallen by 98.7 percent. The vaccine was introduced in England five years later by which point deaths there had already fallen by 99.8 percent. We previously discussed the critical role of vitamin C when fighting a virus, so it's interesting to note the falling rates of mortality due to scurvy during the same time period as access to fresh produce increased.

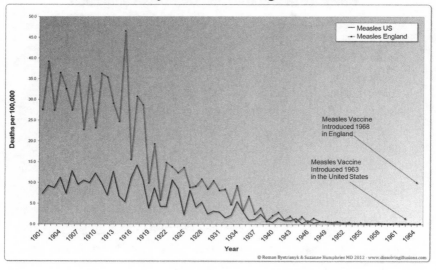

Measles Mortality Rate in US and England 1900 to 1967

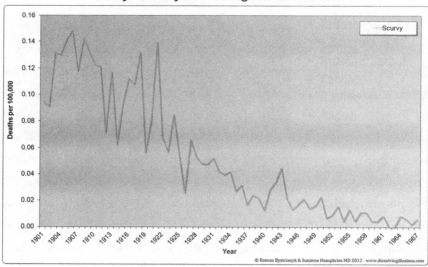

Scurvy Mortality Rate in England 1901 to 1967

There is much more to the story of measles[39] which is beyond the scope of this book but do watch this space for a follow-up book focused on raising healthy children!

Each of the other infectious diseases you've likely thought of as relics of history have an interesting story to tell, and I assure you it's not the one your doctor has been taught. Just to give you a small sense that all is not as it seems I want to let you peer under the hood a little of one of the foundational myths of humanity "combating" infectious disease which is the story of **polio**. The medical establishment will tell you with emphatic authority that polio was a terrible virus which often caused permanent paralysis and sometimes death. They'll mention the hero scientist, Jonas Salk, who invented a vaccine that was responsible for wiping out polio in developed countries; Albert Sabin created an improved vaccine a few years later and now charity organizations are working on eradicating polio from the face of the earth.

In fact, scientists have never really figured out polio since its arrival at the end of the nineteenth century and most of its mysteries remain today.[40] For example, the mode of transmission has never been identified, with many "epidemics" occurring in populations who have no contact with each other; some seemed to be connected to contaminated food. Polio tended to show up in the summer months when children were away from school. It also tended to strike rural populations harder than those in the cities, and animals were sometimes affected. It's not clear why polio emerged and intensified during a period when all other infectious diseases were dramatically declining. It wasn't seen initially in the developing world at all with polio epidemics not showing up in these countries until the second half of the twentieth century. In addition to these mysteries the physiological aspects of the disease are also not understood such as how the virus detectable in the gut passes to the central nervous system and why only a small number of people who have the virus end up paralyzed.

The term *poliomyelitis* comes from the effect seen on the spinal cord in paralyzed patients. In Greek *polios* means gray, *muelos* means matter, and *itis* denotes inflammation. The problem is that there are many causes of paralysis that are still seen today including other viruses such as Coxsackie and ECHO; hand, foot, and mouth disease; Guillain-Barre syndrome; undiagnosed congenital syphilis; lead or arsenic poisoning; and DDT toxicity. Prior to the 1950s, many different diseases were naively grouped under the umbrella of "polio." Once the vaccines were introduced there was a change in policy that required testing for the presence of the poliovirus itself and assessing if paralysis remained after sixty days.

Stepping outside of the medical profession for a minute, was there anything else that changed in the Western world besides the improved living conditions? As it happens during the later nineteenth century a substance called Paris Green became very popular in Europe and the US and was produced by nearly every dye maker in the market.[41] It was made from copper and arsenic, and while it was mainly used for textiles, it found its way into many household products like children's toys, candy wrappers, and wallpaper. Arsenic was already in many medical products, increasing exposures and there was a documented rise in arsenic poisoning.[42] By the turn of the twentieth century, Paris Green had also become a popular pesticide until it was superseded by a new product called lead arsenate (made from lead and arsenic) which was easier to prepare by farmers. It was also valued for adhering to produce longer and thus protecting them from insects. However, testing of produce available for sale proved that rinsing before consumption only removed a portion. The search was on for a safer alternative, but it continued to be used widely until DDT became available after World War II (1945). Of course DDT (considered the glyphosate of its day) turned out to be just as bad and was phased out of use in Western countries in the 1960s. The graph below comparing polio cases with pesticide production (most of which was DDT during this period) is revealing.

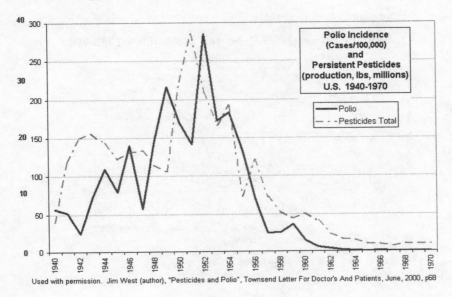

Used with permission. Jim West (author), "Pesticides and Polio", Townsend Letter For Doctor's And Patients, June, 2000, p68

By contrast, in the developing world, insecticides were rarely used in the years after World War II, but their use grew rapidly in the 1980s and continues to expand.[43] While banned in the US and Europe, DDT is used in many countries with India being the single largest manufacturer and consumer. "Polio" continues to be an ongoing problem in India. Scientists do recognize the connection of insecticides to polio-like disease in the developing world[44] but nonetheless, the World Health Organization (WHO) continues to make lofty goals with its Global Polio Eradication Initiative vaccinating millions of children. Although the stated goal has not been achieved, the WHO claim great success in reducing polio cases from 350,000 in 1988 to only 403 in 2013 (a 99 percent reduction). But on further examination it turns out the actual number of reported cases in 1988 was 32,419, with the WHO admitting it increased the number tenfold due to assumed underreporting.[45] However, the next graph reveals a little-known fact that while global polio cases seem to have fallen, acute flaccid paralysis syndrome (AFP) reached 100,000 in 2010 which is three times the number of reported polio cases in 1988.[46]

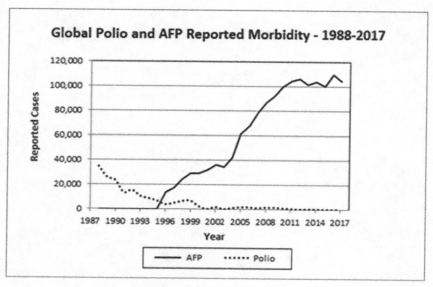

Source: Plotkin 2013—Vaccines (6th edition) as presented in *Turtles All the Way Down*.

There is more to the history of polio than I have been able to cover with this short overview. For those wanting to know more I'd recommend the book *Dissolving Illusions* by Dr. Suzanne Humphries and Roman Bystrianyk[47] which is a compelling history book complete with photographs and written extracts from historical sources. Its vivid depictions of life in the nineteenth and early twentieth centuries will make you marvel at what your grandparents and great-grandparents lived through. It then delves into not only polio and measles but also whooping cough which provides another revealing story of this still widespread disease.

The telling of the smallpox drama uncovers even more bizarre details than the polio narrative.[48] It was actually smallpox that led to the whole concept that the best way to protect humans from microbes was to help them generate antibodies to the offending microbe. But we now know a lot more about the miraculous human immune system including all the many pieces described earlier that constitute our innate immune system which jumps into immediate action when a pathogen shows up and is always at the ready. It is the adaptive immune system (just a small piece of the puzzle, our B and T cells) that "remembers" an encounter with a pathogen in the past and is able to neutralize it a second time. This is why after natural infection with most diseases you are immune for life. However, the adaptive immune system takes a few days to ramp up, clone the right B and T cells, and distribute them. The innate immune system is doing all the work in the meantime and often the infection is cleared without the adaptive pieces coming much into play. It actually takes a lot of effort to "trick" the orchestra into making antibodies when the innate system has been bypassed.

This attempt to circumvent nature leads us to the second myth we need to address head-on to make sure you have the full picture.

In most respects vaccines are just like any other pharmaceutical product we've discussed so far: made by industrial companies looking to make a profit. But there is one glaring difference that makes it important to dig into their history a bit more. When you are sick you have to weigh the pros and cons of any remedy. You might have an infection that is so overpowering your system that you are in danger of losing a leg or worse. Taking an antibiotic at that point is worth the risk of the potential side effects. But vaccines are injected into healthy individuals, often infants and children, and often with no choice in the matter.

A second book I encourage you to read is *Turtles All the Way Down: Vaccine Science and Myth.*[49] It was first published in Israel in Hebrew in 2018 and is now available in English worldwide. The authors have chosen to stay anonymous to ensure the focus is only on the claims of the book (and the extensive online reference document that accompanies it). But the silence that followed led one academic to offer a $4,000 cash reward to anyone who can challenge any of the statements made in the book or even a robust rebuttal to the conclusion drawn at the end of just the first chapter. There have been no attempts.

The title itself is illuminating. It's a clever spin on a story that has circulated for 150 years in scientific circles. Supposedly a scientist had just finished his lecture on the solar system when an elderly lady approached him and said she had a better theory. That in fact the earth was flat and sat on the back of a giant turtle. The jovial scientist kindly asked what was underneath the turtle to which the elderly lady replied *"another turtle." "And what is under that one"* he asked? *"Why it's turtles all the way down,"* she said. Scientists continue to use this story to portray the chasm between wise and rational scientists and ordinary laypeople. The authors of this fantastic book have instead laid out the most airtight case yet that actually, when it comes to vaccines and infectious disease, the roles are reversed. The laypeople concerned about vaccine safety are making the rational evidence-based assertions. Plus the specific claims of the medical establishment assuring the safety of vaccines rests on nothing but turtles all the way down.

The first part of the myth concerns the clinical trials vaccines go through before they are licensed for use. The gold standard is known as a double-blind, randomized placebo-controlled trial. This means one group gets the drug (a vaccine in this case) and the other gets an inert placebo. Randomized means trial participants are randomly assigned to be in one group or the other, and double-blind means that neither the participants (test subjects) nor the researchers know who has the product being tested or the placebo. The problem is that none of the vaccines currently recommended for children (at least those available in the US, UK, or Israel as studied by the authors) has ever been tested against an inert placebo. Instead, the so-called control group receives another vaccine or an injection of the vaccine ingredients without the antigen. But it's the vaccine ingredients that are often the problem.

In addition to the antigen such as the measles virus (or in the case of tetanus or diptheria the toxin that is released by the bacteria), vaccines contain a host of other ingredients like preservatives (often formaldehyde, a known carcinogen), stabilizers, and adjuvants. An adjuvant is necessary to get the immune system to respond—to trick it into reacting when something is injected into an arm that nature would expect to come via the mouth or respiratory system which would alert the many other pieces of the immune system first. Adjuvants are therefore highly toxic by design, usually aluminum or mercury. They are attached to the antigen, say a weakened or dead virus, to ensure the body mounts an attack. The idea is that in the attack to rid the body of the toxin it also makes antibodies to the virus. Sounds good in theory, but the problems are legion.

The most common clinical trials actually compare the new vaccine being studied with a different vaccine that has been assumed to be safe. For example, the DTaP vaccine which includes diptheria, tetanus, and pertussis replaced the older DTP vaccine which was known to cause serious side effects in infants.[50] However, the control group in the clinical trial for DTaP were given the DTP vaccine. So there was no true placebo. The old DTP was developed in the 1930s and 1940s, and there was no control group or any attempt to collect data on side effects at that time. One in twenty-two infants in the new trial was hospitalized but it wasn't considered alarming as it was similar to the control group!

Turtles All the Way Down details each vaccine and the design of the clinical trial involved. By the end of Chapter 1 you'll be surprised there

are any healthy two-year-olds walking around at all. It is only due to God's amazing design that these little bodies can deal with the onslaught they are subjected to. Many of them cannot.

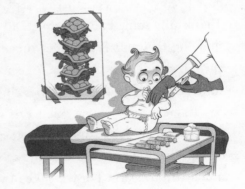

The book goes on to address each turtle of the accompanying parts of the myth including the unsubstantiated and untested vaccination guidelines with multiple vaccinations being given in rapid succession or even on the same day. It looks at the reporting systems set up to track ongoing problems once the vaccine is in the market, and how these systems are deficient by design. It addresses the fallacy of herd immunity, that only about one-third of the available vaccines actually stop you getting infected and being able to transmit the infection to others. This blows up the argument you should inject a vaccine to protect others. It mentions the waning efficacy of most vaccines compared to a natural infection. Whereas God's design was meant for most of these infections to be caught in childhood which leads to mild disease protecting you for life, catching them as an adult is a more serious proposition. Mumps for example is making a comeback often in those who were vaccinated against it in childhood. It can cause infertility if caught later in life. For those readers ready to list the news reports of definitive studies on vaccine safety, the book does a stellar job of dissecting five of the most prominent studies in recent years and how the media advertised false claims.

A whole chapter of the book provocatively questions why the most important studies have never been done by government officials namely comparing unvaccinated children (and adults) to those who have been vaccinated either partially or in accordance with guidelines. Thankfully some brave doctors and scientists have done these studies showing how much healthier unvaccinated children are without the chronic conditions so typically seen nowadays.[51] They have inevitably suffered a large backlash for speaking out.

To be sure, vaccine science is complicated, and I've only been able to touch on a handful of aspects here but hopefully it was enough to convince you that the science is in no way settled. There is much still to learn. For the sake of your own health and that of your family, I would urge you to investigate further. There are many other wonderful books written on the topic, some of which I have listed in Appendix D.

In case you are not in the child-rearing stage of life, I want to leave the history lesson with one more graph—that of influenza and pneumonia deaths in the US since 1900. You will note that the death rate has remained steady for the last fifty-plus years even though annual vaccinations have been available with marketing campaigns to increase their uptake in recent decades. Flu shots are reconfigured every year to keep up with the fast-mutating influenza virus. Aside from containing a large dose of adjuvant (usually mercury), these shots are known for their low efficacy rates. You are far better served by bolstering your miraculous immune system naturally if you want to reduce your fear of flu season.

Influenza/Pneumonia Mortality Rate 1900 to 2017

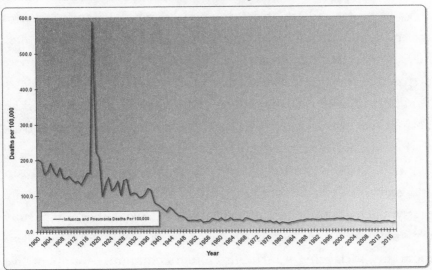

Source: DissolvingIllusions.com

Pandemic of Fear

So then how does SARS-Cov2 and the disease known as Covid-19 play into this scenario? At a surface level people who are malnourished or with underlying disease are always at risk from a virus such as influenza. To give you some context, according to the WHO in 2019, pneumonia and respiratory infections were the fourth-leading cause of death and that year these infections claimed 2.6 million lives which was a little lower than average.[52] There was a small uptick in 2020 but nothing to warrant the fear and panic that ensued. The data gets really murky after that for complicated reasons.[53]

At a more personal level, if you were one of the thousands of people hospitalized with Covid-19, or if you had a loved one hospitalized or even die from a SARS-CoV2 infection or complications, you've been living through one of the hardest times of your life. The tragedy of Covid-19 is happening at the level of public health but also at a very private level. It has led to unfathomable suffering for so many. Doctors, nurses, and other first-responders on the front lines during these difficult times were and are heroes to be celebrated. But I am a seeker of the truth, and I'm here to share with you even those truths that may be painful to hear so you can better manage your health and be more prepared for the next declared pandemic.

For me Covid was a nonevent. Other than having a busier than normal year at work as a global health consultant, and general frustration at the unscientific rules and restrictions that were being imposed, 2020 is remembered in my family as a year full of fun and growth. We had a summer vacation hiking in Montana and life pretty much got fully back to normal around September. Thankfully my kids were at schools that managed to keep them in the classroom and socializing. Our tight church community (of about five thousand people) had services outside through the summer with most midweek ministries continuing with creative solutions to work around the restrictions. Our own weekly small group of fourteen couples met in homes and backyards. All of this was also back to normal by September.

There was plenty of Covid going around and even a few hospital-ized but I'd be the first to head over to the house of anyone I knew with some homemade chicken soup and a bag full of supplements. Others did the same. There was no fear or panic. Just sensible measures taken and a community that pulled together, actions that strength-ened the faith of many. Very few chose to get the experimental shots unless required by a place of work. My own company was going to require it and I was expecting to resign immediately but then they dropped the mandate.

I did succumb to Covid two years later in June 2022 after a long overnight flight to the UK and a particularly busy and stressful week leading up to the flight. Plus I indulged in various sugary treats once I got there, which further depressed my immunity. I was mainly tired with a bit of a cough but treated it with extra supplements, ivermec-tin, and hydrogen peroxide nebulization. No work was missed and no lasting side effects.

The whole sorry saga of Covid has been examined at length by others so I've provided some reading suggestions in Appendix D. It seems very little has been learned in the last hundred years after all.

In the meantime, while the medical establishment wants you to focus on the historical reduction in infectious disease allegedly due to their innovations and at the same time instigating fear in new ones that come along, they have managed to avoid any difficult questions about the massive rise in chronic disease over the last fifty years. Autoimmune disorders, allergies, asthma, developmental, and neuro-logical conditions as well as diabetes and heart disease . . . we'll go there next.

Points to Remember

1. Antibiotics were brought to market long before we understood the importance of our microbiome to overall health. While a blessing in certain acute situations, antibiotics decimate our microbiome leaving us more vulnerable to resistant and more pathogenic bacteria.

2. There are often many other side effects of antibiotics and other antimicrobial medications.

3. Our immune system consists of an intricate orchestra of cells, organs, and systems in the body that all work together to keep us healthy.

4. There are many natural remedies that work in concert with your body to combat infections.

5. Digging into history reveals that the majority of the diseases we have been led to fear had already declined substantially before modern medicines and vaccines came on the scene. Better sanitation, hygiene, refrigeration of food and nutrition take much more of the credit than the modern pharmaceutical industry.

6. The myths associated with vaccination are the most egregious with many layers of poor science involved in the medical establishment's hold on this dogma.

CHAPTER 7

Shedding the Disease

If you asked my doctor, he'd tell you that I have a number of chronic "diseases"—hypothyroidism (underactive thyroid), hypercholesterolemia (blood cholesterol levels higher than considered normal), and eczema. Yet I take no medication whatsoever, not even over-the-counter drugs, feel great most of the time, and have no limitations on my life. My son Ethan was diagnosed with ADHD and Asperger's syndrome when he was five years old. The doctors told us we would have to put him on powerful drugs that could cause all sorts of side effects but without them our son wouldn't be able to function in society. Today Ethan is eighteen years old and one of the healthiest teenagers around. He also takes no medications, has no limitations on his life, and he's the kind of kid who gets straight A's without studying, is effortlessly good at most sports, and designs aircraft and race cars in his spare time. So, what is a "disease"?

Professor Jackie Leach Scully wrote an interesting essay on this topic a few years ago which I encourage you to read.[1] She explains that while the definition of disease changes with the human and cultural context "we must have a reasonably clear idea, first what a disease is, and second, which diseases are most worth the investment of time and money." This highlights the practical matter of labeling a set of symptoms as a certain "disease" so that treatments can be marketed to combat it. The labeling also enables us to track statistics to monitor what is going on in a population and perhaps altruistically address it in a certain way through policy. Quit smoking campaigns of the 1990s are a good example of this once lung cancer was highlighted as being on the rise and the connection was made.

But does the label help you as an individual? You might get a momentary period of relief when the symptoms that have been plaguing you for months or years finally get a name and you feel vindicated that there is, indeed, something identifiable wrong with you. But then you enter the world of the "standard of care," which includes medication, potential surgery, and ongoing testing. You won't be told what is causing the disease. Likely, your doctors will just put it down to "bad luck" or "bad genes." With no known origin, there can be no real cure. So you are expected to hand your future over to the guy in the white coat.

At the same time, *medical gaslighting* has become more widespread these days. This practice of ridiculing patients is more recently connected with people experiencing adverse symptoms since getting a Covid-19 vaccine, but medical gaslighting has been going on for years. Whenever a doctor cannot identify the reason for the symptom, they will insist that there is nothing wrong and it's all in your head. It has been instilled in their training that a vaccine couldn't possibly cause any ill effects, the food you eat is inconsequential, and if nothing shows up in a blood test or imaging then nothing is wrong. They send you home with a pat on the back and a prescription for an antidepressant or antianxiety medication.

The Intersection of Infectious and Chronic Conditions

While government agencies and maybe your health plan have been focusing on infectious disease, it is estimated that around 133 million or

43 percent of all Americans are living with one or more chronic diseases.[2] The CDC puts the rate at 60 percent.[3] This includes more than 40 percent of children and adolescents.[4] The rates have skyrocketed in the last two decades. While an infectious disease tends to be self-limiting, a week or two of discomfort, a chronic disease persists for an extended period of time, months or years, perhaps a lifetime. The economic cost is astronomical in terms of spending on healthcare and lost productivity. At the individual level quality of life can be seriously impacted.

The war on germs that started in the early twentieth century has gotten seriously out of hand. We've discussed the importance of microbes to our overall health in terms of the synergistic nature of our microbiome. We've also seen how the majority of infections are entirely manageable with some common sense and nature-provided assistance. It's also interesting to note that in fact a bout of certain infectious diseases seems to benefit us in the long run. There is plenty of medical literature documenting tumor remissions after a measles infection for example. A large Japanese study found that a history of measles and/or mumps in childhood significantly protected against deadly heart attacks and strokes later in life.[5] Another study found that each additional contagious disease contracted in childhood, such as measles, mumps, rubella, chicken pox, and scarlet fever increased the protective effect against cardiac events as adults by 14 percent.[6] Yet again God's mysteries abound.

What if in our effort to stamp out infectious disease we inadvertently encouraged chronic illness?

If nothing else the Covid fiasco is bringing to light some revealing facts. In the US, simple data from the Bureau of Labor show the number of people unable to work due to disability accelerated exponentially starting in February 2021.[7] In an eighteen-month period there were 3.2 million newly disabled Americans, the majority of which had been fully employed at the time of their disability. The data shows the rate of disability is higher for those who were employed than the general population. For the first time ever, it was actually bad for your health to be working for an employer. Insurance companies typically rate the fully employed as healthier than those who don't work. Hence insurance premiums for your employer are lower than you can get as an individual. But in 2021 and 2022 something changed that affected the employed population more than the rest. Vaccine mandates perhaps?

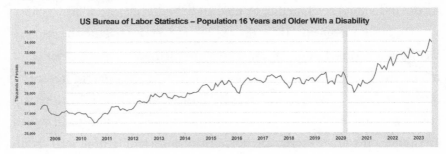

Source: US Bureau of Labor Statistics

The UK has a far better dataset to study. The Personal Independence Payment (PIP) program under the Department of Work and Pensions (DWP) tracks disability payments (PIP claims) by the body system underlying the cause. The next graph shows the massive rise in disability claims due to hematological conditions (disorders of the blood) from February 2021 compared to the preceding few years including 2020. Other conditions tell a similar story though this one is the most striking. I also have personal experience of this category as my eighty-four-year old dad in the UK is affected. In January 2021 he was perfectly healthy riding his bike all over London but after taking his first Pfizer shot his health slowly deteriorated. It got worse with additional shots, eventually being diagnosed with vasculitis (inflammation of the blood vessels) which rendered him hospitalized more than once. His conventional doctors told him it was nothing to do with the shots, so he kept taking them. I was able to take him to a wonderful functional medicine doctor in 2022 who admitted otherwise, pointing to the significant rise in vasculitis he'd seen in the past year. The whole UK dataset is available for anyone to study.[8]

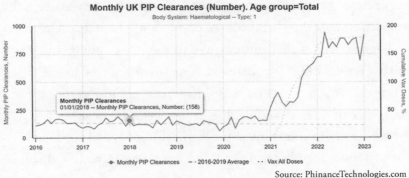

Monthly UK PIP Clearances (Number). Age group=Total
Body System: Haematological -- Type: 1

Source: PhinanceTechnologies.com

It is beyond the scope of this book to get into the travesty of Covid-19 but the massive human experiment of rolling out a single type of pharmaceutical to so many people all at the same time has given us the data we need to see more clearly that modern pharmaceuticals are often causing more problems than they fix.[9]

The ongoing condition known as Long Covid can be considered a chronic disease as many people have been dealing with a variety of debilitating symptoms for over a year (the official definition of chronic disease). Whether the condition arose after contracting Covid-19 with or without a prior vaccination, the pathology is very similar to conditions arising due to a reaction to the Covid-19 vaccine itself. In this case, it doesn't matter what the label is as the underlying cause is likely the spike protein, identified as toxic to human cells, coupled with an existing weakness in the immune system. It highlights the fact that we can't really separate "disease" into the two categories of infectious or chronic (communicable or noncommunicable in WHO speak).

Illness is the body not functioning optimally. The root cause is rarely just a single factor such as a pathogen. Back to germ theory vs. terrain theory. If your body is healthy, you won't succumb to a pathogen. If you are unhealthy to start with, a pathogen (such as a virus or bacteria) could throw you into a chronic condition. Maybe it's the toxin the bacteria excreted (in tetanus for example); or a myco-toxin excreted by mold (a fungi). The toxin could be man-made such as pesticides and all the chemicals we covered in Chapter 4. Ultimately, it's a huge variety of elements day to day, month to month and year to year that results in health or illness as we discussed in Chapter 3.

But this is actually good news. If we can get to the root cause or causes, we can reverse chronic disease and generate health.

I want to help you think differently. Think beyond the labels. You (or your family member or friend) are not a person with X disease. A medical professional has identified a collection of symptoms or something out of whack in the body which meets the criteria of a particular label. In conventional medicine that opens up a list of drugs that have been approved to treat it. Rarely will they reverse or cure it, but the doctor will be there to let you know what the next drug or the next step is when your symptoms progress. There is another way.

While nearly all chronic diseases can be prevented and reversed with the principles discussed in this book—lifestyle and natural remedies, it is useful to understand some underlying features of each condition to help you prioritize your approach. If we don't touch on the specific diagnosis you are concerned about, the principles covered should give you plenty of direction to move forward.

When Your Body Attacks Itself

The three diseases that get the most attention in the developed world these days are cardiovascular disease, diabetes, and cancer. They are the top killers no doubt and we will get to them, but millions more people are suffering from a barrage of miserable and sometimes debilitating "mystery" symptoms. Many people suffer in silence; perhaps you're one of them. Others take months or years of visiting multiple doctors, many of which will tell them there's nothing wrong. But eventually you might get that label of one or more autoimmune diseases.

I want to tell you the story of my good friend Kimi. I met her in 2020 when she and her military husband moved to California and joined our small-group ministry at church. She had a medical port in her chest and would miss group every few weeks. Initially we didn't know her that well, so we never asked many questions, but as time went on, she disclosed she was having a type of chemotherapy for an autoimmune condition. Each time she had the infusions it flattened her physically for a week, and we got used to bringing her family food to help out. As the months went by each infusion week left her more depleted and she had to take steroids to deal with the severe side effects. It was hard to watch.

Eventually we had grown close, and given my work, I asked for more details on her condition. She disclosed she had been diagnosed with something called mucous membrane pemphigoid, and her oncologist insisted she needed these infusions of intravenous immune globulin (IVIG) which has a string of nasty side effects associated with it. She also commented that initially she had been diagnosed with pemphigus vulgaris, but when a new symptom popped up, they changed the label. I probed further into her history as to what caused her to seek a diagnosis in the first place. An itchy throat put her in the hospital when she suddenly became unable to swallow. Tests were generally negative other than basic inflammation. Lots more questions from me on her diet, stress levels (husband in the military periodically deployed!), and other factors. It eventually came out that she'd had breast implants put in years ago. Aha! I thought. Have you considered removing them? Turned out the insurance coverage the US government provides to its military personnel fully covers the $300,000 for the IVIG treatment, but it won't pay $5,000 for the breast implant removal. Something is very wrong with this picture.

Friends immediately stepped in to help with the cost and Kimi went ahead with the breast implant removal. The oncologist was extremely upset when she said she was discontinuing treatment. He told Kimi she was an idiot and refused to help out if she ever had a flare-up in the future. My friend felt almost an instant improvement a week after the outpatient surgery. She has made significant changes to her diet, a new supplement routine, and other lifestyle changes and a year later, no flare-ups. She is still dealing with some of the side effects of the drugs she was on for years, but the future is looking bright.

The most common examples of autoimmune conditions you've probably heard of are multiple sclerosis (MS), lupus, rheumatoid arthritis (RA), Crohn's and ulcerative colitis (types of inflammatory bowel disease we'll collectively refer to as IBD), psoriasis, celiac disease, type 1 diabetes, Hashimoto's thyroiditis, and Graves disease. Chronic fatigue syndrome and fibromyalgia also have an element of autoimmunity. The incidence of these types of conditions has been rising steeply the last two decades with estimates now of well over fifty million people in the US[10] alone diagnosed with at least one (and if you have one autoimmune condition you are at high risk for another). Millions more struggle with various individual symptoms without having yet got a diagnosis. These are warning signs of a disordered immune system and a red flag of what is to come if steps aren't taken to reverse the process. Symptoms include digestive problems (gas, bloating, indigestion, reflux, heartburn, constipation, diarrhea), allergies, asthma, brain fog, depression, skin problems, hair loss, headaches, infertility, joint/muscle pain, sleep problems, and more.

If you (or your loved one) haven't yet received a diagnosis, I'd cautiously suggest the time is better spent researching the likely causes and using the guidance and resources in this book to find solutions. Ideally this would include finding your way to some sort of "alternative" professional such as an integrative, naturopathic or functional medicine doctor who can lend some expertise. But if that is outside of the budget or the health plan coverage available, there is plenty you can achieve on your own.

Let me tell you another secret of the medical industry—there are more than one hundred autoimmune conditions in the diagnostic manual and most of them are not well understood by conventional medicine. Part of the problem is due to the specialization of care as mentioned in the history of Chapter 2. You go to a neurologist for MS, a rheumatologist for RA, a gastroenterologist for celiac or IBD, an endocrinologist for Hashimoto's or Graves . . . and if you have more than one condition, you'll be managing multiple doctors. But these conditions all arise out of an impaired immune system and as we saw in Chapter 6 all of the pieces of your immune system are intricately connected.

There are in fact more similarities than differences between each of these conditions which is why I wouldn't worry too much about receiving a particular label. In all cases it is a matter of an imbalanced immune system mistakenly attacking and destroying the body's own tissue. Autoimmunity can attack any organ, enzyme, hormone, or type of cell depending on your genetic predisposition and your unique epigenetic triggers. The elements involved are what give a particular categorization. A doctor might confidently put you in one of these categories, but this can never account for the infinite complexity of the human body and the sensory input of your past or future day-to-day lifestyle that affects it.

Conventional doctors will paint a pretty bleak picture that you have a lifetime affliction and your only options are a range of highly toxic very expensive drugs with nasty side effects that will treat the symptoms and perhaps arrest further progression. Often these drugs are designed to suppress your immune system, which is going to leave you open to a host of infections and other problems. These doctors may support you cleaning up your diet a bit but will typically scoff at the suggestion that anything in your diet or environment is causing the symptoms.

Here are some key strategies we'll look at that are most useful if you are dealing with a diagnosed autoimmune condition or likely heading for one given the range of symptoms you may be suffering from:

- Address underlying infections
- Fix your food with an emphasis on an anti-inflammatory diet
- Correct nutritional deficiencies
- Consider one safe inexpensive medication called low-dose naltrexone

Everything else we're discussing in the book such as removing toxins, getting enough sleep, and moving your body are vitally important too but these four are particularly critical as an alternative treatment for autoimmune conditions.

Inflammation underlies every chronic disease. Symptoms are your body's cry for help. One area of inflammation is created by chronic infections of pathogenic bacteria, viruses, fungi, or parasites. We're not returning to the discussion in Chapter 6 but it's important to note that these pathogens don't always clearly announce themselves. Others may cause a bout of flu-like symptoms but then you seem to recover and go on with your life. Except they end up hiding dormant in your tissues and create inflammation that unbalances your immune system. Your immune system knows they are there but can't quite eliminate them without help.

One culprit is the **Epstein-Barr** virus. A member of the herpes family, it causes the disease known as "mono" which many people contract in their youth. (It's also known as "the kissing disease"). A recent study has linked Epstein-Barr with the later development of MS.[11]

Another culprit is **Candida**. You might know it as yeast. Most commonly associated with urinary tract infections, candida overgrowth has been linked to asthma, allergies, chronic fatigue syndrome, fibromyalgia as well as lupus and MS. Candida exists in all of us but if our microbiome gets unbalanced for the reasons we've discussed—use of medications, eating too much sugar and processed food, unmanaged stress—it can take over, damaging the gastrointestinal tract.

Lyme disease is getting a lot of attention in the US these days, with diagnoses up over 300 percent in the last fifteen years in rural areas[12] with CDC estimates nearing 500,000 cases annually across the country. Lyme is caused by the *Borrelia burgdorferi* bacteria and is transmitted to humans through the bites of infected blacklegged ticks, also called "deer ticks." There is some evidence that it's now also being spread by other bloodsucking insects like mosquitoes and horseflies. The bacteria looks like a long, thin wiggly corkscrew which microbiologists call a spirochete. Another famous spirochete which has similar properties to Borrelia is the syphilis bacteria. It can also burrow into your tissues and cause a huge range of symptoms if left untreated. Like Lyme it is sexually transmitted and from mother to babies in the womb.

Part of the problem with Lyme is that many people don't realize they have been infected. The symptoms can be vague and often there is an absence of the so called "bull's-eye rash." Conventional medicine relies on standard tests known as the Western blot test and ELISA (enzyme-linked immunosorbent assay) but these have been shown to miss up to two-thirds of cases. Even using this 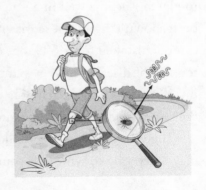 test, one study showed that nearly 40 percent of patients with an MS diagnosis tested positive for Lyme (the B. burgdorferi bacteria).[13]

Conventional medicine will also claim that Lyme is easily managed with a three-week course of antibiotics but this is frequently not the case. The bacteria's ability to hide out and change form, lay dormant, and flare up means it is particularly challenging and much better suited to a multipronged functional medicine approach. Coinfections such as *Babesia* and *Bartonella* may also be passed on by the insects, inflicting damage on the immune system and leave it in a weakened state. Conversely you may be less able to combat Lyme if your immune system has already been compromised by mycotoxins from mold in your house or place of work for example. This all comes back to our discussion on the importance of maintaining a healthy microbiome which is the foundation of a robust immune system.[14]

> **Stevia** (whole leaf extract) has been shown to be more effective than conventional antibiotics against all forms of B.burgdorferi.[15]

Other common triggers for autoimmunity lurk in the food that you eat and I'm going to start with gluten. **Gluten** is a type of protein found in grains. The highest levels are in wheat, barley, and rye but there are smaller quantities of glutens in all grains including corn and rice. As far back as the 1990s scientists were suggesting that sensitivity to gluten was involved in a range of neurological conditions.[16] It's also been shown that gluten sensitivity can lead to lesions in the brain that can be mistaken for MS lesions on scans. Case studies abound of total reversal of diseases such as symptomatic lupus on a gluten-free diet. I myself was once suspected of having lupus long ago when I was still in the grip of conventional medicine. I am now vehemently gluten-free.

There's a number of complications with gluten, which is why you may not yet be convinced it could be a factor for you.[17]

- It is estimated that only one out of seven people with gluten sensitivity actually have any gastrointestinal problems.

- The gluten molecule itself is large and shares some of the same protein sequences as your own tissues such as your thyroid. In the presence of an already enflamed immune system this can lead to a phenomenon called molecular mimicry where your body wants to fight the gluten but also ends up fighting your own cells at the same time.
- It may not be the gluten molecule that is affecting you but the toxic pesticide glyphosate that comes along with the wheat and other grains in countries that are still using glyphosate. (See discussion in Chapter 4.)
- Gluten-free is not the same as low-gluten. It can take three months to calm the system down from even a small bite of birthday cake. If you've tried cutting out just wheat, you are missing a lot of gluten in your diet and you won't see results.

If you're still not convinced, then let me just tell you that gluten has been found to be the main culprit in **leaky gut**. Even if you're doing everything else right, gluten can sabotage all your efforts with a single bite. Gluten triggers the production of a substance known as "zonulin" which regulates the cells lining your intestines and causes the tight junctions between them to loosen.[18] This allows partially digested food to leak through. Your immune system then attacks the food molecules as if they were a harmful bacteria or virus. Leaky gut can then lead to all sorts of food "allergies" and inflammation.

Hard to believe when bread has been such a mainstay of our diet for centuries. But the wheat of today bears very little resemblance to the wheat and grains of old. Corporations have developed new hybrids with forms of glutens that our bodies just don't recognize as natural.

If you are dealing with an autoimmune condition or suspect one based on symptoms, my advice is to cut out gluten 100 percent for a period of six months before you make an assessment. Gluten lurks in pasta and baked goods but also in many other types of processed foods and condiments. Manufacturers use gluten as a preservative and thickener in all sorts of products. You must read labels and be vigilant.

Taking you back to Principle #3 in Chapter 5, I would recommend you follow an anti-inflammatory diet which actually cuts out all grains including rice and corn. Dairy is also avoided (including whey protein) as the casein molecule can be mistaken for gluten and acts similarly in the body. Full-fat coconut milk is a great substitute. An anti-inflammatory diet also avoids legumes and other plants high in lectins like the nightshade family (tomatoes, white potatoes, eggplant, and sweet peppers). You could equally try the ketogenic diet (keto) that has also been touted for autoimmune conditions. It was originally developed for epilepsy which could be considered an inflammatory condition. There's a lot of similarities between the two but keto can be a little harsh on the system. Importantly, focus on fresh fruits and vegetables, fish, meats, and healthy fats. Make sure to include lots of healthy spices like garlic, ginger, turmeric, and cinnamon.

Nutrient deficiencies are likely to need more than an ongoing change in diet depending on how severe they are. As I explained in Chapter 2 under Orthomolecular Medicine, it is a very individual process and could lead to more unbalancing if you're not careful. But to make sure you don't neglect

Sourdough or Ancient Wheat?
For those looking for any "way out" of eliminating bread you might wonder if sourdough bread is an option. Some find fewer digestive problems from organic sourdough because it includes fermented enzymes to help break down the proteins. However, as discussed in the list, absence of digestive issues does not solve the problem of gluten.

What about heirloom wheats such as einkorn, which have not undergone any hybridization? Similar story.

Only you can decide what is right for you. I'm just laying out some facts!

this important aspect of health improvement I've provided a few ideas
for consideration.

- **Vitamin D** is here again! See the discussion in Chapter 6. But
  for autoimmune diseases vitamin D can be used medicinally at
  very high doses. This is due to vitamin D resistance being seen
  in some autoimmune patients.[19] Dramatic improvements have
  been seen in psoriasis, asthma, and RA for example with doses
  at levels around 25,000 to 50,000IU per day.[20]
- All of the **remedies discussed in Chapter 6** are relevant here
  for dealing with the underlying infections. A parasite cleanse
  that contains wormwood and black walnut is a good place
  to start together with grapefruit seed extract. Other herbal
  ingredients can help eliminate candida overgrowth. L-lysine
  can help manage latent viral infections.
- Taking a **daily probiotic** is just plain good sense for anyone
  as a strategy against the insults to our microbiome from
  modern living. But for autoimmunity it is critical to start
  with repairing your gut health as central to a well-functioning
  immune system. Don't just grab a bottle from the grocery
  store though. Research those that are certified to contain a
  minimum of 30 billion organisms by the time you ingest
  them (50bn is even better) with at least ten different strains.
  Probiotics are not a silver bullet though and it is questionable
  how effective they are at making permanent changes to
  your microbiome, but as part of an overall strategy, useful
  nonetheless. Eating fermented foods is an even better
  strategy.[21]
- **Digestive Enzymes** can be useful to ensure you are fully
  digesting all the healthy food you are now eating and
  maximizing nutrient absorption.

- **Omega-3 fish oil or cod liver oil** has many health benefits
  but is particularly effective against autoimmune conditions
  for its anti-inflammatory properties.[22] As usual, be careful of
  your source to avoid contamination with heavy metals such as
  mercury. See Resources for recommended brands.
- **N-acetylcysteine (NAC)** is a form of the amino acid cysteine
  and has a range of beneficial effects especially for chronic
  conditions. It helps the body create glutathione in the liver,
  which is vital for detoxification. It is best known as a remedy
  for hangovers and Tylenol toxicity but has been described as
  "an old drug with new tricks" as scientists keep finding new
  beneficial qualities.[23] Take 500–1,000mg twice a day.

This brings me to another drug that I wholly endorse. Naltrexone. Specifically **Low-Dose-Naltrexone (LDN)**. Like ivermectin, it was discovered decades ago and known for its safety profile but is so cheap that Big Pharma now actively ignores it. Perhaps because it has been found to have such a dramatic effect on a wide range of conditions it is negating the need for the very expensive new drugs they are selling. Consequently, nobody is paying the millions of dollars involved in running placebo-controlled double-blind studies that doctors are trained to rely on in order to prescribe it for certain conditions. Hence you may not have heard of this drug at least in its low-dose form.

Another similarity to ivermectin is that LDN has a number of modes of action so the "side effects" are actually in line with what the body needs to better ameliorate the symptoms of the condition. However, while ivermectin is super safe for personal management and many countries (and at least one US state at the time of writing) allow its purchase without a prescription, LDN is prescription-only and does need to be overseen by a physician due to its mode of action on the brain and potential to interact with other medications.

It is helpful to understand how LDN works so that you can see why it is useful for so many conditions. It is known as an *opioid antagonist*. It binds to the opioid receptors in your brain blocking any other substances or chemical messengers from binding. It is approved to treat opioid and alcohol abuse in doses of 50–100mg. Low-dose naltrexone, on the other hand, is prescribed in tiny doses of 1–5mg a day. So it only binds to the receptors for a few hours and then the magic is in the rebound effect. The biochemistry is a little complicated, but here's a simplified version:

- *Receptor site binding* to both the opioid receptors in your brain and the toll-like receptors (TLRs) in your specialized immune cells (macrophages and microglia—see The Miraculous Immune System in Chapter 6)
- *Upregulation of endorphins* as your body is tricked into thinking it's not producing enough. Endorphins are the body's natural pain relievers.
- *Immune cell inhibition* from blunting the TLRs which suppresses immune cell activation and reduces the production of pro-inflammatory signaling molecules.
- *Decreased inflammation and pain* resulting from the combination of increased endorphins paired with a decrease in pro-inflammatory signaling molecules which further impacts immune function, cell growth and pain response.

LDN has been shown to have a profoundly positive impact on a range of autoimmune and inflammatory conditions including most recently Long Covid. If you want to know more, I'd highly recommend the aptly named book *The LDN Book,* which is a compilation written by different doctors and pharmacists who are experts in their field.[24] There are chapters dedicated to MS and lupus, inflammatory bowel disease, chronic fatigue syndrome and fibromyalgia, restless leg syndrome, depression, autism, and cancer. *The LDN Book* also includes a detailed history of LDN as well as helpful appendices to assist you in discussing it with your doctor and answers to a range of common questions you may have.

I must reiterate though the need for you to individualize your approach as no single remedy is going to "fix" your problem. While these key strategies I've mentioned are all useful in dealing with an autoimmune condition or mystery symptoms that point to autoimmunity setting in, you need to embrace healthy living overall. Going back to our bucket in Chapter 3, you may increase some of the good stuff going in with these strategies but it won't be enough if the bad stuff keeps overflowing. You'll also need a large dose of patience. It took years for your body to get so out of balance, it will take some time to set it right. Don't give up and return to old habits if you aren't seeing changes. Just adjust the details. Something that didn't seem to work for you previously may work now that other aspects have been addressed first.

Metabolism Woes

One of the biggest blind spots I find when talking to people about their health is the foundational role of metabolism and blood sugar control. They just want to know what supplement they can take to improve XYZ. Often they want to cling to a prescription medication which may reduce problematic symptoms, but you know by now that doesn't generate health. Exercise may come up; a willingness to go to the gym, try a new sport or a daily walk with friends. Anything it seems is on the table except for addressing the one thing that is the game changer for your health—how and what you eat.

The label of **diabetes** is given to nearly 500 million people worldwide (that is half a billion) with it being assigned as the cause of death of 2 million a year.[25] This doesn't account for the many millions more who are considered prediabetic (another label) or have undiagnosed *insulin resistance*.

Insulin is a hormone released into the bloodstream when you eat and blood sugar rises. It directs your liver, muscle cells, and body fat to absorb the sugar for energy metabolism or storage. Thus restoring normal blood sugar levels. If there is more sugar than can be metabolized, the brain signals the beta cells of your pancreas to secrete more insulin to help. Over time you build up insulin resistance as your body works overtime to keep up with all the sugar, and ultimately, the exhausted beta cells deteriorate and die-off. Blood sugar levels get out of control and diabetes sets in.

This is known as type 2 diabetes, which used to be called adult-onset diabetes as it took years of poor eating to appear. Sadly it is now being seen in teenagers and even younger. Not to be confused with type 1 diabetes (previously called juvenile diabetes), which is an autoimmune condition where your body actually attacks and destroys the pancreatic beta cells as if they were an invading virus, leaving your body unable to make insulin.

The symptoms of insulin resistance include fatigue, recurrent infections, impotence, excessive thirst and urination, blood sugar swings involving sweating, and palpitations or tremors when you haven't eaten in a while. I used to have to eat every couple of hours or felt faint. It seemed normal to me. I wasn't overweight so didn't think anything of it. Now I know better.

Maybe some of these symptoms start to impact your life or perhaps you get an annual physical and your blood tests show an elevated hemoglobin (Hb)A1C level causing your doctor to label you as diabetic. An A1C test claims to provide a picture of your average blood glucose level over the past couple of months. Under 5 is considered normal while over 7 is considered diabetic enabling your well-meaning doctor to

prescribe a range of pharmaceuticals that address different aspects of
the metabolic process. Some drugs focus on breaking down sugar and
starch in your food, others make your body more sensitive to insulin,
and another category focus on promoting better glycemic control.

 High blood sugar is very bad news to be sure. We'll get into why
a bit later. But addressing this single symptom, and the complex mechanism involved, with a drug has clearly and scientifically been shown
NOT to improve outcomes (i.e., death or other health problems) and
generally does more harm than good.[26]

Here I must take a quick sidebar to highlight the latest Big Pharma
ruse telling us **obesity** is a disease. Technically you are considered
obese if your Body Mass Index is greater than 30. (BMI = your height
in inches, divided by your weight in pounds.) A BMI above 25 will
label you as overweight. But this is an oversimplified measurement
as muscle weighs a lot more than fat so you could be a lean healthy
gym rat and be technically considered overweight or even obese. Being
underweight (BMI below 18.5) is far more detrimental to your health.[27]

But wait, data coming out of the Covid saga showed that obesity
was a risk factor for a poor outcome. True, but it is not necessarily the
obesity itself, rather the underlying mechanisms that lead to obesity
also drive poor Covid outcomes. There are studies connecting obesity
to a vastly increased risk of diabetes. In fact, one study combining
data from the US and Europe found the risk of diabetes in obese men
was seven times higher and for obese women twelve times higher than
normal-weighted people.[28] But not everyone who is diabetic or insulin
resistant is overweight. Let me say that again so you don't miss it—
*you don't have to be overweight to have insulin resistance or full-blown
diabetes.*

However, Big Pharma has utilized the connection of diabetes and weight to drive another major marketing campaign. One of
those diabetes drug categories is called a GLP-1 receptor agonist (for

Glucagon-like peptide). It has the useful side-effect of slowing your stomach emptying making you feel full for longer and helping you lose weight. You might have heard of Ozempic (also called Wegovy at higher doses) or Trulicity. Doctors are now prescribing these drugs for people with normal HbA1C levels but who are considered obese or even merely overweight. Not only is there a significant annual cost of these drugs—you would probably need to be on them for the rest of your life as the weight comes back as soon as you stop taking it—but the side-effects are terrible. Most commonly nausea, vomiting and diarrhea, but also stomach blockages and potentially psychological effects are being studied.[29] They also pose a risk for patients needing surgery as your stomach won't empty within the normally advised fasting window leading to life threatening complications during anesthesia.

Weight-loss should never be an end goal. Good health is the end goal. There are infinitely better ways to manage your blood sugar and reverse insulin resistance which don't involve drugs. If you focus on the principles in this book including how you nourish your body as discussed in Chapter 5, losing weight if needed will be a natural outcome as your body instinctively gets itself back in balance.

The one strategy I do want to highlight here is **Intermittent Fasting**, also known as **Time-Restricted Eating (TRE)**. It's an extension of nourishment principle #2 covered in Chapter 5 but surprisingly powerful for such a simple concept. "Oh that's one of those fads of the day" I'm hearing you cry just like gluten-free diets. Well in fact both of these strategies are rooted in the natural order of our world as it was intended before the distraction of modern convenience. Contemporary hybridization, ultra-processing, and glyphosate has messed up gluten. The ever availability of food has messed up our metabolisms. Back in the day you did a few hours' work in the fields before breakfast. Without electricity the last meal of the day was at dusk.

There are various methods, but I practice TRE with a regular eating window of 10 a.m. to 6 p.m. I'll eat only during these eight hours, leaving sixteen hours fasting overnight. I'll have a glass of water in the morning, especially if I'm exercising. I even skip dinner sometimes and have my last snack around 4 p.m. (with plenty of fiber and good fats) or, if I have a busy morning, I may not get to breakfast until after 11 a.m. It took a bit of work to get to this level of flexibility, gradually pushing breakfast a bit later each week. You might need to start with simply eliminating any snacks after dinner. It's particularly important not to eat anything within three hours of bedtime.

After a few months of keeping to a strict routine I am more flexible now eating a bit earlier or later at weekends, if I'm traveling, or having a meal out with friends. But 10–6 is the baseline I return to on regular days. My blood sugar has dramatically stabilized such that I can even go to the gym or hike a six-mile trail before I've eaten anything which was previously impossible.

Other strategies may work for you such as "samurai-fasting" where you only have one meal a day, often in the evenings. Or maybe you eat normally five days a week but for two days you minimize your calories to 500 or less. As long as they are nutrient dense this can work. I have also found that occasionally going thirty-six hours without any calories at all (just drinking water), essentially skipping one whole daytime window, has a noticeable improvement on my energy and alertness.

These strategies are verified to improve insulin resistance but fasting also resets your immune system and is one of the recognized strategies for dealing with autoimmune conditions and Long Covid.[30]

Without repeating what has been covered in earlier chapters here's some other quick priorities for blood sugar improvement:

- *Stop eating sugar!* Pretty obvious but sugar does not just mean the white powder or even the various additives we discussed under Sweeteners in Chapter 4. Sugar is a broad term I've been using to refer to anything that is quickly converted to glucose in your body. This includes bread, pasta, cereal, rice, cookies, chips, tortillas and just about anything that comes in a packet. If you want to get scientific you could look up foods with a high or even medium glycemic index (avoid those!).

- *Build your muscles.* Maintaining muscle mass improves your metabolism and blood sugar control. Exercise daily making sure as many muscles are involved as possible.

- *Eat more fiber.* This is a natural and safe way to slow your stomach emptying down and keep you feeling full longer. Basically eat more plants which is where the fiber's at. Added bonus is that you'll be cultivating your good gut bacteria which will further improve your health.

- *Useful supplements* to combat deficiencies associated with diabetes include chromium, zinc, magnesium, vitamin C, vitamin D and coenzyme Q10. Berberine at 500mg three times a day has been shown to be as effective as the drug Metformin at improving HbA1C levels.[31]

Interestingly **Stevia** (whole leaf extract), the most popular natural sweetener, has been shown to lower blood sugar levels.[33] Raw organic **honey** has also been shown to be beneficial to diabetics.[34]

- *Herbal remedies* include cinnamon, garlic, and ginger. Curcumin (the active ingredient in turmeric) has been shown to be particularly effective at preventing prediabetics developing full diabetes.[32]

C is for Commercial

Cancer is a disease as old as recorded history. Yet with all of the developments in science and technology we claim the "cure" is still elusive. This is the marketing machine at its best. Billions of dollars have chased the mirage of a cure for cancer when in fact we are just fighting nature itself. There is no magic bullet for cancer. It is simply the pinnacle of a body out of balance. A broken metabolism and impaired immune system are two of the biggest drivers.[35]

An ever-growing list of carcinogens in our modern lives is certainly part of the problem as well. The only time meaningful drops in cancer rates have been seen was in the 1990s with the war on smoking in the US and UK. Smoking remains the key driver of cancer in many other countries. But as we covered in Chapter 4, we are exposed to a multitude of other toxins.

Cancer is characterized by mutating cells that can emerge anywhere in the body. Benign cancers form a mass but aren't life threatening. A malignancy develops when the mutating cells go unchecked by the body's own defense systems and destroy healthy tissue. Cancer is a particularly misleading label as mutant cells can pop up anywhere in the body at any time. Part of the immune system's job is to target them and clean them out. This is called *apoptosis*. Problems arise when this mechanism is compromised.

Conventional cancer treatment relies on the heavy artillery of surgery, chemotherapy, and radiation. These treatments are inherently toxic to healthy cells but the hope is they kill the cancerous cells faster than the damage done to the rest of you. Cancer treatment hasn't changed much in the last hundred years.

There was anticipated promise in the discovery of DNA and the developments in gene sequencing. Finding some genes that contributed to mutations and cancer growth while others that appeared to be tumor suppressors. Scientists then focused on drugs to target these genes with one or two small successes. But once again mother nature is far more complex and initiatives such as the Cancer Genome Atlas Project have documented around six million different mutations involved in various cancers, far too many for any number of wonder drugs to address.[36] Science finally confirms what we've known all along. Man will never be able to outsmart God in the way He has designed this world and humans to live in it.

We *do* have the cure for cancer. We've known it all along. First documented in the 1920s by Dr. Max Gerson, the focus is on activating the body's own natural ability to heal itself by treating the underlying cause of degenerative disease—toxicity and nutritional deficiencies. A high-nutrient diet free from toxins can give the body what it needs to fight cancer. Known today as Gerson Therapy,[37] it advocates for an entirely plant-based diet and high-quality supplements as well as coffee enemas to aid detoxification.

Essential oils with cancer-fighting properties include orange, particularly its d-limonene component (terpene), as well as myrrh and frankincense as mentioned in Chapter 2.

While such treatment is scoffed at by the conventional medical industry, the science is quietly catching up with lines of research now focusing on cancer as a metabolic disease. Doctors would generally agree that cancer feeds on glucose (sugar!) but then for some reason if you're undergoing chemotherapy and losing your appetite, they encourage you to eat whatever you want. In fact it is clear that cancer cells metabolize quite differently to healthy normal cells and they can therefore be "starved." They require glucose and glutamine (an amino acid found in animal products). Studies are showing that addressing metabolic issues with a ketogenic diet (high in good fats, low in carbohydrates, no sugar), and intermittent fasting as I described earlier, often leads to better cancer outcomes.[38] The connection to glutamine explains why removing animal products when given a cancer diagnosis is usually a good idea.

The difficulty with cancer though is that by the time you get a diagnosis your body is so far out of balance there may not be enough runway left for nature to work its magic. This is one of the reasons why *prevention* is always the way to go. Nip any underlying problems in the bud to generate health, as conventional cancer treatment will never improve your health. However, some conventional treatment may be needed to prolong your life to give natural healing time to work.

This ambiguity of cancer falling somewhere between an ongoing chronic condition and an acute life-threatening one means that I do not recommend you try and tackle it alone. You need a doctor to monitor your progress and make sure you are not flying too close to the sun. A word of warning though: unless you find an integrative or functional medicine doctor who specializes in cancer, you will be contending with almost exclusively "category 3" doctors rebuking you for not following their prescribed treatment and warning that you're gambling with your life. The money involved in cancer research and treatment is staggering. The proposed budget for the US National Cancer Institute for 2024 is US$7.8 billion.[39] Cancer drugs are some of the most lucrative products on the market, but as we saw in Chapter 2, on average only one out of four patients respond. Sadly, money drives the "standard of care."

There are countless ordinary people who have successfully gone against the establishment and treated their cancer naturally. But it requires a full commitment to serious lifestyle changes, everything we're talking about in this book. The upside is immense though, coming out the other side healthier and stronger with a new zeal for life. It is a very individual decision that only you can make. See Appendix D for further reading suggestions.

The Heart of the Matter

So that leaves just the last of the "big three" to touch on as we wrap up this chapter. Since I've already attacked the biggest sacred cow in medicine (presenting the case that vaccines usually do more harm than good), I might as well attack the other one—*your risk for heart disease has absolutely nothing to do with your cholesterol level or how much satu-rated fat you eat.*

Okay so leaving that hanging out there to sink in a little before we get to the real cause of heart disease, I want to clarify some labels. As you know, I hate labels, but in this case they help to explain what is really going on in the body. The term heart disease is not of any practical use though, as it covers hundreds of different conditions. The term I'm going to use is cardiovascular disease or CVD for short, though that is also problematic. Yes, your heart is involved as it's responsible for pumping the blood around your body. This blood transports oxygen, nutrition, and immune cells to every nook and cranny through the thousands of miles of arteries and veins we summarize as the vascular system. Pretty vital stuff. You do need to keep the pump in good working order. It's a muscle. Use it or lose it. Exercise, or at least energetic daily movement, is critical. But what we're going to focus on is more accurately called *atherosclerosis* which is a thickening and narrowing of the arteries in your body.

Interestingly, atherosclerosis doesn't occur in the veins. But it can occur in any arteries in your body. Those in your neck, leading to a stroke. Those running into your kidneys causing kidney damage. And blockages in the smaller capillaries (doctors call microvascular disease) lead to neuropathies (loss of feeling in hands and feet) and retinopa-thy—damage to the retina of the eyes. These are common complica-tions of diabetes which help us see how all chronic disease is intimately connected. The CVD label is more commonly reserved for blockages in the coronary arteries, those leading to the heart (apparently they look like a crown around the heart if you were to open up your chest and peer in). I'm going to use the CVD label more broadly.

You probably know that a heart attack is caused by a blood clot in the coronary artery. A stroke is caused by a blood clot in the neck or in the brain itself. What if I told you that the entire process of blood clotting is the main story in CVD and that if we just focus on understanding that process better, our risks for cardiovascular disease make a lot more sense.

Your blood vessels are lined with special cells called endothelial cells, a bit like tiles on your bathroom walls, forming the *endothelium*. These tiles are covered in a substance called *glycocalyx*. It's the same substance covering a fish's scales making the fish slippery when you try and pick it up. Glycocalyx has been found to include a range of proteins such as albumin (made in the liver, a shortage of which is a sign of liver disease— another connection), nitric oxide, and anticoagulants. In healthy blood vessels, the blood easily flows through but if the glycocalyx is damaged or thinned it exposes the endothelium. If those cells get damaged the body rushes in to repair them by forming a blood clot. That is just a temporary plug while new endothelial progenitor cells flood the area to replenish the endothelium. Glycocalyx can also then reform. The blood clot will be dissolved as this repair takes place. The problem arises if damage happens faster than the repair process. If the blood clot hasn't been fully eliminated, another blood clot can form on top of the vulnerable area and eventually you get what we call an atherosclerotic plaque.

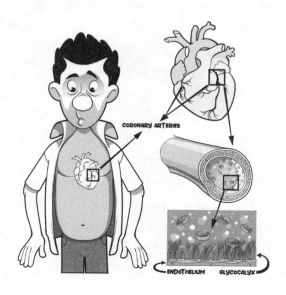

CORONARY ARTERIES

ENDOTHELIUM   GLYCOCALYX

So what causes the damage in the first place? This is the crux of the matter and where attention should be focused. The key culprits are:[40]

- **High blood sugar and diabetes**—the delicate glycocalyx layer is made up of proteins and complex sugars. Elevated blood sugar damages the glycocalyx, thinning it down considerably. This damage is why diabetics are prone to vascular damage in small blood vessels causing poor circulation, neuropathies, retinal damage (to the eyes) and kidney impairment.

> **Glucosamine + Chondroitin + MSM**
> It has been shown that the supplement Chondroitin sulfate and methylsulfo-nylmethane (MSM) usually mixed with glucosamine and typically taken for arthritis, is very helpful in repairing the glycocalyx and hence reduces the risk of heart disease considerably[41] I was very happy to hear this as I'm already taking this supplement to alleviate joint pain.[42]

- **Smoking and other airborne pollution**—here nanoparticles get into the bloodstream and damage the endothelium. It's the reason why chronic obstructive airway disease (COPD) is the number one risk factor for CVD.
- **Bacterial infections**—the most serious form of bacterial infection is sepsis, mentioned in Chapter 6 in our discussion of vitamin C. Bacteria excrete toxins that damage the endothelium and create blood clots all over the body. Survivors of sepsis often have organ damage or lose limbs due to the catastrophic loss of blood to the extremities. However, another source of bacterial infection is closely linked to CVD: Periodontal disease (infections in your gums) can lead to a low-grade leakage of bacteria and exotoxins into your bloodstream

on a daily basis. You may be blissfully unaware of this damage. It is why it is so important to take care of your dental health.

- **Vasculitis and other autoimmune conditions**—vasculitis is essentially the body attacking the endothelium cells as if they were a foreign invader. Kawasaki disease, a form of vasculitis most often seen in children, is a good example of how destructive it can be with heart attacks killing children as young as three with atherosclerosis plaques forming in weeks. Obviously a child this young has no other risk factors. Lupus and rheumatoid arthritis are the other big risk factors according to the data. But as mentioned earlier, one autoimmune label often gives rise to another once the body gets that out of balance.

- **Cocaine**—I don't think anyone needs convincing that snorting cocaine is bad for you but I wanted to include it to highlight the vast damage it does to the cardiovascular system without any other risk factors being required. It's common knowledge that cocaine can destroy the blood vessels in your nose through its acute vascular toxicity and vasoconstriction.[43] It also damages the endothelium and causes blood clots throughout your arterial system.[44]

- **Certain cancer drugs**—due to the fact that many tumors create their own blood supply to grow, drugs like Avastin were developed specifically to prevent the synthesis of endothelial progenitor cells. Avastin was nearly withdrawn from the market due to the massive increase in CVD risk.

- **Cortisol and steroids**—you might have heard of cortisol as the "stress hormone." It's also known as the "fight or flight" hormone. This is because it stimulates the synthesis and release of glucose from the liver to ensure you have the energy to address whatever emergency you are expecting. The problem is if you don't use up that energy you have extra glucose in your blood stream which is then stored as fat. But more importantly it makes you insulin resistant and heading for diabetes—see first bullet. Cortisol also suppresses nitric oxide needed by the glycocalyx and stimulates blood clotting factors in the liver (in case the emergency was a car accident). Prescription steroids like prednisone do much the same thing. The chemical structure of prednisone is almost identical to cortisol. You might know that when you're stressed you are more susceptible to infections. This suppression of the immune system is what prescription steroids are used for, most often in autoimmune disease.

Interestingly enough, clinical tools such as the QRISK[45] used in the UK would agree with this list. The obsession with cholesterol is a mixture of decades-old science (long before we knew of the glycocalyx) and the profits tied up in the billions of dollars spent on statin drugs each year.[46] Cholesterol is so critical to a body functioning well and in fact low cholesterol is more closely associated with increased mortality.[47]

What about high blood pressure you might ask? Well, yes, high blood pressure batters away at your endothelial cells, but it's also a symptom of the mechanisms above. As your arteries narrow the pressure increases. Insulin also raises your blood pressure, another reason to focus on blood sugar management. We don't have time to get into the importance of nitric oxide (NO) to keep your glycocalyx happy but note that being out in the sun triggers NO synthesis, which helps dilate your blood vessels lowering your blood pressure.

Also note how this discussion helps explains why Covid-19 created such a risk of cardiovascular problems. The virus targets the ACE2 receptor found on endothelial cells and in diabetic patients there is already damage to the glycocalyx exposing the endothelial cells. It's been common knowledge for years that a respiratory virus can damage endothelial cells.

Whew! We've covered a lot of ground in this chapter. The intention was to show you that all chronic disease is connected. Focusing on a particular disease label doesn't help you much beyond knowing where to prioritize your interventions. While you can be predisposed to something in particular, it is the intersection of your genetics, those of your microbiome, and all the day-to-day lifestyle factors that will dictate which symptoms show up first.

Just to see if you're paying attention though, there is one more major risk factor for chronic disease that we haven't yet addressed. We have done brief fly-bys, most recently in the discussion of cortisol's role in damage to arteries. Did you catch it? It's chronic emotional or psychological stress. It's clearly a major risk factor as shown in the science, but mental health is such a large topic I have dedicated a whole chapter to it next.

Points to Remember

1. The war on germs may be one of the main underlying drivers of chronic disease with the damage to the immune system from antibiotics and vaccinations.

2. Getting a diagnosis can be useful to help you prioritize interventions but be careful not to succumb to the label of having X disease.

3. The "big three" categories in terms of what is written on the death certificate is cardiovascular disease, cancer, and diabetes. All three are intimately linked to each other and to the fourth category we call autoimmune disease which actually has the most sufferers in highly developed countries like the US and UK.

4. There are more similarities than differences between all autoimmune conditions. If you have one you are at higher risk for another. Ditch the multiple conventional doctors and focus on healing your miraculous immune system.

5. Inflammation underlies every chronic disease. Symptoms are your body's cry for help.

6. Combating insulin resistance by maintaining metabolic flexibility and well managed blood sugar are key.

7. We've had the cure for cancer all along. Reduce toxicity and activate the body's own ability to heal itself through addressing nutritional deficiencies and insulin resistance.

8. What we call heart disease or cardiovascular disease is mostly a result of damage to the blood vessel lining and runaway blood clotting that is part of the repair mechanism. Saturated fat and LDL (known as bad cholesterol) is a red herring.

CHAPTER 8

Mind Your Body to Heal Your Brain

I am no stranger to mental health issues. My brain is always in sixth gear, thinking about several topics at once, finding the links between each, and thinking through the implications three steps down the road. I'm typically in the middle of at least four books in any given week. With a brain as active as mine, I've always had an intensity under the surface which tends to misfire in periods of extreme stress, hormonal cycles, or simply when I am not taking care of myself. I experienced childhood trauma, battled alcoholism, and lived with an active drug user, which created ongoing physical and emotional stress. I also have a son considered to be on the autism spectrum as well as an ex-husband (the active drug user) diagnosed with Asperger's as an adult. And don't get me started on menopause!

For some reason if we're dealing with symptoms such as distress, anxiety, poor memory, irritability, agitation, trouble focusing, hallucinations . . . the list goes on . . . we categorize it as a mental health problem. Mental as opposed to physical. But at the very center of these symptoms is the large organ between our ears we call our brain. We've already seen how our organs and biology are intimately connected to manifest symptoms that impact other parts of our body. The brain is no different.

Do you remember the vagus nerve? Take a quick look back to Chapter 1 to see the illustration of the vagus nerve and how it connects the brain to every other organ in the body. The common example I gave is how you feel butterflies in your stomach when you're nervous or excited.

Here's a few other examples of how our brains and bodies are connected:

- You can quite literally die of a broken heart. It's called Takotsubo syndrome and happens when extreme emotional upset leads to cardiac arrest even in the absence of any underlying cardiovascular disease.[1]
- Cancer risk and outcomes have been found to be based on your personality.[2]
- When you haven't had enough sleep, you are more susceptible to illness. This is separate from physical rest. You could stay up watching TV for two days with your body not moving. But only the total shutdown of your brainwaves into REM and non-REM sleep prevents ill health.[3]
- Emotional stress raises cortisol levels which causes insulin resistance and drives cardiovascular disease.
- Alzheimer's is starting to be called type 3 diabetes due to the connection with blood sugar metabolism and insulin resistance.[4]
- There is a proven link between psychological diagnoses like schizophrenia and the health of your gut microbiome.[5]

As we've discussed throughout this book, the body exhibits its wondrous complications through biology, chemistry, and physics, all of which can be measured to a degree. However, there is an additional realm we need to touch on as it's important to your overall health.

That is *the difference between our brains and our minds*. This fact is part of the reason psychiatry has taken such a terrible path away from the dominion of health.

Our mind is another key piece of evidence we have for the existence of God. How else do we explain consciousness separate to matter? I can close my eyes and imagine the coolest car, but it still doesn't exist. Even a brain scan can't see that car. Maybe it will show a few neurons lighting up but this is simply a conscious thought without any physical input. My brain exists; it just "is." Whereas when I think, I'm always thinking "about" something. I might worry that a stalker is following me down a dark street, however, the stalker may not exist and the situation can easily be proven false. But you cannot prove that thought was not in my brain. My conscious experience is subjective and difficult to explain from a purely physical perspective. Finally, while we can measure the size of my brain, and the extent of its electrical activity, we have a really hard time measuring features such as desires, sensations, emotions, or wills. These are the realm of the mind.[6]

Subjective Labels

I previously expressed my dislike of labels as not being particularly helpful to you as an individual striving for health. But at least in many of those chronic conditions there is a marker that can be measured. If your HbA1C is high you may be tagged with the label diabetic which gives you some insight into your blood sugar being poorly managed, enabling you to prioritize your interventions. You can then monitor your A1C level to see if improvement is being made. With cardiovascular disease you can see plaques or blockages on scans and in cancer you can see a tumor. Accurate measurement gets a little shakier in autoimmune conditions, but there tend to be markers in the blood and some physical manifestations.

Psychiatric conditions on the other hand are diagnosed based on almost purely subjective measures.

The DSM (Diagnostic and Statistical Manual of Mental Disorders) is the definitive reference text for psychiatrists, psychologists, and any health professionals working with mental illness. It is a collection of labels that doctors can (almost arbitrarily) place on individuals and open their prescription pads to particular pharmaceutical medications. These labels include diagnoses such as anxiety, depression, bipolar disorder, attention deficit hyperactivity disorder (ADHD), obsessive-compulsive disorder, schizophrenia, and even personality disorders. Every time the manual is updated, names and symptoms are revised or added. The latest version is the DSM-5, which included the most "diagnostic inflation" yet, as noted by Dr. Allen Frances in his book *Saving Normal*.[7] It controversially added "prolonged grief syndrome," for example, emphasizing that if your grief over the loss of a loved one lasts more than a year, you have a mental illness. There is much concern over the ties to Big Pharma pushing for more labels leading to more patients prescribed one of their products. We'll come back to this "disease-mongering" in a bit.

An interesting study in 2019 by researchers at the University of Liverpool raised alarm over the way psychiatric diagnoses are made based solely on *symptom clusters* which is scientifically meaningless.[8] For example, the study showed there are 24,000 possible combinations of symptoms for panic disorder. There are various diagnoses where two people could share the label but have zero symptoms in common. There is so much overlap in symptoms that two doctors could come to completely different diagnoses for the same patient.

Symptoms are the body's cry for help as we've seen time and again. But why is it that psychiatrists are the only medical professionals that do not look at the organ they treat, i.e. the brain? They tend to operate only on symptoms. Neurologists on the other hand will look at the brain but their sphere of influence tends to be limited to afflictions such as Alzheimer's or Parkinson's disease, noted as "neurological" conditions rather than "psychological." This further propagates the stigma of certain conditions as a moral failing of some kind rather than biological ill health.

So just as we can't really separate infectious disease from chronic disease, we can't separate psychological conditions and mental health from our biological (physical) health. Brain "inflammation" is the common denominator in everything from Parkinson's to multiple sclerosis, epilepsy, autism, Alzheimer's, schizophrenia, and even depression. Unlike the rest of the body though, our brains don't have any pain receptors so we can't feel brain inflammation. It only manifests itself as symptoms, some of which may be in the realm of emotions or behavior.

The final insult is that these labels tend to be lifelong "forever" diagnoses with the implication that they can only be controlled with medication. I used the example that a headache is most certainly not a deficiency in Tylenol or Advil. Similarly, depression is most definitely not a deficiency in Prozac or Paxil. There are many underlying causes of depression. Perhaps you've been eating too much gluten which has caused Hashimoto's thyroiditis. Maybe you have a poor diet and have been taking Prilosec for heartburn leading to a vitamin B_{12} deficiency. Perhaps you don't get in the sun much and have a vitamin D deficiency. Or you took an antibiotic for a urinary tract infection which decimated your microbiome leading to a depletion in brain-loving short-chain fatty acids (SCFAs). Perhaps you ate sushi and got a parasite. Or you hate fish and have an omega-3 deficiency. Maybe you have been eating too many donuts and are prediabetic. All of these situations can lead to symptoms diagnosed as depression.[9]

Another big secret of the medical industry is that once you start a psychoactive medication it changes your brain chemistry and is extremely difficult to discontinue.

Dangers of Medicating the Brain

One in every six adults in the US and the UK now takes psychiatric drugs.[10] Their use has skyrocketed in children as well. Many users are on drug cocktails with multiple drugs taken to address different individual symptoms or combat the side effects of the first. Some have been taking these drugs for decades.

When my son Ethan was diagnosed with Asperger's and ADHD at age five, the recommendation was medication. It was true that he couldn't sit still for five minutes; he had frequent tantrums, particularly if something was out of place or if he was being asked to leave an activity he was enjoying. He couldn't relate to others, had difficulty focusing on tasks like reading, had hearing and touch sensitivities, and his motor was always revved up full speed. The recommended medication (which I declined) was amphetamines. Known as stimulants in medical circles, you might have heard of Ritalin, Adderall, or Vyvanse. Interestingly (or sadly depending on how you look at it), the drug of choice for Ethan's dad (my ex-husband) was meth.

Methamphetamine, also called crystal meth, speed, and a host of other street names, is basically the same stuff. It increases the dopamine and noradrenaline in your brain, which helps with alertness and focus. Dopamine is a neurotransmitter released in your brain during pleasurable activities like eating delicious food or watching a funny movie. It's been said that a meth habit is harder to kick than a heroin habit.

Amphetamines have a long and sordid history with Big Pharma first peddling them after World War II to cure everything from nasal congestion to obesity, anxiety, and depression.[11] Meth abuse is a serious problem at this point. The United Nations estimates there are thirty-four million amphetamine users globally and another twenty million using "ecstasy-type" drugs (another stimulant).[12] Meth addiction destroys your health including weight loss, brain damage, organ damage, and severe tooth decay with users exhibiting irritability, paranoia, hyper activity, increased aggression, and depression to name a few.

Many amphetamine drugs were banned in the 1970s, particularly for weight loss, so Big Pharma had to find another market. They went after our kids rebranding their drugs for ADHD. While marketed as safer formulations, the side effects stated on the package inserts still include appetite loss, insomnia, irritability, hallucinations, depression, and even suicidal ideation. The documentary *Speed Demons: Killing for Attention*[13] is a sobering look at first how a former honors student with a respected legal career suddenly became a mass shooter. It then delves into various other well-known mass shootings and murders across the US including the incident of a ten-year-old deliberately suffocating an infant and a particularly sad case of a father taking the life of his young daughter. In all instances recent prescriptions of these ADHD or "focus" drugs were implicated.[14]

Now that Ethan is on a college campus in another state I have had to have serious conversations with him about the dangers of so-called "study-drugs" where students share their ADHD prescriptions to help cram for a test. With his genetic makeup, less-than-healthy food choices now creeping in, and a tendency to forget to take the supplements that revolutionized his life after his own diagnosis, his susceptibility is a constant concern.

Addiction in the Making?
Binge-Eating Disorder was newly added to the DSM at the protest of many seeing it as a new attempt by Big Pharma to recover their former obesity market. The recommended drug —Vyvanse—is also used for ADHD.

Even more sinister there is a new version of Vyvanse in a chewable form for kids under the age of five who may be unable to swallow pills!

The other powerful drug franchise in the mental health space is of course the antidepressant. A few years ago, Harvard Health estimated that around one in four women in their forties and fifties were taking antidepressants.[15] In total the CDC estimates thirty-six million are on the drugs in the US alone with 60 percent having been on them for more than two years.[16] The most common drugs you may have heard of include Prozac, Paxil, Lexapro, and Zoloft. They belong to a category known as Selective Serotonin Reuptake Inhibitors (SSRI) and are based on the heavily marketed theory that depression is due to a chemical imbalance of serotonin in the brain. The only problem is the science fails to show any connection between depression and abnormalities of serotonin in the brain.[17] When depressed, the amount of serotonin doesn't necessarily drop. It's a far more complex picture with serotonin involved in many processes in the body including mitochondrial energy production, metabolism of sugar and the workings of the immune system. Just like statins and the cholesterol myth, good marketing has been winning out. But while statins do what they claim to do (reduce your blood level of LDL even though that doesn't improve your health and likely makes it worse), the action of antidepressants is dubious. Drug trials show that antidepressants are barely distinguishable from a placebo especially with 30 percent of those not taking the drug advising improvement in their symptoms.[18] Big Pharma has an answer for the ineffectiveness of course. They came up with the label "treatment-resistant depression" suggesting you just add a second drug to the regimen. Ker-ching!

There is very little upside and immense downside from playing with your brain chemistry. In Chapter 2, I mentioned antidepressants being included in a range of drugs known to block the neurotransmitter acetylcholine which can lead to dementia. They are also connected with bone density loss,[19] and one study showed a 620 percent increase in the risk for breast cancer for women who had been on an antidepressant for four or more years as well as a range of other side effects.[20] The US Food and Drug Administration issued a warning against the use of antidepressants in children and adolescents due to the increased risk of suicide.[21] But the biggest problem with antidepressants even for short term use is their addictiveness. Big Pharma downplays the risk with yet another label "discontinuance syndrome" for the unpleasant side effects such as dizziness, nausea, headache, and brain zaps experienced when trying to stop taking them. Brain zaps are the term used to describe what feels like an electric current running through your head. Many patients are simply unable to quit the drugs because of this debilitating side-effect.

As you get into the more severe disorders such as schizophrenia and bipolar disorder you might think the benefits outweigh the harms of antipsychotic medications like Risperdal, Zyprexa, Seroquel, and Abilify. Of course every situation is different and without awareness of the potential root causes and drug-free interventions we'll be getting into for the rest of this chapter, it's understandable to see these drugs as a lifeline. But the side-effects are horrible. Tardive dyskinesia (TD) is the most common, a syndrome of involuntary movement that may not be reversible once the drugs are stopped. This class of drugs cause insulin resistance leading to severe weight gain, diabetes, and cardiovascular deterioration.[22] In one large study of children and young adults these drugs led to a concerning increased risk of unexpected death.[23]

The Big Pharma march goes on relentlessly though—the antipsychotic Rexulti was recently approved to treat agitation in Alzheimer's and dementia patients despite the clinical trial showing little benefit, and there is a fourfold increase in the risk of dying while on the medication.[24]

Getting to the Root Cause

Life is hard. You may be dealing with unreasonable deadlines at work, an abusive boss or partner, financial worries, job insecurity, racism, stressful living situation, physical ill health, death of a loved one, or relational difficulties. These stressors can affect your brain every bit as much as a so-called trauma. What can be considered **trauma** differs by individual depending on their level of resilience, but one definition of trauma is *feeling overwhelmed by events that are beyond your control.* Besides the stressors already mentioned we might add being involved in a natural disaster like an earthquake, suffering a violent attack or a car accident, being exposed to war or combat, physical or sexual abuse, witnessing someone being hurt or killed and a child feeling abandoned by a parent or caregiver. It never ceases to amaze me the harm one human being can inflict on another. Some people actually think the presence of evil in the world is evidence that God doesn't exist. I think the opposite for a host of reasons.[25] The way emotional trauma affects the brain long after the event has passed is one of them—the effect cannot be explained in the physical realm alone.[26]

There are two brain scans that can be used to look at that most complex and important organ which is involved in everything that you do and makes you who you are. A SPECT scan (single photon emission computed tomography) measures blood flow and activity while a QEEG (quantitative electroencephalogram) measures electrical activity. The scans of people who have suffered trauma are markedly different to healthy subjects.[27]

But tough life situations and even trauma don't have to lead to ill health. It's how you deal with adversity that can lead to healing and resilience. I know plenty

Potential Causes of Brain Ill Health

- Emotional trauma
- Head injury
- Toxic insults
- Medication side effects
- Microbiome imbalance
- Food sensitivities (e.g. gluten)
- Nutritional deficiencies
- Blood sugar mismanagement
- Thyroid disfunction
- Disordered immune system
- Social isolation
- Lack of sleep

of people walking around with joy and vitality having dealt with (or currently dealing with) one or more of the examples above.

Physical trauma to your brain through a **head injury** can be equally devastating or worse if left untreated. Your brain is far softer than you realize. Like soft tofu or egg whites. It floats in cerebrospinal fluid housed in your sharp bony skull. It is not only major concussions incurred in a car accident or an American football tackle that hurts your brain. A blow to the head, whiplash, falling out of bed, slipping in the shower, a bicycle crash or assault can injure your brain.

This summer when Ethan and I were visiting his soon-to-be college campus, we decided to take one of those electric scooter rides along the river walkway. They get up to twenty miles an hour and we were having a great time exploring the area. I got a bit carried away with my abilities and was distracted for a moment by some interesting bronze animal statues we passed. Next thing I knew I was hitting the ground with my face. These public scooters do not come with helmets and from a standing position you hit the ground pretty hard. I didn't lose consciousness, but I was stunned for a moment and ended up with a headache, not to mention abrasions across one side of my face. Fortunately I landed on a grassy area rather than the concrete but I realized I had injured my brain and I would need to rest it. I was extremely cautious for the next few days, didn't read or use screens much, drank tons of water and rested as much as possible.

There is plenty of research proving head injuries increase the risk of depression, anxiety, psychosis, suicide, drug and alcohol abuse, ADHD, learning problems, personality disorders, and dementia.[28, 29, 30, 31] Many people don't even remember the injury they may have sustained months or years ago which is why brain imaging is so important.

The brain can also be poisoned through various **toxins** both directly and indirectly. The most common toxins associated with mental health conditions are heavy metals (mercury in your dental fillings, aluminum in vaccines, lead in cosmetics), excessive alcohol, chemicals such as solvents, herbicides, pesticides, recreational drugs such as cigarettes/vaping/marijuana, plastics and additives in food, and mold. Bulletproof Coffee CEO Dave Asprey figured out his mental health problems were being caused by toxic mold and were resolved once he got help from a physician trained to deal with it. He went on to make the documentary *Moldy,* which I highly recommend.[32]

In another case, a couple had been going to marriage counseling for years and were heading for divorce with the husband "diagnosed" with mixed personality disorder plus narcissistic and antisocial features as well as intermittent explosive disorder. None of the treatments were working but in one last effort they went to see Dr. Daniel Amen,[33] an integrative neuropsychiatrist, who looked at a SPECT scan of the husband's brain. The scan revealed holes and a shriveled appearance indicating drug use or some other toxin. It then came to light that the husband worked in a furniture factory exposed to solvents all day which were quite literally dissolving his brain. Taking a six-month medical leave to focus on interventions and then returning to a position away from the solvents healed his brain and his marriage.

Other toxins may be impairing your immune system, disrupting your endocrine system, damaging your DNA, or restricting blood flow, all of which can indirectly harm the brain. Look back to the discussion on cell phones and technology in Chapter 4.

As we've already mentioned a few times, **medication** itself can cause toxic effects on the brain through various mechanisms. These may be medications prescribed for some other ailment or they may be psychiatric medications, covering up one symptom but leading to further brain ill health.[34] Chemotherapy is notoriously damaging to the brain with the resignation to "chemo-brain" almost inevitable. But the effects are more long-lasting than your oncologist may lead you to believe.[35] Drugs used in anesthesia also pose significant risk to your brain with cognitive decline after surgery all too common.[36] The risk may be greatest for those with compromised detoxification systems through an already overflowing toxic "bucket." One reason I'll be talking about training to get in good shape for any required surgery in Chapter 9.

An indirect effect of medication and other toxins is the damage to the **microbiome** in the gut. The gut-brain connection is never more powerful than when dealing with a mental health condition. The bacteria in your gut produce short-chain fatty acids (SCFAs) when they break down fiber and resistant starches in your food. SCFAs play a major role in the health of your gut and nervous system as well as immune function.[37] They are also intimately involved in the synthesis of various neurotransmitters like serotonin, gamma amino butyric acid (GABA), and brain-derived neurotrophic factor (BDNF). Back in Chapter 1 when we looked at the beauty of the vagus nerve, I explained its connection to the "Enteric Nervous System" which is embedded in the walls of your intestines and stomach and known as your "second brain" due to the estimated 500 million neurons it comprises. While the exact mechanisms of action are not entirely clear, disruption in SCFA production has been linked with a range of mental health disorders including schizophrenia, autism, depression, Alzheimer's, and Parkinson's.[38, 39]

The health of your gut, and then your brain, can also be affected by **food sensitivities**. MSG, artificial sweeteners, and other food additives are prime suspects in migraines and conditions with excitable behavior. Red food dye is particularly noticeable as a culprit in ADHD and unmanageable kids. Food dyes like red #40 don't only appear in candy, soda, and lollipops; it gets into flavored yogurts, fruit bars, ketchup, and packaged snacks like Cheetos and Doritos.

In Chapter 7, I explained the evil of gluten and its connection to autoimmune conditions. It is even more insidious in its connection to brain health as often there are no other symptoms other than the neurological one. Gluten has been linked to movement disorders, the degenerative condition ALS (also known as Lou Gehrig's disease), epilepsy, schizophrenia, bipolar disorder, autism, ADHD, and depression.[40] Dr. David Perlmutter, a renowned neurologist says "Gluten is this generation's tobacco."[41] I think sugar may win that prize but gluten is not far behind.

Beyond sensitivity to what you are eating, another major culprit of brain ill health is what you are not eating. **Nutritional deficiencies** are perhaps the biggest contributor to psychological and neurological conditions.

One of the most devastating disorders to encounter is schizophrenia and its various cousins like schizoaffective and bipolar disorders (which looks like schizophrenia in the manic phase). Conventional psychiatrists will admit it is not well controlled with medication and many patients are institutionalized with life expectancy cut short.

A hundred years ago there were many common and often fatal diseases that were due to a simple deficiency of an essential vitamin. Scurvy (vitamin C), beriberi (vitamin B_1 also known as thiamine), and rickets (vitamin D and/or calcium). Another of the classic deficiency diseases was pellagra which was found to be a deficiency of vitamin B_3 more usually known as niacin (scientifically it is known as nicotinic acid not to be confused with nicotine). One of the common symptoms of pellagra was psychosis. In fact schizophrenia was so similar to pellagra psychosis the only diagnostic criteria to distinguish the two back in the 1950s was whether or not the condition responded to standard niacin therapy.

Since the 1950s it has become clear that just as people have different food, sleep, or protein requirements, people need different amounts of critical vitamins to stay healthy. It has also been found that a prolonged deficiency of certain vitamins can lead to a more critical dependency.[42] While regular doses of niacin will avoid pellagra for example, some people, many schizophrenics, appear to have a more severe dependency and need much higher doses to recover and maintain their health. We'll come back to niacin later in the chapter.

Other common nutritional deficiencies that can lead to psychological and neurological disorders include omega-3s (DHA and EPA), zinc, the other B vitamins particularly vitamin B_6, B_9 (known more commonly as folate), and B_{12}. Also, vitamin D pops up here yet again particularly in depression.[43]

You could also have an excess of certain minerals like iron, calcium, or copper so be careful when starting a new supplement routine (as discussed in Chapter 2).

Even if you are not nutrient deficient and without specific sensitivities, you may simply be insulin resistant. Poor **blood sugar management** is another risk factor for brain ill health. It is well known that anxiety and depression are far higher in diabetics than in the general population.[44] We covered some of the risks of high blood sugar in Chapter 7, particularly the cardiovascular damage, but high blood sugar is also associated with brain impairment. We noted earlier how Alzheimer's is starting to be referred to as type 3 diabetes. SPECT scans show that high blood sugar causes decreased blood flow in the brain and a shrinking of the hippocampus (the central part of the brain responsible for emotions).[45] You may have used the term "hangry" to refer to someone who exhibits frustration or anger when their blood sugar has dropped too low maybe after skipping lunch. Addressing this one issue can greatly improve ongoing emotional stability.

My own blood sugar issues were hampered by **thyroid disfunction**. The thyroid is a small gland in your neck about the size of a walnut but yields incredible power. It can be thought of as your overall metabolic regulator affecting every cell in the body through the production of various hormones. The health of your thyroid affects just about every system in the body which is why the symptoms of an unhealthy thyroid are wide ranging and may go unnoticed initially or simply assigned to aging. It is well known that some of these symptoms can be mistaken for psychiatric illnesses.[46] In fact depression can sometimes be the first sign of an underlying thyroid problem. I was fortunate that my doctor had been monitoring my gradually deteriorating thyroid for years at my annual checkups. The problem was when he finally decided I needed treatment I didn't research the so-called "natural" solution he prescribed—a medication innocently called Nature-throid. I took it for sixty days before the brand was discontinued and the pharmacy wanted to contact my doctor for a refill replacement. I was busy and forgot to follow up until I started having cognitive problems, forgetting words, brain-fog, lethargy; it was pretty scary. Turns out I had been taking actual thyroid hormone (from a pig!) but this told my thyroid it didn't need to make the hormones itself anymore. (Remember the use-it-or-lose-it mantra?) I had then stopped cold turkey and my thyroid wasn't prepared to pick up the slack. I now manage my hypothyroid-ism through a completely natural approach that you can read about on EmmaTekstra.com.[47]

More serious thyroid disfunction has been connected with schizo-phrenia, bipolar disorder, borderline personality disorder and other psychiatric conditions.[48]

One of the underlying causes of hypothyroidism is Hashimoto's thyroiditis which is an autoimmune condition. We learned about the amazing complexity of the immune system in Chapter 6 and how malfunctions can lead to autoimmune conditions in Chapter 7. A **disordered immune system** that has to deal with ongoing infec-tions or autoimmunity is another potential root cause of psychiat-ric conditions. Having an autoimmune disease is associated with an increased risk for mood disorders, schizophrenia, bipolar disorder, ADHD, and dementia including Alzheimer's.[49] I explained that Lyme disease is a common underlying infection in autoimmune conditions and mentioned the similarities between the bacteria that causes Lyme and syphilis. Just as syphilis could cause psychiatric problems (dubbed neurosyphilis), there is plenty of evidence that Lyme and other tick-borne infections could be involved in many schizophrenia diagnoses.[50] Underlying dental infections from periodontal disease can get into the brain, and there are several lines of research now looking at how candida (*C. Albicans*), the fungal infection mentioned in Chapter 7, can lead to dementia and Alzheimer's.[51]

As is hopefully obvious by now there is rarely a single cause of any chronic condition, particularly a psychiatric one. Basic lifestyle factors always play a part. Not getting out in the sun or that elusive Open-Air Factor (OAF) discussed in Chapter 6 are more important than you might think. (Social isolation is also a significant issue we'll look at in Chapter 9.) But one lifestyle factor that could be a root cause all on its own is simply a **lack of restorative sleep**. Sleep and brain health are tightly linked and the issues go both ways. Research is clear on many psychiatric conditions leading to insomnia and sleep disorders.[52] But a chronic lack of sleep can itself lead to many of these conditions. Sleeping pills are *not* the answer; medications like Ambien, Lunesta, and Restoril are connected with a more than threefold increased risk of death and terrible side effects like memory issues, confusion, anxiety, depression, and addiction.[53]

Here's a few strategies to make sure you are prioritizing sleep:[54]

- Avoid ingesting anything that can interfere with sleep such as alcohol, caffeine, or certain medications.
- Finish eating and drinking two to three hours before bedtime and avoid anything overly spicy as your last meal.

- Practice good "sleep hygiene" such as a quiet dark bedroom, a little on the cool side. Avoid gadgets and screens near bedtime and choose relaxing activities like a bath or a good book.
- Aim for a consistent sleep schedule every day including weekends that puts you in your bed for seven to eight hours. Ideally follow a sunup/sundown schedule as much as possible and avoid late afternoon or evening naps.

Drug-free Solutions

It is truly amazing what a good night's sleep can do for the ailing brain. But I am not naive enough to think that will solve a mental health condition all by itself. Dr. Amen says in his books "Get your brain right and your mind will follow." Your mind may be kicking and screaming not wanting to comply so we must address both aspects.

Believe me, I know how powerful thoughts are and how disabling they can be. The mind can often sabotage the attempts to get the brain well. For those who have not been afflicted with the worst of these disorders it can be difficult to relate and know what to do. When I am in what I call "the blackness" I have an almost out-of-body experience knowing that I am unwell but struggling to do anything about it. One time I wrote down what it felt like.

The best way I can describe it is walking along beside a large hydroelectric dam on a beautiful sunny day. Everything seems normal then suddenly there's an explosion, the dam has a huge hole and water, a tsunami, is pouring toward me. I know I need to run to avoid the blackness, but my legs don't work. I'm drowning. My brain doesn't work. My body doesn't function. (I often go twenty-four hours or more without eating.) I can see land in the far distance but see no way to get there. I've learned not to struggle; I can sink faster if I do. I wait patiently for a lifeline. I might pray during this time. (I'm usually isolated and immobile at this point.) The thoughts entering my head are extremely negative. Eventually a lifeline is thrown to me, usually in the form of another human being, maybe a kind word, the encouragement to go for a walk; maybe it's a need from one of my kids, my spouse, a friend. It may be a small glimmer in the distance and take Herculean strength for me to go toward that light, but I leap. I am disoriented and skittish, nervous and unsure, but using patience, knowing small steps toward the light is all that is required initially, I can gradually get more secure footing. I have to be mindful of my physical needs as well—drink lots of water, eat something healthy, get some fresh air, get out in nature. I mustn't rush back to "normality," and I mustn't worry

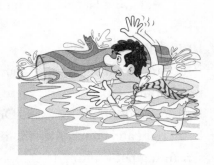

about what I am not doing or what I missed but know that this is where God has me right now for whatever purpose that is.

Your experience or that of a loved one you are concerned about is likely different but I want to emphasize you have options to alleviate symptoms and even reverse the condition, particularly any label assigned. Artificially messing with your brain chemistry should be an absolute last resort. Remember the power of the human body to heal itself? It just needs to be given the right support.

I'm going to touch on a range of solutions to try once you have identified some of your root causes (there are usually more than one) and addressed health issues and solutions mentioned elsewhere in the book. I'll start with some additional interventions you can easily try yourself and then move on to the more specialized options. Make sure you avoid the inclination to find the one thing that will address the particular condition you're dealing with. There is no "pill for every ill." If you find yourself thinking that way then reread Chapter 3 about everything that goes into your bucket of health or illness. *The health of your mind and brain cannot be separated from the health of your body.*

By now you know me well enough that I'm going to start with what you're eating. Like every health issue **nutrition** has the biggest impact. If you refuse to give up the ultra-processed toxic food-like substances that you ingest then I cannot help you. But once you get focused on nourishing your body and your brain as outlined in Chapter 5, you'll be on the right path. Within this context and depending on the severity of your psychological and neurological symptoms compared to other physiologies, you

> **Drug-free Interventions for Mental Health**
> - Nutrition
> - Supplements
> - Exercise
> - Meditation/mindfulness
> - Tapping
> - Breath work
> - Neurofeedback
> - EMDR
> - Stellate Ganglion Block
> - Vagus Nerve Stimulation
> - HBOT

may want to focus on getting good fats into your body. Hopefully you were convinced in Chapter 7 that your cholesterol level and saturated fat are not responsible for heart disease. But LDL (which is actually low-density lipoprotein and not "bad cholesterol") is critical to optimal brain function as it transports cholesterol to your neurons where it is used for various functions such as making neurotransmitters and hormones like testosterone.[55] (You don't find that little nugget in the marketing of statins—*it'll also lower your testosterone but don't worry we have another pill for when your sex life goes downhill!*) Higher dietary fat and cholesterol levels are associated with a lower risk of dementia.[56] The risk of Parkinson's is greatest for those with the lowest levels of cholesterol.[57] Consequently the ketogenic diet (originally developed as a treatment for epilepsy) has been found to be effective for Parkinson's, Alzheimer's, ALS, and autism.

Your brain needs fat, but it also needs short-chain fatty acids like acetate and butyrate which are produced when the good bacteria in your gut digests fiber in plants. So this should be your other focus, getting more plants into your meals. You could also explore the world of fermented (or cultured) foods such as sauerkraut, kefir, certain pickles, and certain yogurts. Most big-brand commercial versions have very little beneficial bacteria, so you may need to supplement with a probiotic. See Resources for recommendations.

Beyond probiotics, the **supplements** you'll want to take will depend on your particular nutritional deficiencies. It was actually Linus Pauling who coined the term *Orthomolecular Psychiatry* and explained that the brain is more sensitive to deficiencies in vital nutrients than any other organ in the body.[58] Much of what we have covered previously on various supplements will be relevant but here's a few more honorable mentions:

- **Niacin (vitamin B₃)** has an incredible history of efficacy against not only mental health disorders but arthritis, cardiovascular disease, kidney disease, autoimmune conditions and more. That's because after vitamin C and D this is probably the most critical substance our body needs as it is converted to nicotinamide adenine dinucleotide (NAD) which is involved in over 400 gene functions.[59] Like vitamin C it is important to keep a consistent blood saturation so it should be taken regularly throughout the day, a minimum of three times a day with meals. Some people are put off by the "flushing" that may occur, a reddening of the skin due to a temporary dilation of blood vessels. It is not harmful and seems to have beneficial properties. Just like the bowel flushing with vitamin C can indicate appropriate saturation, if you don't flush with regular niacin it's an indication you have not yet reached your needed level. Niacin is a very cheap nutrient

and can be easily obtained in various strengths. I wouldn't
waste your money with special formulations that may be less
effective. Niacinamide may be preferred as it can avoid the
flush but doesn't have all the same benefits. You might start
with 100–500mg three times a day (that would be a total of
300–1,500mg) and go up from there if there is no effect. There
is no upper limit so you can't do yourself harm by overdosing.
You may feel a little nauseous and even vomit if you keep
going up but just rachet back at that point. Case studies of
severe schizophrenics have told of doses as high as 50,000mg
a day before they became entirely normal. A more common
formula for psychosis-type conditions (believed to be a form
of pellagra) is 1,000mg three to four times a day taken with a
similar amount of vitamin C.[60]

- **EmpowerPlus Ultimate** is a proprietary formula that includes
thirty-six vitamins, minerals, and amino acids specifically
formulated for optimal brain health using a technique that
makes them ultra-absorbable in one single capsule a day. I
listed the manufacturer Truehope in the Resources section. I
wouldn't normally call out a single formula with such a strong
recommendation, but this product is superior to anything else
I have seen in the market. Part of the problem with mental
illness is that maintaining consistent routines is especially
difficult. So, rather than several bottles and doses to keep
track of, EmpowerPlus is a single capsule with a formula
that has been clinically tested with a large range of mental
health conditions. Their website provides details. I have no
financial ties to this company, but EmpowerPlus changed the
trajectory of my son Ethan's life. Now he's in college though I
have to keep reminding him they only work if you take them,
preferably daily!

- **Melatonin** is an intriguing compound that most people connect with regulating your sleep cycle but it is so much more.[61] It is made by the pineal gland in the brain but also elsewhere in the body and it can be found in mostly plant foods. Darkness triggers melatonin production while light (natural or artificial) reduces it. It is thought the artificial light from electronics is interfering in melatonin production which impacts not only sleep but other mechanisms in the body. Supplementing with small doses such as 1mg taken thirty-minutes before bed can be helpful for short periods.

- **L-Theanine** is an amino acid found mainly in tea plants like green tea. It has a wide variety of healthful properties including antioxidant and anti-inflammatory actions but it is also neuroprotective.[62] It helps focus the brain and decrease anxiety. Ethan took L-theanine in supplement form from age five. I'm British so don't need any encouragement to have an extra cup of tea!

- **Ginkgo biloba** is a potent antioxidant herb that has been shown to increase cerebral blood flow, memory and alleviate neuropsychiatric symptoms.[63, 64] It can also help relieve leg cramps and other muscle pain as well as vertigo and tinnitus (ringing in the ears). Its potency can result in interactions with pharmaceuticals so if you

> **Tinnitus is a sign of brain ill health and not an ear problem**
> Constant ringing in the ears is a more common ailment than you might think. Often attributed to too many years of listening to loud music, the more recent phenomenon of Bluetooth and other electronics in the ears is likely to increase occurrence. But just like you see with your brain rather than your eyeball (Chapter 1) you also hear with your brain. Improve tinnitus by improving your brain health.

are on any medications discuss its use with your doctor first. Take 60mg twice a day.

- **St John's Wort** (scientific name Hypericum perforatum) is another powerful herb that has been used since ancient times to ward off evil spirits. Now it is known as the most powerful natural antidepressant available with far fewer side-effects than medications.[65] However, it can also interfere with pharmaceuticals (such as birth control pills) so make sure to discuss with your doctor if you are going to try it.
- Other herbs like **Gotu Kola** you can grow and eat like spinach for cognitive and neurological health. I take it as a tincture in water. **Ashwagandha** is good for anxiety and stress, **Huperzine A** enhances memory and is good for dementia, **skullcap** quiets the monkey mind and helps with tremors, ticks, and restless leg syndrome. **Kapikachu** is naturally rich in L-dopa (the precursor to dopamine) and is a known natural therapy for Parkinson's.

Supplements are not a panacea, but **exercise** may be! Countless studies have shown how physical movement can improve symptoms of depression, anxiety, and decrease overall stress.[66] Going for a simple walk can immediately lift your mood. Physical activity has been shown to spur the generation of new brain cells, increase the size of your hippocampus and increase blood flow to the brain.[67] Exercise has also been shown to increase the neurotransmitter BDNF mentioned earlier in connection with the microbiome—the gut-brain-body connection at its best. It's long been known that children perform better at school when participating in regular exercise due to the demonstrated "structural and functional changes in the brain determining enormous benefit on both cognitive functioning and wellbeing."[68] We'll come back to movement again in Chapter 9 as critical to overall healthy aging.

Besides going for a walk there are various modalities you can practice in the moment to improve your psychological wellbeing. Three examples I'd encourage you to look into are:

- Meditation
- Tapping (also known as Emotional Freedom Technique, EFT)
- Breath work (particularly Wim Hof methods)

Meditation and other mindfulness practices are considered mainstream these days with many techniques available and apps to assist. They are not just for the new-age business crowd but have clearly been shown to impart a range of mental and physical health improvements.[69] I've struggled to connect with traditional forms of meditation but find **tapping** to be incredible. It uses nine specific meridian points in the body that you gently tap on while you focus on the negative emotion or symptom, addressing the root cause. It sends a calming signal to the brain which has been proven in studies to decrease cortisol levels and bring the body back into balance. It is particularly powerful for addressing past trauma and managing pain.[70]

You may be familiar with **breathing techniques** to address panic disorders, but the way you breathe can have a profound impact on your overall health.[71] A special deep breathing exercise is the first pillar in the *Wim Hof Method* to "realize your full potential."[72] Wim Hof developed his approach after his wife committed suicide, leaving him with four young children to raise. The other pillars are Cold Therapy (iced-water immersion) and Commitment (focus and dedication to practicing the skills). Perhaps considered a little extreme, but trauma and grief are extreme in their profound impact on the body. A radical intervention is often required.

This brings us to the more intensive interventions providing drug-free relief and healing. I can personally testify to the results of

Neurofeedback. It is a noninvasive, interactive treatment that allows patients to retrain their brains to enhance emotional, behavioral, and cognitive health.[73] Ethan underwent neurofeedback at least twice a week for over a year when he was seven to eight years old. The improvements month to month were striking with the initial treatments focused on his hyperactivity and focus, with later treatments dedicated to his social skills.

If your problems can be traced back to emotional trauma then a psychotherapy technique known as **EMDR** (eye movement desensitization and reprocessing) can show incredible improvements in just a handful of sessions.[74] It involves a specially trained practitioner walking you through the trauma while prompting rapid eye movement from side to side or other bilateral stimulation. Believed to be connected to the mechanisms occurring in REM sleep, it enables the patient to positively process the memory and disturbing feelings, transforming the brain at a physical and emotional level. I have had a single session myself on one specific traumatic event and can testify to the almost miraculous difference in how I perceive the event now.

When engaging in psychotherapy of any kind you need to make sure there is an intentionality to the process with a start and expected end. You should select a therapist who has experience with your particular issues and is trained in the relevant techniques. *Internal Family Systems* (*IFS*) is a therapeutic model based on the understanding that our minds are more like members of a family who have different personalities, levels of maturity, excitability, and pain. These "versions" of ourselves can actually split off and take over sometimes in detrimental ways. Understanding these parts and learning to govern them appropriately can be extremely beneficial. There is of course a spiritual aspect to our minds which is best incorporated into our thinking. I'll touch on this in Chapter 9 and Appendix C.

Before we leave psychotherapy, though, I do want to touch on the controversial use of psychedelic drugs to assist in the treatment of trauma and other serious mental health conditions. Here I'm mainly talking about *psilocybin* (the active compound in magic mushrooms) and *MDMA* (more commonly known by its street name ecstasy). Psychedelics such as peyote from a cactus and its active ingredient mescaline have been used for thousands of years for medicinal purposes. They are said to connect the user with the spirit world so we can understand there is something out there greater than ourselves which can be very healing. The misuse of psychedelic compounds has led to their distrust and legislation against them. However, there is plenty of science supporting their careful and controlled temporary use within a medical context.[75] Only you can decide if this approach makes sense for you, but ensure you do your homework and incorporate drug-free solutions as well for best results.

Ratcheting up to a more invasive procedure, a **Stellate Ganglion Block** (SGB) involves injecting an anesthetic into the stellate ganglion which is a bundle of nerves in the cervical spinal column in your neck. The procedure is actually very simple and only takes a few minutes, but the effects have been known to last months or years. Originally developed for pain (similar to an epidural in childbirth) its uses have been expanding since the 1990s to include alleviation of PTSD (also known as PTSI for post-traumatic-stress injury to emphasize its ability to heal).[76]

Vagus nerve stimulation (VNS) is another procedure that addresses the brain-body connection. Here a small device is put under the skin right below the collarbone. It sends mild, continuous impulses to the vagus nerve leading up to the brain.[77] It has been shown to be particularly effective for unresponsive depression and PTSD.[78] As discussed in Chapter 1, keeping the vagus nerve functioning well is critical to many aspects of our overall health. Fortunately, there are many ways to stimulate the vagus nerve yourself including exercise, mindfulness activities like yoga, tai chi, deep breathing, sunlight, and infrared saunas.[79]

The last sample intervention we'll touch on is probably the most expensive but also has some of the most amazing results. **HBOT** (hyperbaric oxygen therapy) is useful for a range of health issues as it essentially saturates the body with concentrated oxygen in a special pressurized container. The increased pressure allows the lungs to take in more oxygen than usual which can then be shuttled around the body to promote healing. If your root cause includes a brain injury, stroke, or intoxication like carbon monoxide poisoning then HBOT should be your first line of defense.[80, 81] It should also be considered for fibromyalgia, chronic infections like Lyme disease, chronic burns and diabetic ulcers, multiple sclerosis, inflammatory bowel disease, and other hard-to-treat conditions.[82, 83, 84]

HBOT is an example of a single intervention with multiple modes of action. This is because it is based on a natural premise—the body needs oxygen to heal. The closer your intervention is to the natural order of the human body and how it was created to operate, the greater your chance of recovery instead of symptom management.

Hopefully you can see now why psychological health is dependent on brain health which is dependent on the health of your overall body. Mental health takes looking after both your brain and your mind. There is no reason you need to lose your faculties when you age. So what is the secret to aging well? Let's conclude with a stroll into our twilight years next.

Points to Remember

1. At the center of all psychological conditions is the brain. It is intimately connected to the rest of your body. Brain health drives mental health.

2. Your mind is separate from your brain however. Successful interventions must address both aspects of the human experience.

3. Psychiatric diagnoses are based entirely on symptom clusters enabling a doctor to place a subjective label on you with the implication of a life-long condition that only medication can treat.

4. There are major downsides of medicating the brain and very little upside. Addiction and further ill health are just the start.

5. It is important to get to the root cause(s) of mental ill health which may be toxins, nutritional deficiencies, or related to other health conditions or lifestyle factors. But it could also be emotional or physical head trauma. It is a good idea to get a brain scan for clues.

6. There are a wide range of drug-free solutions for mental health conditions. Many of which you can try yourself without a professional involved. For more serious conditions there are professionals who specialize in techniques and procedures that aim to cure rather than manage.

CHAPTER 9

Aging Well

We're all aging. From the moment we are born to the day we take our last breath. Aging is advertised as leading to ill health and being undesirable and un-useful when in fact it should be the best time of your life. So what does it mean to "age well"? Getting to retirement with no major disabilities? Reducing the time between life-limiting disability and death?

As we learned from our blue zones discussion, life expectancy in the United States is low compared to other developed countries. What's more it's actually been falling since 2014 while other countries have been improving. But average life expectancy doesn't come close to the whole picture of good health. Many people are fit and healthy into their nineties (even in the US). Remember Dan Buettner's Blue Zones? These centenarians are not in old-age homes confined to their bed or wheelchairs.

Mary MacIsaac was the oldest living person in Canada when she died in 2006 at age 112. She had cross-country skied until she was 110 and was photographed playing the piano with her great-grandson just before she died.[1] In 2008 Kaku Yamanaka died in Japan at age 113. Jean Calment of France holds the record as the longest-living person, dying in 1997 at age 122.[2] She was born in 1875; think about that for a moment! These supercentenarians (living beyond their 110th birthday) have something else in common—nearly all people who live this long are free of major disease when they die including dementia. Doesn't it sound like the best way to go—peacefully in your sleep, living life to the maximum right up to the end?

It is entirely possible. Dr. James Fries explained why back in 1980 with his groundbreaking paper on aging and what he referred to as the compression of morbidity.[3] Dr. Fries planted the earliest seeds for the concept we now call functional medicine; the idea to focus on functionality rather than disability or disease (commonly referred to as morbidity). How can we delay the onset of any disease or symptoms as far as possible and compress the time living with it before reaching the age of natural death. The paper discussed the idea that from a young age our organs build up a reserve beyond what is needed for average everyday living. So our heart, lungs, liver, kidneys etc. can go into overdrive when faced with a temporary threat such as a toxin, injury, illness, or other stressor. Once the emergency is over, organ function returns to its baseline level with no adverse consequences. However, as we age, we use up this organ reserve, all the more if we keep subjecting our organs to stressors. The rate at which we use up organ reserve determines our biological age which is independent of our chronological age. I know people in their fifties who are biologically more like seventy. They look and feel old. I also know people who are chronologically in their seventies who have the biology of a fifty-year-old.

Nowadays we have far more computing power available, which has led to digital models called **epigenetic aging clocks**. These aging clocks are used to quantify the aging process and measure biological age based on a myriad of inputs including everything we've been discussing in this book looking at DNA methylation patterns at the cellular level. There's nothing particularly revolutionary being discovered in terms of what lifestyle factors cause faster biological aging. However, if you are into self-measurement and want to pick only the factor that will slow your aging the most to work on perhaps it's for you.[4]

The most recent study published in April 2023 proves that our organs actually age at different rates.[5] The study showed how the age of certain organs has the biggest impact on your overall biological age. For example, if your heart is biologically younger than your chronological age then your other organs will share this youthful vitality.[6] Using a tool called the "organ age clock" the researchers were able to profile sixteen chronic diseases where advanced biological aging of the primary organ involved in the disease extended to multiple systems. In other words, they proved what we covered all the way back in Chapter 1, that the body is an intricate system that operates as one. It's an interesting paper with helpful illustrations and diagrams but I can't help thinking yet again that it's just science catching up to God's amazing design.

Now you may be surprised that this data junkie is not interested in finding out my biological age and monitoring its progress over the years to come. I'd rather just live my life with intentionality and purpose, being mindful of my bucket and striving for more positive than negative influences. But another theory of aging is worth touching on as a simpler way to think about aging day-to-day.

The term **"inflammaging"** was introduced in a 2018 article published in *Nature*.[7] Researchers determined that what really accelerates the degenerative process is inflammation. While some inflammation is a normal, healthy feature of our immune response, it is only supposed to last for a short duration. We mentioned in Chapter 7 that ongoing inflammation underlies nearly all chronic disease. You can think of it as anything negative going into your bucket is likely to increase inflammation. Whereas the positives are going to turn inflammation off or at least dial it down.

Getting Older

Aging itself is not a risk factor for disease. A doctor may put you in a higher risk bracket due to your chronological age but that is due to these concepts of organ reserve and inflammaging both of which can be managed with a healthy lifestyle.

Let's take the fallacy of **osteoporosis** and osteopenia as an example. These were defined as diseases by the WHO in the 1990s based on the arbitrary formula of a bone mineral density that is 2.5 and 1 standard deviation (respectively) below the peak bone mass of an average young adult (age thirty) as measured by an X-ray device known as DEXA (dual-energy-x-ray absorptiometry).[8] A standard deviation is simply a statistical term used to quantify the extent of the spread of results for the group as a whole. For a start if you take a group of thirty-year-olds they are all going to have very different bone densities based on genetics and lifestyle. But then it is a huge leap to assume an eighty-year-old should have the same bone density as a thirty-year-old. Completely illogical.

To further understand the myth, bone density as measured by DEXA does not equal bone strength (or risk of fracture). In fact, in some cases, having a higher bone density can indicate the bone is actually weaker. Glass for example has a high density but is extremely brittle and shatters easily. Wood on the other hand, which is closer in nature to human bone than glass or stone, is far less dense. But wood is extremely strong compared to glass or even stone, capable of bending and stretching with the same forces that impact bone in a fall.

A 2015 scientific review published in the *Journal of Internal Medicine* entitled "Osteoporosis: The Emperor Has No Clothes" noted:

Current prevention strategies for low-trauma fractures amongst older persons depend on the notions that fractures are mainly caused by osteoporosis (pathophysiology), that patients at high

risk can be identified (screening) and that the risk is amenable
to bone-targeted pharmacotherapy (treatment). However, all these
three notions can be disputed.[9]

It goes on to explain and prove each of the three problems.

Another great marketing campaign by Big Pharma has made drugs like Fosamax, Boniva, and Prolia a multibillion-dollar cash cow despite growing evidence their side effects are far worse than the so-called disease, including gastrointestinal problems such as esophageal cancer,[10] atrial fibrillation,[11] bone pain and even a greater risk for fractures.[12] It's also been a boon for the DEXA machine makers as Big Pharma campaigned to make them standard equipment in doctor's offices.

Maintaining your bone strength and avoiding falls is almost entirely in your control. Chronic inflammation is the biggest driver of weakened bones as bone renewal is inhibited. If you address the chronic diseases covered in Chapter 7 you will be improving your bone health at the same time. Natural remedies focused on your bones include optimizing your vitamin D, K2, and magnesium levels, consuming plenty of protein and healthy fats, and including strength training in your weekly routine. We'll come back to the importance of exercise for balance and bone strength a bit later.

Another condition associated mainly with aging is **hearing loss**. It is the third most common chronic health issue in the US; nearly twice the number of people who have diabetes or cancer are afflicted with hearing loss. But a recent study found that up to 18 percent of teenagers have measurable hearing loss most likely due to loud music, earbuds, and headphones.[13] People of all ages need to protect their ears from loud music, garden equipment, electric tools, and even kitchen appliances. Unsurprisingly it has been found that your intake of nutrients impacts your risk of hearing loss.[14] An increase in carotenoids, vitamins A, C, E, and folate (vitamin B_9) which are found in fruits and vegetables, as well as omega-3 fatty acids found in fish,[15] can all improve the situation.[16] Hearing loss isn't inevitable. In addition to improving blood flow to the inner ear, nutrients also protect the brain which is actually doing most of the hearing.

For me I fall into the trap of thinking I'm just getting older when I feel a twinge of **pain** doing activities that never used to bother me. A sore knee here, a backache there. It's estimated that over 50 million people in the US alone deal with chronic pain every day.[17] 17 million of them with high-impact pain that limits their life or work activities on most days. Knees, hips, and backs are most common. More complex conditions such as fibromyalgia, shingles, diabetes-caused neuropathies, arthritis, and other musculoskeletal conditions abound. It's estimated that the healthcare industry in the US spends nearly one trillion dollars a year on treating pain.[18] This is more than heart disease, cancer, and diabetes combined. But for all their high-tech treatments such as spinal surgery, nerve blocks, and ablations, not to mention all the drugs, there is very little to show for their services. Chronic pain is notoriously difficult to treat, but that's because conventional doctors don't focus on the root cause. Age has nothing to do with it.

Healthcare Keeps You Sick

Doctors can be mystified with chronic pain as often there is no physiological reason for it. People with amputated limbs complain of pain in their missing leg. The cause of a headache or migraine can involve a range of underlying factors that do not involve the head. Pain is a symptom. It is very real. But the complexity of the human body requires a holistic approach to gain health, and freedom from pain is often a side-effect. In contrast the healthcare industry focuses on expensive overtreatment and the pursuit of quick fixes.

One of the worst interventions the healthcare industry peddles is the painkiller drugs. Who wouldn't want a quick fix from pain but at what cost? We covered the problems with the over-the-counter painkillers in Chapter 2 as well as Vioxx and Celebrex that are particularly damaging to the heart. But I would be remiss if I didn't spend a little time on the opioid crisis, which has its roots almost entirely at the feet of Big Pharma.[19] In 2022 it was reported that 96,700 deaths in the US annually are due to drug overdoses and of these 72 percent are due to opioids.[20] The most common prescription drugs involved in opioid overdoses is oxycodone (such as OxyContin) and hydrocodone (such as Vicodin). These are powerful drugs chemically similar to heroin making physiological addiction very difficult to avoid. If you think it couldn't happen to you just watch the award-winning miniseries *Dopesick* which chronicles the rise of OxyContin and the criminal marketing schemes of its manufacturer Purdue Pharmaceuticals. The dramatization tells the story of a doctor, based on a real person, who was initially resistant to the marketing claims that an opioid drug had a minimal risk of addiction. He finally agreed to try it on a patient who was happy to be out of pain, which increased the doctor's confidence it was truly a miracle drug. But ultimately, he loses countless patients to overdoses. He even succumbs to junkie behavior himself after a car accident left him in pain and the hospital pushed it on him.

The events depicted in *Dopesick* including the monetary payments to doctors who prescribe opioids and the associated criminal case won against Purdue Pharmaceuticals are now a matter of public record. But doctors and dentists continue to prescribe these potent drugs as a first line of defense when in fact they should be the last resort. The dentist tried to hand me Vicodin when my then sixteen-year-old son had his wisdom teeth taken out. I declined. One day of ibuprofen, ice, and rest was all he needed. The number of teenagers who get prescribed these opioids for sports injuries and minor accidents is truly horrifying.

Don't be misled to assume your pain is worthy of such an intervention. There are many alternative approaches for pain such as:

- Improving your nutrition to avoid inflammatory foods (gluten, anything processed) and increase whole fruits and vegetables plus incorporating anti-inflammatory spices like turmeric and ginger.
- Adding supplements such as high-dose niacin (proven to reverse arthritis), as well as glucosamine (usually formulated together with chondroitin sulfate and methylsulfonylmethane, MSM).
- Movement is perhaps the last thing you want to do when in pain but this is one example proving the body is not a machine—it actually improves functionality the more you use it.
- Acupuncture as discussed in Chapter 2. Heat and light therapies can also be helpful. I'm quick to get in a hot bath if my back is a little sore.
- Tapping or other types of meditation or mindfulness practices.
- Essential oils like peppermint and frankincense if the pain is localized.

Your doctor may also be quick to recommend **surgery**. I had once suffered greatly from Thoracic Outlet Syndrome which is essentially trapped nerves in my shoulder causing radiating pain down my arm and numbness in my fingers. The orthopedic specialist wanted to surgically remove my top rib to solve the problem! I elected for physical therapy, which returned me to full mobility in a few months. I am aware of the weakness now and make sure to do the appropriate exercises to avoid a relapse, happily retaining a full complement of ribs.

Surgery is truly amazing in what it can accomplish within the human body. As a teenager I wanted to become a brain surgeon often watching live surgeries on TV. Surgery has been compared to playing God. But just because something *can* be done doesn't mean it *should* be done. Anytime you take a knife to open up the human body you are exposing yourself to all sorts of risks.

My friend Marie has been suffering from MS as long as I've known her, coupled with anxiety and a huge range of food allergies. We got chatting recently about when all these symptoms started as she is finally ready to address them holistically. It was around the time of some "routine" gallbladder surgery twenty years ago that also corrected a hernia left over from a C-section. In sharing the story, she suddenly remembered she had a body scan years later which revealed a titanium staple had been left inside her. She had completely forgotten but acknowledged that's when all her symptoms first started.

Aside from human error, a sample of risks you might encounter whatever type of surgery you are having include shock, hemorrhage, wound infection, deep vein thrombosis, pulmonary complications, urinary retention and reaction to the anesthesia or other drugs received.[21] No surgery should be considered routine. Gallbladders for example are amongst a handful of organs that doctors are taught to be "unessential," i.e., that we can live without them. But God's design is perfect. You will never return to optimal health if a well-designed organ has been removed. Alternative approaches should always be attempted first. The doctor recommending surgery may not the best candidate to discuss another path though. You should seek an opinion from a professional with a different tool kit.

A recent study published in the *International Journal of Surgery* notes:

Globally, a staggering 310 million major surgeries are performed each year; around 40 to 50 million in USA and 20 million in Europe. It is estimated that 1–4% of these patients will die, up

to 15% will have serious postoperative morbidity, and 5–15%
will be readmitted within 30 days. An annual global mortality of
around 8 million patients places major surgery comparable with
the leading causes of death from cardiovascular disease and stroke,
cancer and injury.[22]

In Chapter 1, I noted that pharmaceutical drugs are actually the third leading cause of death in the US and Europe. A 2013 study estimated that at least 210,000 deaths a year were attributable to preventable harm in hospitals with the authors suggesting the number may be nearer 400,000 and that nonlethal serious preventable harm is ten to twenty times as much.[23]

Okay, but what if you had an accident and surgery is truly unavoidable? Once you've asked your surgeon a whole bunch of questions, try and give yourself at least three months to prepare. You should view surgery as hard on your body as if you had to run a marathon. You would train right? Here's a few tips to train for surgery:

- If overweight, you should shed a few pounds.
- Kick any bad habits like smoking or drinking excessive alcohol.
- Boost your nutrition by focusing on whole foods; skip the junk.
- Review all medications and supplements that might interfere with the surgery or healing process.
- Increase your exercise routine. At a minimum walk every day.
- Communicate your wishes such as decisions for before and after surgery including necessity of pain medications.
- Gather social support to improve your mental health as we'll get into later in the chapter.

Outpatient procedures are also quick to be pushed on unsuspecting patients without a discussion of the pros/cons and alternatives. I mentioned my high genetic risk for breast cancer in Chapter 3. It might surprise you to know I haven't had a mammogram in over ten years. The risks just outweigh the benefits. Firstly, they involve a high dose of ionizing radiation which is known to harm human tissue. Women who have had radiation treatment for breast cancer for example are known to be at an increased risk of heart disease and lung cancer in the decades after their treatment.[24] Plus there is a significant risk of overdiagnosis. Mammography picks up a wide variety of abnormalities

Top 10 questions to ask your surgeon
1. Is surgery the only option for my condition?
2. What are the potential risks and complications?
3. What is the success rate?
4. What is the expected recovery time?
5. What are the short and long-term effects on my overall health?
6. What are the anesthesia options and risks of each?
7. How many of these exact surgeries have you performed?
8. Are there any lifestyle modifications I should make before the surgery?
9. What can I expect in terms of pain management afterward?
10. What are the costs involved?

many of which may be slow growing or resolve if left alone such as the "stage zero" breast cancer known as *ductal carcinoma in situ* (DCIS). In the present paradigm once cancer is detected it is treated with surgery, chemo, and radiation. A systematic review published in the *British Medical Journal* in 2009 estimated that the overdiagnosis rate was 52 precent such that one in three women offered screenings ended up overdiagnosed.[25]

There are far better alternatives such as thermography (using infrared cameras) that is noninvasive, doesn't even touch the body, and poses zero risk. There are also various blood tests available such as the ONCOblot test used to detect the presence of a protein ENOX2 shed from cancer cells[26] and the RGCC test which looks for Circulating Tumor Cells (CTCs) in the blood.[27] Plus good old-fashioned body awareness and self-exams. There is plenty of online information and even apps that can guide you through a monthly self-check.

Colonoscopies are another major income source for doctors. As I'm over fifty I was encouraged to get one. I've declined. I have no symptoms, eat a healthy diet full of fruits and vegetables, avoid toxins as much as possible; it makes no sense. They are not without risks with far more incidents of accidental perforation, major bleeding and infection than you might have assumed.[28] Only you can decide if they make sense for you but do your research. There are other options to monitor your colon health such as a fecal immunochemical test, fecal occult blood test or a stool DNA test.[29] The RGCC blood test previously mentioned looks for any type of cancer. Your doctor may argue that a colonoscopy enables polyps to be removed immediately but not every polyp turns into cancer. When those that do are present, a particular microbial signature can be found in the colon; an imbalance of bad microbes instead of good. Stool samples that look closely at your microbiome may well be the best indication of cancer risk.[30] Protecting your microbiome is probably the best solution to reduce the risk of colon cancer. Improving your nutrition and avoiding pharmaceuticals is key.

Other tests you may not need and could cause more harm than good include:

- Bone Density Scans[31]
- Coronary Calcium Scans[32]
- CT Scans and MRIs (which deliver seventy times more radiation than an X-ray)[33]

- Prostate Cancer screening[34]
- PAP Smears[35, 36]

The Choosing Wisely[37] initiative provides resources to help you have a conversation with your doctor about which tests and procedures make sense, and which do not.

Back to pharmaceuticals, the mainstay of conventional healthcare, a new study published in October 2023 has revealed that Americans now spend about half their lives on **prescription drugs**.[38] The analysis estimated that a baby boy born in 2019 would on average spend 48 percent of his life on medications, whereas a girl born in 2019 would do the same for 60 percent of her life. A man who was already aged twenty-five in 2019 will spend 59 percent of his remaining years on medications whereas a twenty-five-year-old woman will spend a whopping 71 percent of her remaining years taking drugs. This has got seriously out of hand and benefits no one but the giant medical industrial complex sponsored by Big Pharma. It's certainly not making anyone any healthier.

Polypharmacy (taking multiple drugs) is a particular problem in your later years. Amongst sixty-five-year-olds in the study nearly half were taking five or more drugs. The researchers noted polypharmacy raises the risks of negative effects including falls, cognitive impairment, hospitalization, lower quality of life, and mortality.

For the small percentage of you not already taking a prescription drug, Big Pharma is trying to

The Anti-Aging Maestro
NAD (we met in Chapter 8) is a crucial molecule in the body playing a role in energy metabolism, DNA repair, and the process of cell survival or death.[39] Niacin (vitamin B_3) and its various forms is a precursor to NAD. While it's found in many whole foods, it's a critical vitamin to supplement. Mary MacIsaac (the oldest Canadian) was said to have credited her long life with her daily niacin regimen.[40]

entice you with a new category called *Senolytics* using the marketing machine to focus on aging itself as if it were a disease. Senolytic drugs act by destroying senescent cells—damaged cells that have stopped dividing but refuse to die. It's been demonstrated that clearance of these cells can treat age-related diseases and expand health spans.[41] What you may not hear is that nature has provided natural senolytics such as quercetin and fisetin which are found in—surprise surprise—fruits and vegetables.[42] Are you getting it yet?

Habits Build Health

Seriously though, don't just stop taking any pharmaceuticals your doctor has prescribed. You'll need to get yourself healthy first now that you are armed with an understanding of what it takes, and then work with your doctor to gradually wean yourself off the chemicals. But before you throw away the pillboxes, how about you fill them up with supplements? My husband and sons are really bad at remembering to take their vitamins. So many people complain supplements aren't helping them but when you dig into their habits they only take them occasionally.

Habits are the small decisions we make and actions we take throughout the day. They are repeated behaviors that you do almost automatically. Your habits make you who you are. Habits build character but habits can also build health.

I am a creature of habit. I am by nature very disciplined and focused. But your personality may lend itself to a more fly-by-the-seat-of-your-pants approach. I welcome that. I love a weekend or vacation where I can totally switch off and just see how it goes. If you're in peak health and it's working for you, fantastic. But if you are serious about improving your health, you need to set goals and make a plan. You need to get intentional about your health and form healthier habits.

While eating well is obviously critical, your growling stomach will tell you to eat, so the focus may be exchanging a bad habit (like an afternoon doughnut) for a good habit (like some nuts). Adequate hydration, however, definitely takes some work. By the time you feel thirsty you are way past dehydrated. You need to intentionally force yourself to drink water throughout the day and monitor how much you are drinking until you build up to an automatic habit.

Supplements can be thought of as expendable or only needed when you feel a cold coming on. But they are a vital health habit particularly as we age. If you already take medications, it might be a simple switch. But if you don't currently have to remember to consume some-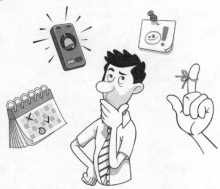thing that didn't arrive on your plate it can be quite an effort to remember. The first few weeks may take sticky notes, reminders on your electronic calendar, or texts from your spouse or best friend. But it is possible to incorporate a complete supplement routine no matter how busy your life is. I travel extensively and it has become part of my pretravel ritual to count out the number of each supplement I need for the trip. I use the little plastic pill bags so I don't have to take all the bottles with me. (As you might imagine, I take several different supplements!) It's become second nature to throw down a few supplements with every meal. Remember we're trying to re-create what you could have naturally gotten from food as your body expects, so take supplements with a meal as much as you can.

With our modern lives full of toxins and stresses that humans didn't have to deal with a hundred years ago, it is nearly impossible to meet your nutrient needs through food alone. Ditch the medicines and embrace daily supplementation. Your body will thank you for it.

Another critical habit in the nutrition vein is food planning. If you're not a planner—get over it! This one is nonnegotiable. At a macro level you need to plan the next few days' meals and snacks for when you go grocery shopping. You might resolve to try one new vegetable a week. (Review Chapter 5.) At a more micro level you need to figure out what exactly you are going to eat. Appendix A provides some food hacks to get you started as I know this is a tough one for many people. You also need to get in the habit of carrying snacks wherever you go so you don't get caught out in a food desert. If you're going to be away from home for an extended period plan where you will find healthy food.

Sleep habits are often the hardest to change. Do you stay up watching TV or scrolling through social media long into the night? My son Ethan hates to go to bed before 3 a.m. He'll force himself to do it if he has an early class the next day, but it doesn't come naturally to him. I'm at the other end of the spectrum. I love sleep. 10 p.m. is my strict bedtime, sometimes earlier. If I'm up past 10 p.m. perhaps on a night out with friends, it feels really weird. Resolving to get to bed at a reasonable hour and give yourself the opportunity for seven to eight hours of sleep is vital to age well. It is a myth that you need less sleep as you age. (We looked at the necessity of sleep in Chapter 3 and again in Chapter 8 regarding brain health.) It's not that your *need* for sleep reduces as you age but that your ability to physiologically *generate* sleep is impaired usually due to underlying ill health.[43]

Sleep Patterns

The natural rhythms of sleep may become more obvious as we age. Sleep cycles of REM/NREM sleep last around 90mins; you need 5 of them per night. If you briefly awaken in between to head to the bathroom it's okay. Keep to low night-lights and make sure the path to the bathroom is clear to avoid falls. As long as you slip back to sleep quickly there is no need for interventions.

Part of the complexity of sleep involves your circadian rhythm. Every living thing has an internal biological clock that is influenced by light and dark and regulates your internal processes. When it gets dark in the evening your body creates the hormone melatonin which helps you fall asleep. When the sun comes up you wake up and feel more alert. If your circadian rhythm is out of whack due to poor habits, it can take some time to get it back on track. Regulating your mealtimes can help, perhaps delaying breakfast for a couple of hours and avoiding snacks after dinner. For those night owls you'd benefit from some early morning sun a few days in a row. As you age you may find yourself unable to stay awake past 8 p.m. and then wide awake at 3 a.m. In this case you can work on getting afternoon sunlight to reset your circadian clock.

While we're on the subject of the outdoors, even if the sun isn't out, being outside for ten to twenty minutes a day would be another great habit to get into. We discussed the benefits of nature in Chapter 1. "Biophilia" is the scientific word coined in the 1980s to explain the inherent human need to interact with nature. Our increasingly indoor lifestyles contribute to a slew of negative health effects. Many scientific studies have confirmed the wide-ranging health benefits of being outdoors although the hypotheses for why differ.[44] I take the theological stance that it is due to the connection it brings us to something bigger than ourselves. Taking a moment to appreciate the wonders of nature can show us that we are simply creatures within the great cosmos created by God.

It doesn't matter the activity, whether you are just sitting on your front door step watching the world go by or sitting in the back of a pickup truck gazing at the constellations on a clear night. If you really can't get outside, then hopefully you can spend some time by an open window. Indoor houseplants can bring some of the same benefits.

I am a huge nature-lover and go outside every opportunity I get.

You heard about my camping escapades. But every day I find some excuse to get outside for a while. If it's not gardening or filling up my various bird feeders, I'll just steal ten minutes to take my breakfast or lunch outside. If I have some extended reading to do, I'll plop myself in a chair outside to do it. Almost any afternoon, if I have been house-bound in my office, I'll take a fifteen-minute walk around the block. Rain or shine. Of course exercising outside is combining two of the most healthy habits.

There is a mountain of evidence that your level of physical activity has a direct impact on your longevity whatever your genetic predisposition.[45] In Chapter 3 we looked at why Your Body Needs to Move and in Chapter 8 the specific effects on the brain and mental health. But exercise doesn't need to feel like a chore. It's one of the more enjoyable new habits you can add to turn your health around. Combining it with nature gives immediate positive input whether it's a walk, a bicycle ride, a round of golf, some pickleball. Indoor pursuits also count such as yoga, dancing, various exercise apps and videos, and of course any type of gym. Strength training or resistance training which aims to build muscle or at least prevent muscle loss has been further shown to improve longevity and should be included at least twice a week.[46] Stretching and balance exercises that can be done at home with nothing but a chair can be easily added to the mix. These solutions are far cheaper and healthier than resorting to osteoporosis drugs in the hopes of avoiding fractures as we age. (A word of caution to the gym rats who think exercise gives them license to eat anything—no amount of exercise will outrun a poor diet from a health perspective.) How much formal exercise you need to add will depend on your current fitness level, how much general movement you already incorporate into your week and any physical limitations. You need to move rigorously every day. But you can start slow and build up your intensity and activities gradually.

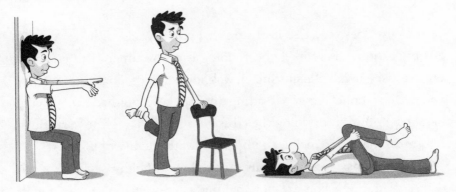

Some of this habit-creation may seem daunting to you right now, especially the idea of adding more formal exercise. So you may want to focus on *micro-habits*. Adding a new major habit can be overwhelming and prone to failure. A micro-habit is taking a first tiny step that is too small to fail. Mastering a micro-habit can then lead to another and another . . . and before long you have transformed your life. Here's some examples:

- Park your car at the far side of the parking lot to give yourself a bit of a walk to your destination.
- Drink a glass of plain water as soon as you wake up.
- Pick a reasonable bedtime and stick to it.
- Leave your phone outside the bedroom at night. Buy an old-fashioned alarm clock if necessary.
- Buy some nuts and carry them with you for snacks.
- Leave your sneakers by the front door to remind yourself to go for a walk.
- Buy a good-quality multivitamin and add it to your breakfast routine.

Intentional Hobbies

One of the best habits you can develop to keep your brain sharp is to learn something new every day. Just as your body needs exercising, your brain does too. Use it or lose it. Even if you're still working in a complex job, you've likely been doing it a long time. The best mental exercises involve acquiring new knowledge or doing an activity you haven't done before. Reading (particularly nonfiction), playing Scrabble or bridge, or doing the crossword puzzle is a great start. But a hobby can have a tremendous impact on your quality of life.

Hobbies may seem frivolous, but the word hobby can be used to describe anything you are not making a living at. It can be a calling, provide deeper meaning to your life, and contribute to your identity. Hobbies are a fantastic stress reliever although in some cases you may have to remind yourself it is only a hobby and perfection is not required. A hobby takes you away from the mundane pressures of life, it declutters your brain allowing you a certain amount of mindfulness as you focus on the activity at hand. Certain hobbies can engage your creative side and stretch your imagination. Learning a new language or a musical instrument has been shown to make visible improvements in your brain structure and health.[47, 48] A hobby compels you to take some time for yourself, particularly important for caregivers and those juggling work and family commitments seven days a week. The best thing about hobbies is that anyone can start a new hobby at any age or time of life. Plus, you don't have to be very good at it. Just find some enjoyment and curiosity.

I have many activities I find enjoyable but never actually classed them as hobbies. I think because I dip in and out of different activities throughout the seasons of my life. I love to take photos of nature, landscapes, animals, birds, and interesting plants. I have a decent camera but have never taken a class. I love to garden, grow vegetables, and entice unusual birds to my backyard. For a couple of years, I raised wild monarch butterflies. I grew plenty of milkweed, their plant of choice, when I heard there was a shortage along their migration route which includes Southern California. Eggs were laid and caterpillars

showed up. I wanted to keep them
safe so I bought some net enclosures
and would move them under the
protection once they got to a certain
size. My son Ethan was really into
bugs at the time, and it was a fun

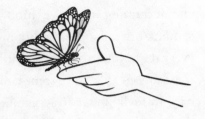

hobby we enjoyed together. It was fascinating to watch them eventually spin their chrysalis and ultimately emerge as beautiful butterflies.
One summer I released over forty into the wild which gave me a sense
of contributing to their survival. Monarchs are incredible creatures as
they migrate thousands of miles away, but their offspring somehow
know to come back to the same place where their parent was born.[49]
The unfathomable magic of DNA.

For a different season when my younger son was into trains, I built
him an N-gauge model train set working on tiny little buildings and
painting cars and bridges one Christmas holiday. I had a whole town
designed and spent hours laying out the roads, bridges, and farm areas.
I joked that I was going to become a hermit one day and have a whole
basement with a giant layout (I still might!). I love to golf, hike, ski, go
off-roading, go-karting, Jet-Skiing. . . . I wouldn't call any of them a
hobby as I don't get to do them all that often, but they keep me active
and engaged when I get the chance. Food may be considered a hobby
for me. I spend a lot of time researching new recipes and ideas. I've
recently got into culturing my own goat milk yogurt with a particularly high probiotic count. It's been interesting learning to ferment at
exactly the right temperature for thirty-six hours to ensure a successful
batch.

The other two activities I've taken up most recently and possibly
most intentionally are kickboxing and pickleball. I chose kickboxing because I needed to add some more intense exercise to my weekly
routine. I go three times a week to a gym where there are nine stations of

circuit training you move through for three and a half minutes each. The
stations use all sorts of equipment and the full-body exercises change
every day. Not only does it work out my body, it works out my brain as
the exercises all involve some combination of punches and kicks and you
have to really focus to remember the order and keep good form. I am
thoroughly spent when I leave there. I was put to shame one day recently
when I fell into the trap of thinking for a moment I may be too old for
kickboxing. Just then a lady showed up who proudly told me she was
turning eighty-one that week and had only started three months earlier!

As a former tennis player I gave in to pickleball for purely social
reasons but I now really love it.[50] The very best hobbies are those you
can do with other people.

Wired for Connection

Just as humans are divinely wired to interact with nature, we are
divinely wired to interact with each other. Glance back to Chapter 3
and the description of Italian Hospitality in the Pennsylvania town of
Roseto. It turned out the only distinguishing feature of Roseto that
insulated its inhabitants from the typical health issues seen in the surrounding area was their social connections.

Science continues to quantify and try to make sense of the phenom-
ena with study after study showing how powerful social connections
are to good health and how detrimental loneliness is.[51] One study even
showed loneliness is associated with an increased risk of Parkinson's
disease.[52] Shockingly (or not!) Big Pharma is even trying to make loneliness a clinical finding amenable to pharmaceutical intervention.[53]
Loneliness isn't necessarily simply the absence of friends but it does
have a relatively straightforward solution. The cure for loneliness is an
emotional connection to others. People we can be ourselves with, share
our innermost feelings with and walk through the ups and downs
of life with. A close friendship like this needs to have mutual trust,

acceptance and care or concern. God talks about friendship all over the Bible. In fact He commands it.[54] Not surprising since He designed us that way.

If you're looking for more secular proof, the classic bestselling book *Bowling Alone* provides an interesting perspective on what the author calls Social Capital.[56] The chapter connecting the quality of your social relationships to health and happiness goes into much depth with over twenty scientific references associating strong social connections with better physical and mental health. Originally published in the year 2000, it speculated on the future impact of the internet. Rereleased and updated in 2020, there is a new chapter which addresses the rise of social media. While not all bad it does acknowledge that mental and physical health is positively impacted by in-person interactions, but the effect is negated with online interactions. Social media usage is correlated with poorer psychological wellbeing.[57]

> **Physical Touch is a Powerful Anti-inflammatory**
>
> Touching is far more than a sign of love or friendship. Physical contact has been proven to be vital for optimal health. Even basic touch such as a hug, pat-on-the-back or hand-holding has been shown to trigger a cascade of biochemical reactions that boost immunity, lower blood pressure and reduce stress.[55] So hug your friends and don't let the flame die out on intimate touch with your spouse.

It has definitely gotten harder to make real friends in our modern world. We might mistake likes and connections on social media as friendships, but only in-person connections optimize the health benefits of interaction. With the new social constructs of "your truth" and "my truth," verbalizing your beliefs with openness and sincerity can be considered a microaggression. So it's best to invest in friendships that encourage a positive sharing of ideas and are mutually respectful and curious. You also want to surround yourself with

people who are investing in their health like you are and inspire you
to healthy habits.

Even if you have a spouse or other family members living with
you it's important to cultivate close friendships outside of that circle. If
your spouse has died and you're living alone it is even more important
to commit to spending regular time each week connecting with others.

If you recently retired from work and found that was where
all your connections happened, perhaps you could look into a new
hobby or something you used to enjoy before work took up too
much time.

If you're not sure where to start you could look into volunteering
opportunities. Even beyond the social connection, altruism has been
scientifically shown to reduce markers of inflammation throughout
the body.[58] People more inclined toward helping others tend to experience a healthier and longer lifespan. Grandparents who spend time
looking after their grandchildren live longer on average than grandparents who do not.[59] There are limits though. If you're a long-term
caregiver to a loved one you are more likely to become socially isolated
and experience worse health yourself.[60] Balance is key.

I am not a naturally social person, preferring the company of my
husband, my kids, and one or two particularly close friends. But I have
reaped many rewards from actively participating in my church and
the small-groups we belong to there. (A small-group being a sub-con-
gregation usually connected to a specific ministry.) For example, the
last few years we have been in a group of twelve to fourteen married
couples at our church who all have older teenagers or college-age kids
and are therefore facing the same challenges we are. We have a meal
together every Wednesday and discuss the previous weekend's sermon
or a special marriage-related teaching delivered within our sub-minis-
try. We dig into what we have learned and how to apply it to our lives,
while getting to know each other at a much deeper level in the process.

Most of us didn't know each other before being thrown together into this particular small group. We have extremely varied backgrounds and day-to-day lives. But after just four or five years together, we have become closer than family. We share holidays and leisure time together and maintain an online group text of prayer requests and day-to-day connections. There isn't a single need in this group that goes unanswered by everyone else. Sickness, a spouse deployed overseas, car troubles, house repairs, moving assistance . . . the commonality being the understanding that God has a purpose for our lives.

Spiritual Purpose

Aristotle was the first to propose the concept of eudaimonia: "eu" from the Greek for good, and "daimon" translated as spirit. It describes the notion that living in accordance with one's spirit, which we can take to mean character and virtue, leads to a good life. More recently, psychologists categorize human happiness into two types. Hedonistic happiness or wellbeing is attained from the pursuit of pleasure, avoiding pain, and experiencing sensory enjoyment. The second is referred to as eudaimonic wellbeing, which is achieved through the pursuit of purpose and one's intrinsic value. Interestingly a scientific study showed that these two types of happiness result in very distinct patterns of gene expression.[61] People with high levels of hedonistic wellbeing showed an increase in inflammation and decreased gene expression related to antiviral responses for example. People with high levels of eudaimonic wellbeing exhibited the opposite, with enhanced anti-inflammatory and antiviral capabilities.

Leisure time is not all it's cracked up to be. Yes, it's important to have a hobby but endless rounds of golf or Pilates classes does not necessarily lead to optimal aging. There is actually no concept of retirement in the Bible. Retirement is a relatively new invention. In Dan Buettner's blue zones, many of the men were found tending their sheep, inspecting their vineyards and one centenarian was still riding his horse wrangling cattle. I started out my career thirty years ago as a pensions actuary consulting on pension plan design and financing. At that time, it was common to have a retirement age of sixty but this has gradually been pushed out to sixty-five or older. Some careers like airline pilots have mandatory retirement ages. Just because you may not have the energy or physical/mental capability to continue in your original career, doesn't mean you should give up on being useful. It's important to have a purpose when you get up in the morning.

Purpose has been defined as "the psychological tendency to derive meaning from life's experiences and to possess a sense of intentionality and goal directedness that guides behaviour."[62] Purposeful people have been found to have less cognitive decline, better sleep, live longer and be healthier overall.

Mindset is critical. An interesting experiment was first carried out by a Harvard psychologist in 1979 and has been recently repeated in Italy.[63] They are known as the counterclockwise experiments. In each case a number of older adults (aged seventy-five plus) were sent on a one-week retreat and were told to pretend at all times that it was twenty years earlier. The organizers went to great lengths to re-create the time period with appropriate media, reading material, and activities. They were even given ID-cards with their younger selves on them. They underwent extensive testing before and after the retreat of their physical strength, posture, vision, cognition, and memory. In every measure they had substantially improved. Even their before-and-after photos demonstrated the enormous effect mindset has on our bodies and our health.

The importance of our mindset demonstrates that we are more than our biology, even more than our social connections. We are all spiritual beings created with divine purpose. Having a sense of purpose but also a moral code to live by provides a robust foundation from which to thrive. Whether it's a connection to God, to the planet, to past generations or to future generations, our lives matter. Without some sort of spiritual connection many people can experience emptiness which can lead to mental and physical ill health. Throughout life but particularly in your twilight years, it's important to maintain a positive mindset and engage in spiritual practices such as prayer, worship and being of service. These habits are so powerful they can override factors contributing to poor health and ensure that you truly enjoy this best time of your life.

Points to Remember

1. Aging itself is not a risk factor for disease.
2. The typically advertised aging problems such as bone health and hearing loss are better managed with healthy natural interventions under your control.
3. Explore the many alternative remedies for pain. Turn to medication only as a last resort.
4. Surgery should never be considered routine. It is inherently fraught with risk. Always get a second opinion from a professional with a different toolbox.
5. Use conventional healthcare sparingly. Even outpatient procedures like mammograms and colonoscopies have risks. Explore alternatives.
6. Build healthy habits like taking supplements, a robust sleep schedule, getting outdoors daily, and an exercise routine. Start small with micro-habits for quick wins.
7. Learning something new keeps your brain sharp. A hobby can be a useful strategy to expand your horizons.
8. Social connections are critical to your mental and physical health. Cultivate close friendships.
9. Figure out your purpose and live it every day.

EPILOGUE

What Now?

I didn't write this book as an interesting discourse on the state of the medical industry. I wrote it to empower you to take matters into your own hands and follow your own health journey. I don't know you or your current state of health so I'm not going to prescribe what your next steps should be. But I am going to provide a few thoughts to help you navigate what to do with your newfound enlightenment.

There was a concern I was covering too much information for one book. In fact, I had planned an additional chapter on the implications for raising healthy kids but that proved to be a step too far. (Check out EmmaTekstra.com for updates on a whole separate book!) The fact is the human body is infinitely more complex than we are led to believe. Factor X almost never causes disease Y. Scurvy, beriberi, and pellagra are three exceptions (caused by an acute ongoing deficiency of vitamins C, B_1 and B_3 respectively). Even particular viruses or bacteria cannot cause the disease they are associated with unless the body's defenses fail in some way. Conventional medical thinking hasn't improved much over the last hundred years with this one-for-one association. At the same time, conventional medicine discounts that simple nutrients are critical to a body functionally well. No man-made pharmaceutical full of chemical additives will replace you supporting your body to function as God intended. Surgery should be considered a last resort.

The body is not just the sum of its physical parts though. Rather than "health" which I find a little limiting, I like to think of the goal as *human flourishing* and it looks something like this:

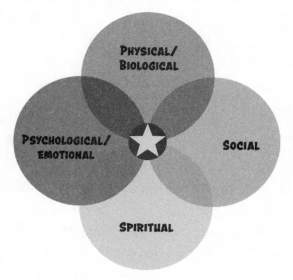

All four parts are required, and all four parts intersect and affect each other. A weakness in one area will affect all others:

- Your biological or physical health includes your metabolic health, your immune system, your musculoskeletal integrity, your nutrient and molecular balance.
- Your psychological or emotional health includes your temperament, your resilience or coping skills, your attitude, perceptions, and outlook.
- Your social health includes your connections and relationships at work, school, family and in the community.
- Your spiritual health includes your purpose, your belief in something bigger than yourself, your reason for being.

You may choose to focus on one of these circles to improve first. Perhaps the one you see as your biggest weakness or the one most affecting everything else. Or you may prefer to focus on a particular chapter in the book or even a subsection of a chapter that most resonated with you. It really depends on where you are right now with your health. Are you pretty healthy and just want to stay that way? Do you have a few nagging symptoms that you'd like to resolve? Do you have a diagnosis and are under a doctor's care and intuitively know there must be a better way?

The best journey for you is always going to be the one that suits your personality and lifestyle. For example:

- Do you love to cook? Studying nutrition and new recipes may be the place to start.
- Are you an outdoorsman, love gardening or nature in general? Maybe herbalism is for you.
- Do you like to spring-clean and organize your house? Maybe start with looking into reducing your toxic load.
- Are you into nice smells? You could explore the world of essential oils.
- Are you on a lot of medications and want to reduce/eliminate them? An orthomolecular solution is probably the place to start—a quality supplement routine.
- Are you simply sedentary and realize you need to move more? Start walking every day and investigate what other exercise or sports opportunities you might enjoy.
- Are you lonely and need to improve your social connections or start a new hobby? You could start a book club using this as your first text to drive a health revolution in your circle!

Clearly a little planning is important. I don't want you to feel overwhelmed and just put this book on a shelf. You could also think through how you best form new habits. Do you first need more information on your particular ailment? I'm someone who likes as much information as possible and you can't convince me of anything without some data. Go the Further Reading I've provided in Appendix D and pick out your next read that goes into more depth on your particular situation. Perhaps you need a friend or partner to join you on your journey. The buddy system is a great way to stick to any new goal. Are you into technology and quantifying your progress? You may want to utilize one of a myriad of app-based solutions—although note my comments on precision medicine below. Do you need a carrot? Promise yourself a reward when you have achieved a certain goal or set an audacious goal requiring dedication to achieve it, such as a marathon or fun run depending on your starting point. Perhaps a stick works better for you? Unfortunately sticks tend to be not of our choosing such as a heart attack, a cancer diagnosis, or your doctor announcing you need medication. Or perhaps your impetus is a life change such as retiring from a job, welcoming your first grandchild, or moving location.

Whatever your situation, listen to that little voice inside you and just make a start. Take one step. Add one micro-habit that's in the right direction.

You're in it for the long haul. Don't try to change everything all at once. Be intentional and set realistic targets. I started on my own health journey over a decade ago and I'm still striving for improvement and make tweaks regularly. My sons, now in their late teens, have to make their own decisions and follow their own health journeys. No one can do it for you.

Your relationship with the healthcare industry will probably be your biggest change. See it for what it is, a profit-making enterprise. Sometimes you'll need a medical doctor. If you're having a heart attack you need to head to the emergency room; I can't help you. If you're having trouble breathing, coughing up blood, or have an unusual pain or lump you need to get it checked out. I want you to use doctors for what they do know and just use them sparingly for what they don't. In fact I hope some of you go to the doctor more. Those of you who are scared what the doctor might diagnose or tell you to do can now understand you are just going to get their opinion. You don't have to do what they say. They might diagnose a label and offer a pill or surgery, but you can simply apply your critical thinking skills and the information in this book to decide what to do about it.

There are app-based solutions for just about every condition these days. No one solution is going to have the exact answer for you as you are a unique individual with a unique lifestyle and situation. There are indeed massive advances in big data and machine learning techniques that can assess many aspects of your bodily processes, microbiome, and genetics. Some claim to be able to figure out the exact supplements you need, or food combinations you should eat, or number of steps to take each day. They call it the promise of *precision medicine*. While some of them may point you in the right direction in terms of priorities, foods that are better or worse for you, or goals to set, I have to advise caution if the overall goal is human flourishing. Never forget that God is in charge. No matter how complex the algorithm, it will never outdo God or your own intuition. Make sure your app doesn't take the enjoyment out of God's prescription for nourishment of heart, soul as well as belly. And that the importance of relationships, interaction with nature and finding your purpose are incorporated in your plan. As Albert Einstein is reported to have said:

Most things that matter cannot be measured, and most things that can be measured, don't matter.

If your situation is complicated or you are on a lot of medications, you will probably need a professional partner to get you on the right path.

In this case I urge you to find an integrative or functional medicine professional. If you are employed check what your health plan covers or supplemental services your employer might offer. If conventional medical care is all that is covered and pushes you toward drugs and surgery then hand your employer this book and tell them to especially read *Appendix B: A Word to HR Managers and Corporate Sponsors*. Conventional medical care will only lead to higher healthcare costs and sicker employees. Supporting employees to seek care that will reverse disease and drive health is a win-win for all.

If budget is a barrier, I suggest you note what you currently spend out of pocket on healthcare and lost productivity. Investing in a healthy future where you're flourishing at your peak is a worthy endeavor and likely to generate much larger returns than other items I bet you spend money on today.

I will leave you with my **10 Principles for being a Healthy Human**:

1. Nourishment is a priority. Think about every mouthful.
2. Move your body every day.
3. Reduce toxic exposures. If it didn't exist 100 years ago, be wary.
4. Commit to uncompromising sleep.
5. Prioritize and optimize your relationships.
6. Believe in a power bigger than yourself. Find His purpose in your life.
7. Avoid medications and embrace supplements and natural remedies that work with your body.
8. The sun is your life force. Get outside in nature every day.
9. Water is magical. Drink more of it.
10. Use your critical thinking skills at all times. Only you and God know what your body needs.

APPENDIX A

Food Hacks to Get You Started

Whether you're a gourmet chef, live on fast food or anything in between, it can seem daunting to upgrade your nutrition. Here I've outlined a few ideas to get you started. Like any of my 10 principles to be a healthy human, you just need to take a first step in the right direction. Once you get comfortable with one new habit you can add another.

Some of you may prefer a full 30-day meal program, of which there are legions available, many of which are very good. But I prefer to teach you to fish. Slowly build habits that will become your new baseline and fit with your particular lifestyle and culture. You only need a few staple recipes to fall back on to start improving your nutrition.

Better Breakfasts

As the first meal after your fast to repair and restore, it is important to launch your day with plenty of good protein and fat for strong energy levels. For the first week or two I'd recommend focusing only on improving your breakfast routine. Remember we are aiming for at least a full twelve hours of fasting. If you have to get up early to go to work, consider taking breakfast with you. A smoothie tends to travel well. The ingredients can be prepared the night before. A batch of my crustless mini-quiches can also be prepared at the weekend and a couple grabbed and reheated each morning. A hearty omelet is truly the breakfast of champions.

Breakfast Smoothie

You'll need a blender of some kind.

> *Ingredients* can be adjusted to your taste. Experiment!
> - Base: Nut milk such as almond or coconut
> - Low-sugar frozen fruit, such as raspberries (¼ cup), or an unsweetened acai smoothie pack
> - Fat: ½ an avocado or heaped tablespoon of almond or peanut butter
> - Protein: 3 tablespoons hemp seed and/or scoop of protein powder*
> - Greens: Handful of spinach and/or parsley, moringa, spirulina etc.
>
> *Directions*
> - Put all ingredients in blender and blend well.

* Check ingredients of protein powder carefully. Avoid "isolates" and other chemicals. Plant-based are best.

Hearty Omelet

You'll need a skillet or egg pan.

> *Ingredients* can be adjusted to your taste and for variety.
> - Teaspoon of grass-fed butter for cooking
> - 1 shallot, peeled and chopped finely
> - 1–2 inches of zucchini, chopped
> - ¼ cup sliced mushrooms (optional)
> - 1–2 asparagus spears, chopped (optional)

- Handful of arugula (or spinach/kale—I like arugula with eggs for its peppery taste.)
- 2 organic pasture-raised eggs
- ½ an avocado

Directions
- Heat pan and melt butter on medium heat.
- Add shallot, zucchini, asparagus, and any other vegetables that need cooking. Sauté for 2–3 minutes.
- Lightly whisk eggs with a fork and add to pan.
- Continue to heat on medium. Flip over as necessary to cook both sides, another 1–2 minutes until eggs are almost solid.
- Add arugula to the egg for a final warming. Serve with avocado.

Crustless Mini Quiches

These measurements make about 12. Well worth the extra effort.

Dry ingredients
- ½ cup almond flour
- ½ cup hemp seed hearts
- 1 cup shredded Parmesan cheese
- ¼ cup flaxseed meal
- ½ tsp baking powder (aluminum free)
- ½ tsp oregano (optional)
- ½ tsp basil (if using dried, fresh is even better!)
- ½ tsp parsley (if using dried but I prefer a handful of fresh parsley chopped finely)

Wet ingredients
- 6 eggs, whisked
- ½ cup organic cottage cheese
- ⅓ cup thinly sliced green onions/scallions or chives (optional)

Directions
- Preheat oven to 375°F.
- Mix together dry ingredients in a bowl.
- Separately mix together wet ingredients.
- Combine ingredients. Mix well. Scoop mixture into muffin cups.
- Bake for 25 minutes.

Plan Your Snacks

Once you've got breakfast figured out it's time to think through emergency snack food. The biggest derailer from trying to eat well is when life gets in the way and you find yourself caught out in a hurry or stuck in a food desert. The easiest snacks are those you can carry around, leave in your car, or grab at short notice. Nuts and seeds are your friends here. Make sure they are organic, without any additives like sugar or flavorings (other than sea salt, natural garlic, or chili powder for example) and preferably sprouted for easier digestion. Refer back to Chapter 5 for details. Jerky or what my son calls "meat bars" can also be useful if organic, grass-fed, wild-caught, and without additives. There are hundreds of other types of ready-made "bars" including the healthy-sounding granola bar. Don't be fooled by the shiny packaging. Make sure to carefully read the ingredients. The Resources section has some recommended brands.

I'll give you one recipe here for my famous turmeric seed loaf. One genetic trait of my British upbringing that has been impossible to overcome is the need for an afternoon cup of tea and something yummy to get me through to dinnertime. This recipe is versatile, secretly healthy and also makes a great breakfast on the run or post workout snack.

Turmeric Seed loaf

It's worth the effort—I promise!

Ingredients

- 2 cups almond flour
- ½ cup raw organic walnuts or pecans
- ¼ cup shredded coconut
- ½ cup raw pumpkin seeds
- ¼ cup raw sunflower seeds
- ¼ tsp salt
- 1 tsp ground turmeric
- ½ teaspoon baking powder (aluminum free)
- 3 eggs
- 2 egg whites
- 3.25 oz coconut oil melted (½ cup is 3.7oz, so just a bit less)
- 2 tbsp organic pure maple syrup
- ½ large banana, mashed

Directions

- Preheat oven to 325°F and line a small loaf tin with baking (wax) paper (3.5 × 12inch).
- Combine almond flour, nuts, seeds, salt, turmeric, baking powder, and coconut in a large bowl.
- In small bowl, whisk together the remaining ingredients. Add wet mixture to dry mixture and combine well.
- Pour the batter into the prepared loaf tin and bake for 45–50 minutes or until a skewer comes out clean.
- Allow to cool in the tin before slicing. Serve plain or with a little (grass-fed) butter or pure fruit jam.

Super Salads

So now you're looking at lunch, probably the hardest meal to upgrade particularly if you're working all day or juggling kids and activities. If you ignore your lunch upgrade and resort to fast-food or store-bought options you could be derailing your overall health improvement with knock-on effects of a bad meal. I discuss eating out a bit later, but for now I'm going to exhort you to focus on super salads for lunch. If you're really sure that you're fine with bread then you could adapt this recipe into a sandwich but a big bowl of salad gives you more options. Buy some food containers (preferably glass) and a freezer bag and commit to making your lunch as a baseline habit.

Versatile Super Salad

Switch it up and experiment with the ingredients and dressings. No two days need to be the same, but ditch the iceberg lettuce!

Ingredients

- Protein: Wild-caught canned mackerel (sardines, anchovies, and salmon also work). Shredded chicken or meat left over from last night's dinner is a bonus option.
- Greens: Arugula is my staple. Romaine also works. Add some fresh parsley.
- Bitter greens: Radicchio and/or endive
- Cucumber
- Jicama
- ½ avocado
- Other good fats: Olives plus pecans, walnuts or seeds

Dressings (choose one)

- Extra-virgin olive oil (EVOO) mixed with organic honey mustard
- EVOO with balsamic vinegar

- EVOO with apple cider vinegar, add some ground garlic, ginger, paprika
- Equal parts tahini and sour cream with a little lemon juice, coconut aminos, and spices

What's for Dinner?

I find that dinnertime is where a family's culture really shines through. I don't want to mess too much with staple family meals that you are most comfortable with particularly if you are already in the habit of sitting down together to eat. If you're reheating pre-bought TV dinners in the microwave I definitely want you to explore alternatives. But there is a lot you can upgrade just by tweaking the ingredients of existing go-to meals you are already making.

As an example, if spaghetti Bolognese is a family favorite then upgrading the ground beef you buy to organic grass fed, selecting a tomato sauce that has no additives and adding a whole bunch of additional vegetables to the sauce can boost the nutritional value considerably. Onions, zucchini, garlic, mushrooms, even finely chopped kale and fresh parsley can all go unnoticed in a good pasta sauce. You might look into organic brown rice pastas instead of traditional wheat-based.

If you are facing major health issues or struggling with poor digestion, leaky gut or a depleted microbiome you may need to focus on a more therapeutic meal plan for a while. Here I'm giving you two staple recipes which will make your body and cells do the happy-dance. My sweet potato hash would be welcomed in several blue zones. Easily adjusted with whatever ingredients you have on hand I have often eaten versions of it several times in a single week. If my gut is impaired for any reason (like a recent conference trip where I accidentally ingested gluten and suffered the consequences) I'll resort to soup for my evening meal to give my gut a little less work to do as I wind toward my nighttime fast.

Sweet Potato Hash

Mix and match the ingredients (all organic) and experiment with spices.

Ingredients

- Sweet potatoes: I like to use a combination of white Hannah sweet potatoes and Japanese purple sweet potatoes.
- Butternut squash
- Mushrooms: any kind such as shiitake, portobello, cremini, maitake
- Bone broth, coconut milk, or coconut aminos for liquid
- Zucchini
- Plantain, optional
- Cauliflower
- Edamame (whole soybeans) or leftover chicken/beef
- Spices: ground turmeric, pepper, garlic, ginger, cinnamon, paprika
- Kale (I like lacinato for its thick leaves, which are easily chopped)
- Ghee or coconut oil to coat pan

Directions

- Heat a skillet on the stove and add a tablespoon of ghee or coconut oil.
- Chop sweet potatoes and butternut squash finely (pieces no bigger than 1 centimeter) and add to the pan. Cover with a lid. Cook on medium for 3–5 minutes.
- Add in chopped zucchini and mushrooms.
- Add a tablespoon or so of liquid so the vegetables don't stick to the pan and the potatoes can steam a little.
- If including plantain, slice and add to pan. Keep mixing. Add more liquid if necessary.
- Break up cauliflower into small florets and add to pan.

- Add edamame or other precooked protein.
- Add plenty of spices. My favorite combo is salt, pepper, turmeric, garlic, and cinnamon.
- When mixture is close to cooked (probably not more than about 8 minutes of cook time) add the chopped kale or other greens for the final minute.

Leftover hash also makes a great breakfast. Just reheat and add some eggs to the pan for a tasty scramble or omelet.

Gut-Healing Soup

You'll need a blender of some kind. These measurements make a meal for one. SIBO friendly.

Ingredients
- 1 tablespoon coconut oil
- 1 carrot
- ¼ cup chopped zucchini
- ½ cup bone broth: I use grass-fed beef broth prepackaged from Thrive Market but you can also purchase frozen or make your own. Chicken and turkey broth also work.
- Spices: turmeric, ginger, salt, pepper, cinnamon
- ⅓ cup chopped kale
- ¼ fresh parsley
- ⅓ cup coconut milk

Directions
- Melt the coconut oil in saucepan.
- Add chopped carrot and zucchini.
- Add bone broth and spices. Simmer for 20 minutes.
- Add kale and coconut milk. Heat on low for 5 more minutes.
- Blend in high-speed blender.

If you are not following a SIBO diet you could add other vegetables like onions or leeks, butternut squash, and cauliflower. I'd also add generous amounts of garlic to your spices. Cauliflower can make it creamy so you may not need the coconut milk in this case.

Out and About

Once your taste buds wake up to real food, you're going to find yourself seeking better options when you're out with friends, on a date, or just on the move. Seek out restaurants with fresh local ingredients. They do exist. It might take some homework. If the meat, poultry and fish is lower quality you may do best by opting for the plant-based options with simple sauces. If the main selection is grilled chicken or fish, ask for some extra veggies.

The big global brands of fast food should be completely off the table if you are getting serious about your health. The negative additions to your bucket far outweigh any meagre nutrition you might glean to get you through the hunger pangs. It's just not worth it. There are newer "casual dining" options in many locations which have improved the possibilities when you're out and about. Here you generally move along a line and can select from fresh ingredients often sourced locally. Just ask questions about the contents of any sauces or salad dressings.

Treats and Desserts

I am a foodie remember. I LOVE dessert and treats. There are plenty of incredibly tasty options for satisfying desserts when you need an indulgence or for a special occasion. Piecrusts made from almond flour and coconut oil, chopped dates or bananas for sweetness, raw cacao for healthy chocolaty goodness . . . there are many amazing options that have nothing to do with corn syrup or other fake ingredients. But I'm trying to focus on staple recipes to get you started with new habits that you can learn as a foundation to a healthier future. My chocolate mousse and chia pudding are easy to make and healthy enough for daily consumption especially if boosted with protein powder for an extra kick or post exercise snack.

Chia Pudding

Ingredients

- 1 teaspoon chia seeds
- 1 tablespoon hemp seeds
- 1 scoop (healthy) protein powder (optional)
- 1 cup unsweetened almond/coconut milk
- ½ cup berries and/or ½ banana, sliced
- Sprinkle of cinnamon (or nutmeg)

Directions

- Mix all the ingredients together in a glass jar with lid or covered bowl.
- Refrigerate at least 3 hours.
- Enjoy!

Chocolate Mousse

Always a crowd favorite but remember cacao has caffeine in it so there is the potential to disrupt sleep if eaten late at night.

Ingredients

- 3 large ripe avocados
- ½ cup raw cacao powder
- ½ cup pure maple syrup
- ½ cup full-fat coconut cream (no additives)
- ½ tsp sea salt

Directions

- Blend all ingredients in a high-speed blender until soft and creamy.
- Poor into serving bowls.

- Top with blueberries or strawberries.
- Chill for at least 20 minutes.
- You can also freeze this recipe to make into Popsicles or chocolate ice cream.

APPENDIX B

A Word to HR Managers and Corporate Sponsors

With over twenty-five years in Corporate HR Consulting, I have to provide a few words to those of you with influence beyond your own families and communities. People are struggling. Consultants throw around words like "quiet quitting" and "presenteeism" to emphasize many employees are not working at their full potential. Lack of engagement, reduced productivity, and general dissatisfaction are common discussion points in HR conference rooms. I would call it a general lack of human flourishing across the four realms of Physical, Emotional, Social and Spiritual health.

All four realms are interconnected and you can't denote these dimensions as wellness or wellbeing as something apart from health or healthcare. Often a company has separate teams responsible for the health plan (a benefit) and for wellbeing (coming under the umbrella of employee experience or the company culture). This drives a disconnect between one team promoting pharmaceuticals and surgery while the other team acknowledges that what you really need is lifestyle management and social connections.

Corporate wellbeing strategy often also incorporates a financial dimension. The strategy then features elements relating to Physical, Emotional, Social and Financial wellbeing in equal parts. The idea is if you can teach people how to better manage their budget or save for a rainy day, they will gain financial resilience and not be so stressed out when something unexpected happens. It is true that stress due to financial problems can negatively impact physical health. But if you take a visit to the blue zones (see Chapter 3) you'll see that many of the poorest people in the world are flourishing. I can also testify that in my own tight community, those with financial difficulties still have the joy and resilience I associate with human flourishing if their social, spiritual and emotional health is good. Even if their physical health is failing, the financial aspects aren't a factor in their daily outlook.

Think about that for a moment. As an employer, your human capital is part of your bottom line. Often you can't afford to pay workers any more than you already are. And workers that are always focused on their finances are never going to have enough. When the focus is their purpose, their relationships, being of service and having a curiosity about the world, finances diminish in importance.

From a corporate profitability standpoint though, healthcare costs are rising year after year while employees continue to get sicker. Productivity is reduced not just from the sickness days but from distracted employees on the job dealing with their illness or that of a loved one. Managers who are battling poor mental health affect the work environment for their whole team, which has knock-on effects throughout the organization. Physical health and healthcare provision cannot be divorced from the overall notion of wellness or wellbeing.

Rather than putting all the focus and resources on conventional medical care attempting to eek out some cost savings through specialized networks, centers of excellence, promoting off-patent (generic) drugs and passing more of the cost onto employees, it needs a wholesale paradigm shift in how employers support the health and wellbeing of their workforce. It starts with a different kind of health plan. One that puts the health of the participant above the profitability of the healthcare industry. It would lead with lifestyle management, provide nutrition counseling, cover high-quality supplements and seek the root cause of any symptoms rather than promoting pharmaceuticals and surgery.

It is true some employees may prefer to take a pill than make any lifestyle changes. But assuming everyone feels that way is simply wrong. In my experience once you outline the full story as presented in this book, the majority of people would opt to avoid conventional medical care as long as they received adequate support to embark on the alternative.

The system is currently rigged against them though. If their health plan only covers pharmaceuticals and surgery, that's what they'll accept. They usually have no idea there is another way. If they do find out, they quickly discover they can't afford the out-of-pocket expenses of a functional medicine consult and there are no subsidies for the vitamins and supplements that will turn their health around.

These days there is a wide range of innovative start-up companies now offering various forms of functional medicine sold as wellness solutions. For an initial monthly fee usually under $200 for example, employees with certain specific conditions like diabetes or an auto-immune label can get access to these resources to coach them back to health. Often the employee is on a high-cost drug that the health plan is heavily subsidizing. This enables these new vendor solutions to demonstrate significant ROI (returns on the investment) of 2,3, even 4:1 savings by addressing nutrition and lifestyle factors to reverse the condition and get the employee off the medications.

I welcome these solutions but their availability is not enough to move the needle on employee health or runaway healthcare costs.

Employers need to lead with these solutions, not tack them on as an extra aimed at employees who are already sick. True "prevention" is not flu shots and statins which only add to the negative burden on a body. Nor is it the early detection of disease with mammograms and colonoscopies. Prevention is education, good nutrition, understanding what actually drives disease, and what it takes to be a healthy human. In short, prevention is promoting human flourishing across the four dimensions.

Here are some sample questions to discuss with your advisers:

- What are the biggest cost drivers in our health plan? The top 10 drugs being used, the most common surgeries, certain chronic conditions? Are there better ways our employees could be tackling the indicated health issues?
- Is our health plan incentivizing poor behavior? Can we make adjustments that will drive employees to behaviors that will improve their health?
- Do we have alternative options available to employees for those who want to take a lifestyle-driven approach to their health? Are these programs being utilized?
- Are we tackling mental health in our employees and managers optimally?
- Are we doing enough to help educate our employees on health topics? Is our messaging around preventive care optimal?
- Does our company culture encourage behaviors that impact our employees' health and wellbeing? Such as long hours, performance assessment only related to numbers, and individual rather than team achievement?
- Are there members of senior management who can help drive a change to a culture of human flourishing?

APPENDIX C

Spiritual Addendum

We cannot ignore the fact that to achieve optimum human flourishing as I defined in the Epilogue requires a spiritual dimension. I gave an overview of Spiritual Purpose at the end of Chapter 9 focusing on the human need for purpose in life and the importance of mindset. Here I'd like to expand a little on those concepts. The peace that comes with fully knowing the truth about the universe, what God expects of us and where we will spend eternity can do more for your health than anything else we have discussed in this book. Just like a small child thrives in the total trust and security of their parent and the parameters provided, like not sticking fingers in the electrical outlet or trying to cross a busy road alone. Such a child has a firm knowledge their needs will be taken care of and at the end of the day they will be tucked up in a warm bed. Children who don't have these foundations struggle to function well.

Everyone has beliefs whether you consider yourself a religious person, an atheist, a scientist, or a skeptic. We all have a worldview even if we are not consciously aware of it. But while everyone is of course entitled to their own worldview, some are better than others, particularly those that actually fit with reality.

Back in Chapter 1 we noted that in the 1950s doctors encouraged the belief that cigarette smoking was good for us. In Chapter 2 we learned of the changing beliefs around germs and remedies such as mercury and arsenic. While we are free to choose any worldview we want, it must be acknowledged that all worldviews are not equally healthy for us.

In his book *The God-Shaped Brain: How Changing Your View of God Transforms Your Life* psychiatrist Dr. Tim Jennings documents the impact various religious views have on the brain. Essentially, he proves that viewing God as promoting love, forgiveness, compassion, reasoning, critical thinking, and the pursuit of truth and evidence are healing to the brain. Whereas viewing God as inciting fear, intolerance, conflict, resentment, undermining reasoning, shutting down thinking, and coercing others are damaging to the brain. Interestingly, believing there is no God (that life just spontaneously occurred) falls somewhere between the first two views in its effect on brain health as long as the humanistic view includes altruism, honesty, and freedom of conscience. Often someone takes this humanistic view because they believe the only alternative is God as a punishing dictator. This interpretation of God has arisen from a distortion in human history and the false belief that God's laws function like human laws—imposed rules that require the rule giver to inflict punishment for rule breaking. But God's laws are very different to human laws. God's laws are simply reality.

My own worldview changed over a number of years. You can read about my journey on my website (EmmaTekstra.com/blog). While many people will tell you they believe what they believe because they had a spiritual experience or they were raised that way or a major event in their life changed them, what is most important is the truth. The absolute truth, or reality itself. So instead of my experience, I'm providing a brief overview of what I've learned, the evidence available, and some further reading and resources for you to investigate further. It took me several years of studying the evidence and questioning apparent contradictions or confusions to be finally convinced of a few foundational truths that I will touch on:

- There is a God who created the universe and every living thing in it.
- The Bible is the actual Word of God and an accurate history book with ongoing instructions for us in every situation.
- Jesus died on a Roman execution cross and was resurrected three days later to prove He was who He said He was, God's son.

Science Makes No Sense without God

As I've mentioned throughout the book you can't separate the facts about God and the universe from the facts about the human body or anything else in science. Physics, chemistry, biology, or any other scientific discipline simply doesn't make sense unless you consider the possibility there really is a God and He created everything in the universe. Albert Einstein searched for the elusive theory of everything but just like the elusive cure for cancer we discussed in Chapter 7, it's been staring us in the face the whole time.

If you type "**The Big Bang Theory**" into a search engine these days, you get several entries for a TV show that ran from 2007 to 2019. The show was created by legendary writer/producer Chuck Lorre and was actually very good. I confess to watching every episode (perhaps recognizing my son Ethan in the brilliant but socially incompetent physicist Sheldon Cooper) but I digress. I find it interesting (satisfying!) that the scientific big bang theory has been upstaged by a TV show! If you go a bit further in your search you may find commentary on this theory (yes, it is a theory that has not been proven) along the lines of it being a workable explanation of how the universe came to be. One site calls it "our best guess." The mathematics that go into the theory include Einstein's general theory of relativity and a few other equations of particle physics. The general idea being that about fourteen billion years ago the conditions existed for matter to suddenly occur. At a point in time and space, known as the singularity, there was an explosion resulting in a sea of protons, neutrons, and electrons (tiny particles) that as they cooled started combining to form atoms and the elements such as hydrogen and helium. Digging further you will find some conflicting theories regarding space dust and then if you get into the details of how the planets were formed, you'll find a few more theories including the *core accretion model*, which states that particles are driven by the force of gravity (but where did gravity come from?) and essentially clump together. Then some more cooling and the formation of tectonic plates that cover the earth's core and leads to volcanoes and earthquakes that we still experience today. Water was then conveniently deposited through collisions with cosmic bodies (comets and asteroids).

This can all sound very plausible until you start asking questions like "Where did the original matter come from?" These scientists are trying to tell us that everything came from nothing, and we haven't even begun to talk about lifeforms yet. It seems to me they are working really hard to try to disprove God at all costs.

Meanwhile, the **First Law of Thermodynamics** (i.e. proven) tells us that mass and energy can be neither created nor destroyed, it can only change form. So if no natural process can create or destroy energy then neither the universe nor the basic laws of physics can explain the existence of our solar system. The most reasonable explanation is that something or someone outside the laws of physics and outside the universe created it.

The **Second Law of Thermodynamics** tells us that the entropy of a closed system (entropy can be thought of as a measure of chaos, disorder, or randomness) will increase or remain constant over time unless an outside force acts on it. Think of a jigsaw puzzle with 1,000 pieces. You pour all the pieces out of the box onto the kitchen table and then walk away and forget about it for a hundred years. If no one has come near the kitchen table in all that time, is it more likely to have been completed or even partially completed or still be a muddled mess? Do you think there is any time period you could wait to see if it became more ordered? This is the same unlikeliness of our extremely ordered solar system happening by chance.

One of the best vacations we took in recent years was to Ecuador. We spent five days on a ship traveling around the Galapagos Islands. The islands were made famous by Charles Darwin when he visited in 1845 and laid the groundwork for his **Theory of Evolution by Natural Selection**. Consisting of over a hundred islands and islets, nineteen of which are large but only four are inhabited with people, it is truly a unique place. There were about a hundred tourists on our ship. Every day we went to a different island to explore but always went back to the ship to eat and spend the night, as the majority of the islands are preserved with no structures on them. Sometimes we got to swim and snorkel in the oceans around an island. Every morning we would start off with a nature talk explaining what we were going to see on the excursions. We had wonderful local guides who had to complete onerous university training to be allowed the privilege of being a Galapagos naturalist.

It quickly became apparent that the theory of evolution was being taught as fact which led to some interesting discussions with these guides. On one excursion I remember our guide Natalie dutifully explaining how the islands had been formed around five million years ago. Then later that day we were hiking through an area in the middle of one of the islands looking at tortoises and iguanas and she announced that the area was totally underwater just twenty years ago. (So it took only twenty years for the land to raise up this last ten feet but apparently needed five million years to raise up the previous thirty feet!)

The animals are wonderful; mainly because they live in a protected habitat so are unafraid of humans. But I saw only evidence for God's hand in creation rather than the unsubstantiated theory of evolution. The sea lions looked exactly the same as those we see near the ocean in Southern California. The marine iguanas are unique, they swim and eat underwater, but they are clearly still iguanas. Snorkeling in the water, the fish, octopus, sea turtles, and sharks are all identifiable as in many other spots around the world. The tortoises are giant, but they are still clearly tortoises. There's also geckos, snakes, and lizards on land that seemed pretty common to us. How did they get to this remote set of islands 1,000km from the nearest land mass of Ecuador?

It was the birds that really impacted Charles Darwin, especially those finches. Our naturalist explained that there are thirteen species of finches in the Galapagos across the different islands. While they are all very similar in shape, size and color, the differences include diet, habitat, beak size, and shape. Adapting to the environment over generations can be seen all around us but that is not what the theory of evolution claims. The diversity in the bird life on the Galapagos is remarkable (especially when compared to a relatively limited set of land animals). The blue-footed booby was our favorite. A very tame and vocal fellow with bright blue legs and feet. Often seen on marketing materials about the Galapagos. There are also red-footed boobies and several other species of boobies that can be found around the world in other coastal dwellings. Not so unique to the Galapagos.

Scientists agree that *microevolution* occurs as the variation within species like the finches. Or like the dogs in your neighborhood. From miniature poodles to English bulldogs to those huge Great Danes;

there's immense variation but you recognize them all as dogs. Even within the human species there is great diversity if you consider the features of humans found in Asia to Africa, Aboriginal to Caucasian, and everything in between. However, Darwin's theory is based on *macroevolution*, the concept that successive changes from microevolution eventually leads to larger changes over greater periods of time. So large that one kind of creature, such as a fish, eventually grew legs and walked out of the water to become a reptile. This requires entirely new bodily features, legs instead of fins. The problem is the science simply doesn't add up.

The first snag is that mutations are random, not purposeful— the result of mindless undirected chance. You might have heard the term penicillin-resistant bacteria and been prone to think the bacteria "evolved" some form of resistance to make them survive. But in fact, scientific experiments have proved that the penicillin-resistant bacteria have always been there in the population before they have encountered penicillin. This has enormous implications for our health. In the case of our finches, we can agree that on certain islands where there were only seeds to eat, those that had a beak more capable of breaking up seeds, survived and became fitter while those offspring with less well-suited beaks might have grown thin and died before they had the opportunity to mate. The parent finches didn't look at the food available and somehow will their offspring to grow the type of beak that would work best.

The next obstacle is that evolution requires that the random mutation confers some sort of benefit on the creature so they are better able to survive. But if evolution occurs gradually, how would a mutation that creates the start of a wing be beneficial? An extra stub sticking out the side of a body but doesn't yet enable flight, seems like a disadvantage? We also see that mutations are always within limits. Dogs are still dogs. Finches are still finches. Over fifty years of research on fruit flies covering hundreds of generations, subjected to all sorts of mutation agents, has resulted in a whole lot of mutant fruit flies. Even more ambitious is the Long-Term Evolutionary Experiment started by evolutionary biologist Richard Lenski in 1988. Over thirty years of growing E. coli in his lab, six generations a day, the equivalent of 150 years of human history every twenty-four hours, over 70,000 generations documented, but guess what? All those flasks still contain E. coli. There is no sign of any other strain of bacteria showing up, let alone another class of organism.

There is actually a ton of evidence for the existence of God if you only choose to look for it. The diversity of the evidence amongst many different disciplines makes it a particularly irrefutable case once reviewed objectively. See Appendix D and Resources for more.

God Speaks through the Bible

There is a whole fascinating history as to how we got the Christian Bible in English or whatever your preferred language is.

Some people may argue that the Bible was put together by various church leaders attending certain councils in the fourth century deciding which books would be considered canonical and which were to be excluded. If we examine history in detail, however, we find that is simply not the case. The vast majority of the New Testament (NT) has been considered scripture since the first century. Particularly those books that contain clear evidence proving they are eyewitness accounts and were written down in the first century within decades or less of Jesus's life and resurrection.

Focusing on these NT books for a moment we can investigate the claim of them being eyewitness accounts. It includes the four gospels of Matthew, Mark, Luke and John, Luke's follow-up to his gospel— the Book of Acts, and Paul's writings such as Romans, Corinthians, and letters to Timothy for example. It is interesting to note that no one has ever disputed the author of these mentioned books. Church leaders of the later first century and second century were already referring to these gospels and letters in their own writings that we also have copies of.

To start putting together a timeline we can focus on the most significant historical event in the region and in Jewish and Roman history—the destruction of the temple in Jerusalem in the year 70 AD. Before the destruction there was a three-year siege by the Roman army that devastated the Jewish people and was written about extensively. There is no mention of these two events anywhere in the gospel writings. Jesus predicts the destruction of the temple in Matthew 24:1–3 but it is not mentioned anywhere in the NT to have happened even though such a description would have validated Jesus's prediction. This provides strong evidence that these books must have been written before 70 AD so we are already within about thirty years of Jesus's death and resurrection in 33 AD.

We also know from history that Paul died in Rome in 64 AD and Peter, the following year. Even though the deaths of less important figures are recorded such as Stephen (in Acts 7:54–60) and James, the brother of John (in Acts 12:1–2) the deaths of Paul and Peter are not included. This suggests they had not yet occurred.

Luke explains that his gospel was his first account and the Book of Acts followed (Acts 1:1–2) and when we first meet Paul, when he was known as Saul (in Acts 7:58), he is described as a young man. In Paul's first letter to Timothy he quotes as "scripture" both Deuteronomy and the gospel of Luke (1 Tim 5:17–18). He quotes the other gospels regularly in his other writings. Luke also quotes the gospels of Mark and Matthew repeatedly. He freely admits in Luke 1: 1–4 that he was not an eyewitness himself but a historian looking into the accounts of first-person eyewitnesses. Luke was a physician who was a companion of Paul's.

Mark's gospel is widely believed to be the oldest, the first account written down. John Mark (his full name) was a disciple of Peter and a cousin of Barnabas (Colossians 4:10). The later writings of Papias, who lived 60–130 AD, referred to Mark as "the interpreter of Peter." We can also note how Mark mentions Peter most prominently and also avoids mentioning the less-flattering incidents concerning Peter (covered in other gospels) probably as a sign of respect. Based on these and other evidence Mark's gospel is actually understood to be Peter's eyewitness account. Mark omits some key details and leaves some characters unnamed in his account. This suggests he was protecting them from persecution by Jewish leaders lending weight to the fact they were still alive when he wrote his account.

Other evidence to support the gospels being eyewitness accounts can be found in studying the words themselves. For a start they each use words like "witness" and "testimony" regularly as if knowing the importance of documenting the events they have seen with their own eyes. Eyewitness accounts to any crime or incident always differ. In fact if two witnesses ever provided exactly the same testimony we'd be suspicious they had colluded to get their stories straight. Perspectives differ and are colored by an individual's personal experiences and interests. While there are many similarities between the four gospels there are also many differences, both in the language used, some of the details, and the personal perspective.

As an example, Matthew 8:14–16 explains Jesus healing Peter's mother-in-law in Capernaum and then waiting until evening to begin healing others. Mark 1:21 explains that it was the Sabbath, which fills in a gap in the narrative for us (as to why they waited). There are many such examples of filling in gaps to get a complete picture from studying all four gospels together.

Moving beyond the internal evidence of the NT itself, we can look at external evidence to trace the chain of custody to make sure that the eyewitness accounts written down in the early years following Jesus's life is the same accounts that we read in our Bible today. In the first and second century we can trace the disciples of the apostles and of Paul and read their writings that quote the original narratives and confirm the key points of Jesus's life and teaching. John was the youngest of Jesus's disciples and was the only one not martyred for his faith. He lived to be over ninety years old and died a natural death. John taught Ignatius and Polycarp, who in turn taught Irenaeus who taught Hippolytus as just a sample. Peter taught Mark who had various disciples who became church leaders and so on.

These leaders were scattered around the world and sometimes words were changed in the copies of scripture produced, some by accident, some to enhance clarity or understanding. But the "textual criticism" of later church leaders and Bible translators were able to compare manuscripts from different locations and identify what was most likely the original text. In fact our modern translations do an even better job of this as technology has enabled us to look at so many more versions all at once.

So we can actually be very confident that the words we are reading in our modern New Testament are actually the words of some of the original eye witnesses who saw firsthand the life and works of Jesus.

Taking the Bible as a whole, it is a library of sixty-six books (thirty-nine in the Old Testament and twenty-seven in the NT) written by about forty different authors from a wide range of backgrounds in three languages covering a time period that spans 1,500 years. The consistency and unity of message and how all parts neatly dovetail together is remarkable. For example, the prophets in the OT document over three hundred prophecies regarding the Messiah himself, about who he will be and the events around his appearance. (Micah 5:2 and Isaiah 53 are often quoted but there are many more). Jesus fulfilled every detail. Once you start looking it is very difficult to deny the supernatural nature of the Bible and that's before you get to any of the other evidence such as the geographic and political prophecy it contains or comparison to archeological findings. The best way to test this is to read it for yourself. I've provided some resources but I might suggest you start with reading the book of Proverbs and marvel at the ancient wisdom that is still so relevant today. The book of Romans is my favorite book as it most clearly explains God's intentions for us humans and how we get to heaven. The book of Luke is another good place to start clearly covering Jesus's life and ministry.

The Bible is God's way of communicating with us. Like letters from a loved one you would be excited to read to get to know them better. God wants a personal relationship with every one of us directly. But He intends the Bible to be understood as a whole. In the introduction to this book, I warned you not to skip ahead to find the parts most relevant to your current health situation. I urged you to read through the Foundations in Part I before moving onto the Implications in Part II as everything connects together. You could read one sentence or paragraph of this book out of context and head down a very wrong path. Much more critically, the Bible can be misunderstood if you just focus on one verse here or there without understanding the context it was written in, the intended audience and what was happening in the culture at that time. Scholars have figured all this out from non-biblical sources. Then you can consider what are the moral truths being taught that are still relevant today. And only then can you start to apply it to our lives now. I promise you there is nothing going on in our culture in the twenty-first century that God hasn't seen at some point in the past.

I mentioned in Chapter 1 that you'd be amazed how much science is in the Bible. For example, in the oldest book of the Bible Job, estimated to have originated around 1500 BC when it was commonly believed that the earth sat on a large animal or giant, it says "He hangs the earth on nothing" (Job 26:7). Science didn't discover this until 1650 AD. Another Old Testament book, Isaiah, states "It is He who sits above the circle of the earth" (Isaiah 40:22). The book of Isaiah is estimated to have been written between 740–680 BC at least three hundred years before Aristotle suggested the earth might be a sphere. The book of Hebrews in the NT was written two thousand years ago long before microscopes and the discovery of atoms, but it says "the things which are seen were not made of things which are visible" (Hebrews 11:3). There are many more examples.

You'd also be amazed how every circumstance you find yourself in and issue you are facing is miraculously covered in the pages of scripture. There are still mysteries that God has determined our human brains can't handle. Like the concept of a triune God—one God in three persons: the Father, the Son (Jesus), and the Holy Spirit. Scholars can prove it is so but cannot fully explain how it works. But that's okay. All will become clear when we get to heaven.

So how do we get to heaven? I'm glad you asked. I can tell you it is not dependent on your good works. God's standard of good is too high for any human to attain. God is perfect and holy. For us to be righteous enough to be in His presence we'd have to be perfect too—never think a bad thought; never snap an impatient word at our spouse or kids; never tell a white lie to make life easier for ourselves; never covet what someone else has . . . Instead, God in His unbounding love for us sent His son Jesus to live a perfect life and then be sacrificed in our place. Anyone who puts their full trust in God and therefore His son Jesus will go to heaven and live out eternity in God's presence. This fact is known as "*the gospel*" which translates as "the good news." It's good news because the bad news is that those who die without having placed their trust in God go to the place we call hell. Other terms are used in scripture such as in the book of Revelation "the lake of fire" where there is "weeping, wailing and gnashing of teeth." This knowledge is what drives real Christians to speak of their faith to loved ones even when it causes conflict as the price for being ignored is so great.

In the meantime, if the Bible really is true then God's instructions for how we should live will undoubtedly lead to the highest level of human flourishing. In a book about health & longevity this fact alone should cause you to pause and reflect.

Resurrecting Truth

The third foundational truth that must be grasped is possibly the hardest, but it is actually the most critical. The main problem people tend to have with the claim that Jesus rose from the dead lies in the fact that it would be classed as a supernatural event—a miracle. We're not talking about a heart that stops momentarily or a doctor reviving someone after a few minutes or even someone with no discernible brain activity who is kept functioning with machines and later wakes up. The biblical account is very clear that Jesus was fully dead and three days later was alive interacting with hundreds of people for over a month.

We must come to the evidence though with no bias. If we start with the assumption that miracles can't happen there is only one conclusion we can reach. We don't know how it's possible for a monarch butterfly to return to the garden where its great-grandparents were born but through modern tracking devices, we know it happens.

So then with a completely unbiased thought process we can look at all the possibilities and decide which seems the most reasonable from the evidence we have. To narrow down the possibilities we can start with certain facts that nearly all skeptics agree on as part of the historical record. It is generally accepted that Jesus died on a Roman crucifixion cross and was buried in a tomb. Three days later his tomb was found empty, and no one has ever produced his body. The disciples believed that they saw Jesus resurrected as we know from their eyewitness accounts and other non-Christian writings. Finally, it is agreed that Jesus's disciples were transformed by what they saw and went on to teach others and ultimately many of them died for what they believed.

One possibility is simply that the disciples were wrong, that Jesus hadn't actually died in the first place. However it is clear that Jesus was heavily beaten and abused before being crucified, so much so he couldn't carry his own cross and in his weakened state seemed to die quicker than the other condemned prisoners. While the legs of the other prisoners were broken so as to speed their death that day, the guards found that Jesus was already dead so didn't need to break his legs (John 19:33). Even more interesting, the guards pierced his side with a spear to check and not only didn't he flinch but both blood and water were noted as coming out of him (John 19:34). While early church leaders had questioned this account, we now recognize, from our modern understanding of the human body, that Jesus had most likely suffered from circulatory shock given what he'd been through, causing water to accumulate around his lungs, a pleural effusion, which was released when his side was pierced. We also know that Roman guards would face death if they allowed a prisoner to survive crucifixion so it was highly unlikely they would make such a mistake particularly with a high-profile prisoner.

Another possibility is that the disciples lied about Jesus's resurrection. This would require quite the conspiracy with over five hundred people noted to have seen and interacted with Jesus over forty days. But it doesn't account for the empty tomb which was heavily guarded by Roman soldiers or the transformed lives of the disciples which would be hard to follow if they knew it was a lie.

A third possibility proposed by skeptics is that the disciples were actually delusional due to their intense grief from losing their teacher and mentor. But it again doesn't account for the empty tomb and hard to believe that so many people would have the exact same hallucination.

A fourth possibility is that everyone was fooled by an imposter claiming to be Jesus resurrected and then the disciples unknowingly advanced the lie. But it is hard to believe there could be an imposter that knew Jesus's mannerisms and teaching style better than the twelve disciples most close to him. Even one of those initially skeptical, Thomas, who had only heard from others, was later convinced when he saw for himself including additional miracles "this imposter" was able to do during those forty days. And it still doesn't account for the empty tomb.

A fifth possibility is that only one or two disciples actually had the "visions" of Jesus and they influenced everyone else. However, this doesn't account for the number of separate sightings of Jesus by different people groups described in great detail, nor of course the empty tomb.

A sixth possibility is that the legend of Jesus was amplified and distorted over time but the early dating of the original eyewitness accounts show the characters depicted were still alive and therefore could have disputed the claims if untrue. The earliest church leaders include reference to the resurrection as a key pillar of the Christian faith.

While we can see major problems with six possible explanations against the resurrection, there is only one reasonable explanation that seems to address all of the evidence. That is that the disciples were accurately reporting that Jesus rose from the dead. This accounts for the empty tomb, the observations by eyewitnesses, and the transformed lives of the apostles.

Taking another path, we might think through why Jesus is so special that not only did his arrival set the start of the Common Era—our calendar used across the world re-started from the year of Jesus's birth—but the widespread impact Jesus has had on all aspects of life independent of religious endeavors. There is no other person in history who has had such a wide impact. Not a religious leader, not a military leader, not a movie star or musician, no leader of a country, or any other statesman. Jesus has had an impact in every corner of the globe, and he lived at a time when there was no internet and no printing press. In fact, most people were unable to read the written word in his day. If you delve into the history of other religious systems almost every one of them either modified their system in line with the account of Jesus (if they originated before the Common Era), mentioned Jesus in some way in their teachings to acknowledge his existence, or merged Jesus into their system.

There is a lot more to the astonishing impact of Jesus but to sum up this foundational fact I'm quoting from the wonderful book *Person of Interest* by former cold case police detective J. Warner Wallace:

> *Jesus was born in a tiny irrelevant town in the Roman Empire and raised in another small village. He had to walk from one place to the next, and as an adult never travelled more than two-hundred miles from the town where he was born.*
>
> *He had none of the resources people use today to make an impact: no social media platform, no podcast audience, no clever videos and no website. He didn't even have the resources people used in the first century to make an impact: he never held political office, never ruled a nation, never led an army, and never authored a book.*
>
> *His family was insignificant. The locals suspected he was an illegitimate son, his mother was a poor peasant woman and his father couldn't afford much. Jesus didn't receive an expensive education, never married, never had children, never owned a home of his own, and didn't possess much more than the clothes on his back.*
>
> *As an adult his own brother was suspicious of his ministry, a work that ended after three short years. Public opinion turned*

against him, most of his followers abandoned him, one disciple betrayed him, and another denied him. He was rejected by the religious, hunted by the powerful, mocked and unjustly persecuted by his enemies. He suffered an unfair trial, was publicly humiliated, brutally beaten and unduly executed in the most horrific way. Even then, the few followers who remained had to borrow a grave to bury him. Yet this is the man who changed history. . . .

Implications for Human Flourishing

So maybe you *believe* the Christian story and/or *believe* in God but belief is not what God is asking of you. Even Satan believes in God (James 2:19). God is asking you to respond, to put your entire *trust* in Him. That means you no longer live for yourself and what this world expects of you but you make God the Lord of your life. Not the copilot as bumper stickers like to say. It won't be all butterflies and rainbows. Jesus never promised "your best life now" as misguided preachers like to advertise. The world is still full of evil and difficulties due to fallen humans but with God as your guide you will have a solid and unshakeable foundation that will bring peace and purpose. If you embrace this way of life particularly one that revolves around a Bible-teaching church, being of service, and growing in your faith (understanding of God and of reality) the science-based ideas for physical and mental health will make so much more sense and be easier to put into practice.

So while it is nice to live a long and healthy life here on earth unencumbered by health issues, what is far more important is what happens when you die as we all will die eventually. You can certainly wait to embrace God on your death bed and if genuine, you will be welcomed, but this shouldn't be a decision you put off. None of us know the date and time we will take our last breath. Eternity is not worth risking. Besides, as the science is now able to show us, having the right worldview that corresponds to reality is simply good for your health. You won't succumb to the destructive emotion of fear, particularly fear of germs or other humans, no matter the latest shenanigans of governments or authorities. You will be firm in your full knowledge of the truth that God is in charge, and nothing is a surprise to Him. You'll rely on your God-given intuition and critical thinking skills to know what is best for you and your family. You'll understand how to interact with this world and the other living things God has provided to nourish and sustain us. You'll feel a love for all of humanity, recognize your need for human company and gladly embrace the rich tapestry of differences and opinions. In short, you will experience a level of human flourishing that only comes when you are walking with God.

APPENDIX D

Further Reading

The most important takeaway I hope you have learned from this book is that your health is in your hands and your hands alone. You MUST educate yourself in order to make the best decisions. Critical thinking requires data, information, knowledge. I deliberately wanted to give you the big picture—the wood instead of the trees. This breadth was needed for a better understanding. It was important to teach you to fish. Now you need to dig into those aspects of health and healthcare that interest or concern you the most or are most relevant to your current situation. I've provided a small selection of books that expand on various topics I had covered chapter by chapter. There are many more. I don't agree with everything in these books, but they are a good place to start.

Chapter 1: The Human Eyeball

J. Warner Wallace. *God's Crime Scene: A Cold-Case Detective Examines the Evidence for a Divinely Created Universe* (David C Cook, 2015).

Stanley Rosenberg. *Accessing the Healing Power of the Vagus Nerve: Self-help Exercises for Anxiety, Depression, Trauma, and Autism* (North Atlantic, 2017).

Chapter 2: Medicine for the Soul

Richard Gordon. *The Alarming History of Medicine* (St. Martin's Press, 1994).

Paul Starr. *The Social Transformation of American Medicine: The Rise of a Sovereign Profession & the Making of a Vast Industry* (Basic Books, 2017).

Melody Petersen. *Our Daily Meds: How the Pharmaceutical Companies Transformed Themselves into Slick Marketing Machines and Hooked the Nation on Prescription Drugs* (Picador, 2009).

Andrew Weil, MD. *Health and Healing: The Philosophy of Integrative Medicine and Optimum Health* (Houghton Mifflin Harcourt, 2004).

Dana Ullman, MPH. *The Homeopathic Revolutio: Why Famous People and Cultural Heroes Choose Homeopathy* (North Atlantic, 2007).

Eric Zielinski, DC. *The Healing Power of Essential Oils* (Harmony, 2018).

Jeffrey S. Bland PhD. *The Disease Delusion* (HarperCollins, 2014).

Chapter 3: Don't Blame Grandpa

Dan Buettner. *The Blue Zones: 9 Lessons for Living Longer from the People Who've Lived the Longest* (National Geographic, 2012).

Robynne Chutkan, MD. *The Microbiome Solution: A Radical New Way to Heal Your Body from the Inside Out* (Penguin Random House, 2015).

Matthew Walker. *Why We Sleep: The New Science of Sleep and Dreams* (Penguin, 2017).

Chapter 4: A Toxic Planet

Stephanie Seneff, PhD. *Toxic Legacy: How the Weedkiller Glyphosate is Destroying Our Health and the Environment* (Chelsea Green, 2021).

Joseph Mercola, DO. *EMF*d: 5G, Wi-Fi, and Cell-Phones: Hidden Harms and How to Protect Yourself* (Hay House, 2020).

Chapter 5: A Body Needs Nourishment

Mark Hyman, MD. *Food: What the Heck Shall I Eat?* (Little, Brown & Company, 2018).

F. Batmanghelidj, MD. *Your Body's Many Cries for Water: You Are Not Sick, You Are Thirsty! Don't Treat Thirst With Medications* (Global Health Solutions, 1997).

Michael Pollan. *The Omnivore's Dilemma: A Natural History of Four Meals* (Penguin, 2006).

Chapter 6: It's Flu Season Again

Robert F. Kennedy Jr. *The Real Anthony Fauci: Bill Gates, Big Pharma, and the Global War on Democracy and Public Health* (Skyhorse, 2020).

Thomas E. Levy MD, JD. *Rapid Virus Recovery: No Need to Live in Fear* (MedFox, 2021).

Thomas E. Levy MD, JD. *Curing the Incurable: Vitamin C, Infectious Diseases, and Toxins* (MedFox, 2011).

Ann Louise Gittleman PhD, CNS. *Guess What Came to Dinner? Parasites and Your Health* (Avery, 2001).

Suzanne Humphries, MD, and Roman Bystrianyk. *Dissolving Illusions: Disease, Vaccines, and the Forgotten History* (2015).

Anonymous. *Turtles All the Way Down: Vaccine Science and Myth* (Skyhorse, 2018).

Brian Hooker, PhD, and Robert F. Kennedy Jr. *Vax-Unvax: Let the Science Speak* (Skyhorse, 2023).

Ronnie Cummins and Joseph Mercola DO. *The Truth About COVID-19: Exposing the Great Reset, Lockdowns, Vaccine Passports, and the New Normal* (Florida Health, 2021).

Colleen Huber, NMD. *Neither Safe Nor Effective: The Evidence Against the Covid Vaccines* (2022).

Pierre Kory, MD, and Jenna McCarthy. *The War on Ivermectin: The Medicine That Saved Millions and Could Have Ended the Pandemic* (Skyhorse, 2023).

Chapter 7: Shedding the Disease

Edward Dowd. *"Cause Unknown" The Epidemic of Sudden Deaths in 2021 and 2022* (Skyhorse, 2023).

Amy Myers, MD. *The Autoimmune Solution* (HarperCollins, 2015).

Terry Wahls, MD. *The Wahls Protocol: A Radical New Way to Treat All Chronic Autoimmune Conditions Using Paleo Principles* (Avery, 2014).

Linda Elsegood. *The LDN Book: How a Little-Known Generic Drug—Low Dose Naltrexone—Could Revolutionize Treatment for Autoimmune Disease, Cancer, Autism, Depression, and More.* (Chelsea Green, 2016).

Stephen Harrod Buhner. *Healing Lyme: Natural Healing of Lyme Borreliosis and the coinfections Chlamydia and Spotted Fever Rickettsiosis* (Raven, 2015).

Mark Hyman, MD. *The Blood Sugar Solution: The UltraHealthy Program for Losing Weight, Preventing Disease, and Feeling Great Now!* (Little, Brown Spark, 2012).

Datis Kharrazian, DC, DHSc, MMSc. *Why Do I Still Have Thyroid Symptoms? When My Lab Tests Are Normal* (Elephant, 2010).

Mark Sloan. *The Cancer Industry: Crimes, Conspiracy and The Death of My Mother* (End All Disease, 2018).

Chris Wark. *Chris Beat Cancer: A Comprehensive Plan For Healing Naturally.* (Hay House, 2018).

Aseem Malhotra, MD. *A Statin Free Life: A Revolutionary Life Plan to Tackle Heart Disease—Without the Use of Statins* (Yellow Kite, 2021).

Malcolm Kendrick, MD. *The Clot Thickens: The Enduring Mystery of Heart Disease* (Columbus, 2021).

Chapter 8: Mind Your Body to Heal Your Brain

Allen Frances, MD. *Saving Normal: An Insider's Revolt against Out-of-Control Psychiatric Diagnosis, DSM-5, Big Pharma, and the Medicalization of Ordinary Life.* (William Morrow, 2014).

Bessel van der Kolk, MD. *The Body Keeps the Score: Brain, Mind and Body in the Healing of Trauma* (Penguin, 2014).

Daniel G. Amen, MD. *The End of Mental Illness* (Tyndale, 2023).

David Perlmutter, MD. *Grain Brain: The Surprising Truth About Wheat, Carbs, and Sugar—Your Brain's Silent Killers* (Little, Brown & Co, 2013).

James Nestor. *Breath: The New Science of a Lost Art* (Riverhead, 2020).

Mark Gober. *An End to Upside Down Medicine: Contagion, Viruses, and Vaccines—and Why Consciousness Is Needed for a New Paradigm of Health* (Waterside Productions, 2023).

Paul Thomas, MD and Jennifer Margulis, PhD. *The Addiction Spectrum: A Compassionate, Holistic Approach to Recovery* (HarperOne, 2018).

Chapter 9: Aging Well

Ann Louise Gittleman, PhD, CNS. *Radical Longevity: The Powerful Plan to Sharpen Your Brain, Strengthen Your Body, and Reverse the Symptoms of Aging* (Hachette Go, 2021).

Robert D. Putnam. *Bowling Alone: The Collapse and Revival of American Community* (Simon & Schuster, 2000).

Margaret Heffernan. *Willful Blindness: Why We Ignore the Obvious at Our Peril* (Bloomsbury, 2011).

Appendix C: Spiritual Addendum

Timothy R. Jennings, MD. *The God-Shaped Brain: How Changing Your View of God Transforms Your Life* (IVP, 2017).

Ray Comfort. *How to Know God Exists: Scientific Proof of God* (Bridge-Logos, 2007).

J. Warner Wallace. *Cold-Case Christianity: A Homicide Detective Investigates the Claims of the Gospels* (David C Cook, 2013).

Gregory Koukl. *The Story of Reality: How the World Began, How it Ends, and Everything Important That Happens in Between* (Zondervan, 2017).

Norman L. Geisler and Frank Turek. *I Don't Have Enough Faith to Be an Atheist* (Crossway, 2004).

Erwin W. Lutzer. *Seven Reasons Why You Can Trust the Bible* (Moody, 1998).

Marvin L. Lubenow. *Bones of Contention: A Creationist Assessment of Human Fossils* (Baker Books, 2004).

Resources

Here are a few resources to get you started with various aspects of good health covered in the book. I have tried to provide a range of ideas to suit different needs and lifestyles. I don't necessarily endorse every product or agree with everything stated on these websites, but they are a good place to start and apply your critical thinking skills to see if they are a good fit for you. They may also give you ideas for what else may be out there.

I have no financial ties to any of these companies. They are entirely my own independent recommendations. More resources, including some movies and documentaries, can be found on my website, EmmaTekstra.com.

Alternative Healthcare
- Institute for Functional Medicine. *IFM.org*. Find information and a practitioner near you.
- Personalized Lifestyle Medicine Institute. *PLMInstitute.org*.
- International Society for Orthomolecular Medicine. *ISOM.ca*. Find a practitioner and a wide range of resources.
- Homeopathic Education Services. *Homeopathic.com*. Books and courses.
- Whole Health Now. *WholeHealthNow.com*. Global homeopathy resource for professionals and patients.

- American Association of Naturopathic Physicians. *Naturopathic.org.*
- Naturopathic Medicine Institute. *NaturopathicMedicineInstitute.org.*
- Thera Wellness Solutions. *TheraWellness.us.* Purchase energy medicine device and find practitioners around the world.
- American Herbalists Guild. *AmericanHerbalistsGuild.com.* Find information and a practitioner near you.
- International Academy of Biological Dentistry and Medicine. *iabdm.org.* Find information and a practitioner near you.
- Grass Roots Labs. *GrassRootsLabs.com.* Lower-cost lab tests you can order yourself.

Detoxification

- Environmental Working Group. *EWG.org.* Consumer information on products such as food, cosmetics, water, and sunscreen with helpful databases and guides.
- Center for Science in the Public Interest. *cspinet.org.* Information on additives in food and other healthy living topics.
- Campaign for Safe Cosmetics. *SafeCosmetics.org.* Advocacy and information.
- Shield Your Body. *ShieldYourBody.com.* Products to help protect you from EMFs.
- Aquasana. *aquasana.com.* Water filtration products including whole house/business.
- Multipure. *multipure.com.* Smaller water filters.
- IQair. *iqair.com.* Information and products dedicated to air pollution, monitoring, and purification.
- Touchstone Essentials. *thegoodinside.com.* Zeolites products for cellular and whole-body detox particularly from heavy metals.

Faith

- Focal Point Ministries. *FocalPointMinistries.org*. Find sermons, explanations, and teaching resources as well as live radio broadcasts.
- Answers in Genesis. *AnswersinGenesis.org*. Find explanations for many scientific questions.
- Cold Case Christianity. *ColdCaseChristianity.com*. Evidence and resources for the Christian faith as told through the eyes of a police detective.

Food

- Good Food on a Tight Budget Guide. *https://www.ewg.org/goodfood/*.
- Cornucopia Institute. *Cornucopia.org*. Nonprofit watchdog organization monitoring organic brands in the marketplace.
- Food Matters. *FoodMatters.com*. Great recipes and inspiration. Sign up for their weekly newsletter.
- Thrive Market. *thrivemarket.com*. Online store with healthier brands at great prices with ability to search by diet. Make sure to read food labels carefully as not everything is healthy.
- Wild Fork Foods. *wildforkfoods.com*. Healthy animal proteins flash frozen with home delivery. Not everything is organic, grass-fed, or wild caught, so shop carefully.
- Butcher Box. *butcherbox.com*. Grass-fed organic animal products straight to your door.
- Wild Pastures. *Wildpastures.com*. More grass-fed organic regeneratively farmed animal products and wild-caught seafood straight to your door.
- Paleo Valley. *PaleoValley.com*. Nutritious on-the-go snacks such as beef sticks and superfood bars as well as coffee, EVOO, and beef tallow for cooking.

- Walden Local. *waldenlocalmeat.com*. Buy in to a share of whole animals with member specials delivered locally.
- Local Harvest. *Localharvest.org*. A nonprofit directory of farms and farmers markets across the US sortable by zip code.
- Local Catch Network. *Localcatch.org*. Find fresh, local, sustainable seafood near you.
- Bluebird Grain Farms. *bluebirdgrainfarms.com*. Whole grains that are organically grown, harvested and milled on their certified organic farm including einkorn, an ancient heirloom wheat low in gluten and often suitable for those who are gluten intolerant.
- Cultured Food Life. *Culturedfoodlife.com*. Information and products to make your own fermented foods.
- Field Forest. *fieldforest.net*. Products to grow your own mushrooms.
- The Food for Everyone Foundation. *growfood.com*. Resources to grow your own food for high yield in small areas and grow-boxes.
- Sample healthier food brands available in stores:
  - Primal Kitchen sauces. *primalkitchen.com*
  - Simple Mills baked goods. *simplemills.com*
  - Tanka bars and snacks. *tankabar.com*
  - Bulletproof coffee. *bulletproof.com*
  - Purity Coffee. *puritycoffee.com*
  - Force of Nature meat products. *forceofnature.com*
  - EPIC meat bars and snacks. *epicprovisions.com*
  - 4th & Heart ghee (clarified butter). *fourthandheart.com*
  - Go Raw sprouted seeds and snacks. *goraw.com*
  - Artisana nut butters. *artisanaorganics.com*
  - Siete tortillas and chips. *sietefoods.com*

- Safe Catch canned seafood. *safecatch.com*
- Wild Planet canned seafood, beef, and chicken. *wildplanetfoods.com*

Herbs and Botanicals

- Kauai Farmacy. *KauaiFarmacy.com*
- Mountain Rose Herbs. *MountainRoseHerbs.com*
- Starwest Botanicals. *Starwest-Botanicals.com*
- Pacific Botanicals. *PacificBotanicals.com*
- Napier's Dispensary. *Napiers.net*

Household Products

- Xtrema. *xtrema.com*. Pure ceramic pots and pans.
- Truly Free. *trulyfreehome.com*. Cleaning products without toxic chemicals.
- Relax Far Infrared. *relaxsaunas.com*. Saunas and heat lamps.

Information Sources

- PubMed. *pubmed.ncbi.nlm.nih.gov*. Biomedical studies and research published by life sciences journals across the world.
- Dr. Talks. *drtalks.com*. Information and webinars on a wide range of health, wellness, and medical topics.
- Choosing Wisely initiative. *choosingwisely.org*. Resources to support decision-making on tests and outpatient procedures.
- Weston A. Price Foundation. *westonaprice.org*. Diet and nutrition information.
- GreenMedInfo. *greenmedinfo.com*. Evidence-based natural medicine information.
- Children's Health Defense. *childrenshealthdefense.org*. Latest information on toxins and effects; particularly how to protect our children.

- Mercola. *mercola.com*. Articles on holistic health and related matters.
- World Council for Health. *worldcouncilforhealth.org*. Global coalition of health-focused (rather than industry-focused) organizations.
- National Vaccine Information Center. *NVIC.org*. Accurate information on all types of vaccines.

Mental Health

- The Tapping Solution. *thetappingsolution.com*. App with tapping exercises (EFT, Emotional Freedom Technique).
- Wim Hof Method. *wimhofmethod.com*. Information and courses on breathing and other techniques.
- Sharp Again Naturally. *sharpagain.org*. Dementia treatment and support.
- reCODE Protocol. *apollohealthco.com/solution/recode/*. Alzheimer's treatment.
- EMDR Institute. *EMDR.com*. Information and to find a practitioner.
- Multidisciplinary Association for Psychedelic Studies. *MAPS .org*. Information and resources regarding use of psychedelics to heal mental illness.
- The Stellate Institute. *thestellateinstitute.com*. Stellate ganglion block (SGB) treatment for trauma.
- Stella Center. *Stellacenter.com*. SGB and other treatments for trauma and serious mental health challenges.

Personal Care Products

- AnnMarie Skincare. *annmariegianni.com*
- Purity Woods. *puritywoods.com*.
- Babo Botanicals. *babobotanicals.com*
- Dr. Bronner. *drbronner.com*
- Xlear brands. *Xlear.com*

Solutions to Chronic Health Conditions

- LDN Research Trust. *ldnresearchtrust.org.* Information on a wide range of conditions low-dose naltrexone is effective for. Find a prescribing doctor and pharmacy near you.
- International Lyme and Associated Diseases Organization. *ilads.org.*
- IGeneX. *igenex.com.* Testing for tick-borne infections.
- RealTime Labs. *realtimelab.com.* Specialty tests available worldwide for mycotoxins, and environmental pollutants. Marketed as "testing for the undiagnosed."
- Surviving Mold. *survivingmold.com.* Resources and to find a practitioner.
- MS Hope. *MShope.com.* Natural treatment for multiple sclerosis.
- The Gerson Institute. *gerson.org.* Natural cancer therapy.
- Chris Beat Cancer. *chrisbeatcancer.com.* Healing cancer online coaching program.
- The Doctor's Farmacy. *drhyman.com/blog/category/podcasts/* Information and guidance from leading functional medicine specialist Dr. Mark Hyman.

Supplements

- Fullscript. *Fullscript.com.* Supplement dispensing platform enabling access to high-quality supplements from leading brands. May need to be attached to a practitioner's account.
- iHerb. *iherb.com.* Curated selection of supplements and other wellness products from around the world.
- Sample quality brands with broad range of products widely available:
  - Designs for Health. *designsforhealth.com*
  - Garden of Life. *gardenoflife.com*

- Jarrow Formulas. *jarrow.com*
- Pure Encapsulations. *pureencapsultions.com*
- Thorne Research. *thorne.com*
- Global Healing Center. *globalhealing.com*. Specialty products from Dr. Edward Group.
- Quicksilver Scientific. *quicksilverscientific.com*. Specialty products from Dr. Christopher Shade. Particularly through liposomal delivery for superior absorption.
- True Hope Nutritional Support. *truehope.com*. Micronutrient supplements focused on brain health.
- Microbiome Labs. *microbiomelabs.com*. Specialty products focused on microbiome health.
- Four Sigmatic. *foursigmatic.com*. Protein powder and supplements focused on the power of mushrooms.
- Real Mushrooms. *realmushrooms.com*. Organic mushroom supplements.
- Beekeeper's Naturals. *beekeepersnaturals.com*. Specialty products from bees.

Notes

Chapter 1: The Human Eyeball

[1] Pierre Kory, MD et al. Review of the Emerging Evidence Demonstrating the Efficacy of Ivermectin in the Prophylaxis and Treatment of Covid-19. https://covid19criticalcare.com/wp-content/uploads/2022/11/FLCCC-Ivermectin -in-the-prophylaxis-and-treatment-of-COVID-19.pdf.

[2] Samuele Zilioli et al. Endocrine and immunomodulatory effects of social isolation and loneliness across adulthood. *Psychoneuroendocrinology*, Volume 128, 2021, https://doi.org/10.1016/j.psyneuen.2021.105194.

[3] Cho KS, et al. "Terpenes from Forests and Human Health," *Toxicology Research*. 2017 Apr;33(2):97–106. Doi: 10.5487/TR.2017.33.2.097. Epub 2017 Apr 15. Accessed at https://www.ncbi.nlm.nih.gov/pmc/articles/PMC 5402865/.

[4] Hansen MM, et al. Shinrin-Yoku (Forest Bathing) and Nature Therapy: A State-of-the-Art Review. *International Journal of Environmental Research and Public Health,* 2017 Jul 28;14(8):851. Doi: 10.3390/ijerph14080851. Accessed at https://pubmed.ncbi.nlm.nih.gov/28788101/. Also see Hunter MaryCarol R., et al. "Urban Nature Experiences Reduce Stress in the Context of Daily Life Based on Salivary Biomarkers," *Frontiers in Psychology*, vol. 10, 2019. Accessed at https://www.frontiersin.org/articles/10.3389/fpsyg .2019.00722.

[5] Yau KK, Loke AY. Effects of forest bathing on pre-hypertensive and hypertensive adults: a review of the literature. *Environmental Health and Preventive Medicine*, 2020 Jun 22;25(1):23. Doi: 10.1186/s12199–020-00856–7.Accessed at https://www.ncbi.nlm.nih.gov/pmc/articles/PMC7310560/.

[6] Koh GC, et al. Tuberculosis incidence correlates with sunshine: an ecological 28-year time series study. *PloS One*, 2013;8(3):e57752. Doi: 10.1371/journal .pone.0057752. Epub 2013 Mar 6. Accessed at https://www.ncbi.nlm.nih .gov/pmc/articles/PMC3590299/.

7   McDonnell SL, et al. (2018) Breast cancer risk markedly lower with serum
    25- hydroxyvitamin D concentrations >60 vs <20 ng/ml (150 vs 50 nmol/L):
    Pooled analysis of two randomized trials and a prospective cohort. Accessed at
    https://www.grassrootshealth.net/wp-content/uploads/2018/08/McDonnell
    -2018-breast-cancer-GRH.pdf.

8   Holick MF, Chen TC. Vitamin D deficiency: a worldwide problem with
    health consequences. *The American Journal of Clinical Nutrituion*, 2008
    Apr;87(4):1080S-6S. doi: 10.1093/ajcn/87.4.1080S. Accessed at https:
    //pubmed.ncbi.nlm.nih.gov/18400738/.

9   Blowing Smoke: Vintage Ads of Doctors Endorsing Tobacco, CBS News.
    https://www.cbsnews.com/pictures/blowing-smoke-vintage-ads-of-doctors
    -endorsing-tobacco/3/.

10 Shah K, et al. Does vitamin D supplementation reduce COVID-19 severity?:
    a systematic review. *QJM*, 2022 Oct 25;115(10):665–672. Doi: 10.1093
    /qjmed/hcac040. PMID: 35166850; Accessed at https://pubmed.ncbi.nlm
    .nih.gov/35166850/.

11 Francis S. Collins, *The Language of God: A Scientist Presents Evidence for Belief,*
    (Free Press, 2006).

12 NIH: The Human Genome Project. See a history at https://www.genome
    .gov/human-genome-project.

13 Sender R, et al. (2016) Revised Estimates for the Number of Human and
    Bacteria Cells in the Body. *PloS Biology*, 14(8): e1002533. Accessed at https:
    //doi.org/10.1371/journal.pbio.1002533.

14 Ibid.

15 Simon, JC., et al. Host-microbiota interactions: from holobiont theory to
    analysis. *Microbiome*, 7, 5 (2019). https://doi.org/10.1186/s40168–019-0619–4
    https://microbiomejournal.biomedcentral.com/articles/10.1186/s40168
    –019-0619–4.

16 Charles Darwin, *On the Origin of Species* (London: J.M. Dent & Sons Ltd,
    1971) p. 167.

17 White, M.P., et al. Spending at least 120 minutes a week in nature is associated
    with good health and wellbeing. *Scientific Reports*, 9, 7730 (2019). https://doi
    .org/10.1038/s41598–019-44097–3 https://www.nature.com/articles/s41598
    –019-44097–3.

18 Totolici G, et al. The role of vitamin D in the onset and progression of
    diabetic retinopathy. *Romanian Journal of Ophthalmology*, 2022 Jul–
    Sep;66(3):214–218. Doi: 10.22336/rjo.2022.42. https://www.ncbi.nlm.nih
    .gov/pmc/articles/PMC9585492/.

19 Boivin DB, et al. Disturbance of the Circadian System in Shift Work and
    Its Health Impact. *Journal of Biology Rhythms*, 2022 Feb;37(1):3–28. Doi:
    10.1177/07487304211064218. Epub 2021 Dec 30. Accessed at: https:
    //www.ncbi.nlm.nih.gov/pmc/articles/PMC8832572/.

20 NIH: SPARC program overview and links can be found at https://common
fund.nih.gov/sparc.

Chapter 2: Medicine for the Soul

1 Various statistics about the healthcare and pharmaceutical industries can
be viewed at Statista.com. Start here: https://www.statista.com/topics/6701
/health-expenditures-in-the-us/#topicOverview.

2 Ibid.

3 Greene JA, Herzberg D. Hidden in Plain Sight; Marketing Prescription Drugs
to Consumers in the Twentieth Century. *American Journal of Public Health*,
2010 May;100(5):793–803. Doi: 10.2105/AJPH.2009.181255. Epub 2010
Mar 18. https://www.ncbi.nlm.nih.gov/pmc/articles/PMC2853635/. Also
see Almasi EA, Stafford RS, Kravitz RL, Mansfield PR. What are the public
health effects of direct-to-consumer drug advertising? *PloS Medicine*, 2006
Mar;3(3):e145. Doi: 10.1371/journal.pmed.0030145. Epub 2006 Mar 28.
https://www.ncbi.nlm.nih.gov/pmc/articles/PMC1420390/.

4 Tyagi, U., Barwal, K.C. Ignac Semmelweis—Father of Hand Hygiene. *Indian
Journal of Surgery*, 82, 276–277 (2020). https://doi.org/10.1007/s12262–
020-02386–6. There is also a great narrative on Dr. Semmelweis in the book
Dissolving Illusions, Disease, Vaccines and the Forgotten History by Suzanne
Humphries and Roman Bystrianyk.

5 For a detailed history of the medical profession in the US, see the extensive
history book by sociologist Paul Starr *The Social Transformation of American
Medicine: The Rise of a Sovereign Profession and the Making of a Vast Industry,*
(Basic Books, 2017).

6 Chernow R. *Titan: The Life of John D. Rockefeller, Sr.* New York, NY (Random
House Publishing, 1998).

7 A. Flexner, Medical Education in the United States and Canada. The Carnegie
Foundation for the Advancement of Teaching, Bulletin no. 4, (1910) https:
//www.ncbi.nlm.nih.gov/pmc/articles/PMC2567554/pdf/12163926.pdf.

8 The repercussions of the Flexner report continue to reverberate today. For
example, see Johnson C, Green B. 100 years after the Flexner report: reflections
on its influence on chiropractic education. *Journal of Chiropractic Education*,
2010 Fall;24(2):145–52. Doi: 10.7899/1042–5055-24.2.145. https://www
.ncbi.nlm.nih.gov/pmc/articles/PMC2967338/. Also, Stahnisch FW, Verhoef
M. The Flexner report of 1910 and its impact on complementary and
alternative medicine and psychiatry in north America in the 20th century.
Evidence-Based Complementary Alternative Medicine, 2012;2012:647896.
Doi: 10.1155/2012/647896. Epub 2012 Dec 26. https://www.ncbi.nlm.nih
.gov/pmc/articles/PMC3543812/.

9   The concept of medical freedom where patients are free to choose the type of care they receive is not new. The National League for Medical Freedom was actually founded a hundred years ago. We can learn much from its history. Petrina S. Medical Liberty: Drugless Healers Confront Allopathic Doctors, 1910–1931. *Journal of Medical Humanities*, 2008;29:205–230. https://link .springer.com/article/10.1007/s10912–008-9063–3.

10 Paul Starr, *The Social Transformation of American Medicine.*

11 For a detailed description of living conditions and how hygiene was the biggest single factor in reducing infectious disease, read *Dissolving Illusions, Disease, Vaccines and the Forgotten History* by Suzanne Humphries and Roman Bystrianyk.

12 Interestingly, there have been no new classes of antibiotics developed since the 1980s. We'll explore infectious disease in detail in Chapter 6.

13 Birn AE, Fee E. The Rockefeller Foundation and the International Health Agenda. *The Lancet*, 11 May 2013. https://www.thelancet.com/journals /lancet/article/PIIS0140–6736(13)61013–2/fulltext.

14 Birn AE. Backstage: the relationship between the Rockefeller Foundation and the World Health Organization, Part I: 1940s–1960s. *Public Health*, 2014 Feb;128(2):129–40 https://www.sciencedirect.com/science/article/abs/pii /S003335061300396X?via%3Dihub.

15 Bealle M. *The Drug Story; A Factological History of America's $10,000,000,000 Drug Cartel: Its Methods, Operations, Hidden Ownership, Profits and Terrific Impact on the Health of the American People.* (Columbia Publishing Company, 1949) While out of print it can be viewed at various online sources such as https://babel.hathitrust.org/cgi/pt?id=uc1.$b39371&seq=16.

16 I also recommend you watch *The True History of Medicine: How Healthcare Became Sickcare,* a full-length documentary written and narrated by Dr. Rick Kirschner. It is available for free at https://talknatural.com/documentary.html.

17 Chernow R. *Titan: The Life of John D. Rockefeller, Sr.*

18 Wilson D, Harvard Medical School in Ethics Quandry. *New York Times*, March 2, 2009. Accessed at https://perfumechowk.blogspot.com/2009/03 /harvard-medical-school-in-ethics.html.

19 As an example a summary of the MD path at Harvard Medical School can be reviewed at https://meded.hms.harvard.edu/pathways.

20 Mindrum, Michael R. Time for another revolution? The Flexner Report in historic context, reflections on our profession. *Coronary Artery Disease*, 17(5):p 477–481, August 2006.

21 One example article of many is Schofferman J. The medical-industrial complex, professional medical associations, and continuing medical education. *Pain Medicine*, 2011 Dec;12(12):1713–9. Doi: 10.1111/j.1526–4637.2011 .01282.x. Epub 2011 Dec 6. PMID: 22145759. Another is an essay appearing

in the *British Medical Journal* in 2021: Fugh-Berman A. Industry-funded medical education is always promotion—an essay by Adriane Fugh-Berman. *British Medical* Journal 2021; 373 :n1273 doi:10.1136/bmj.n1273.

22 For a more thorough discussion of the current pharmaceutical industry read Melody Petersen's *Our Daily Meds; How the Pharmaceutical Companies Transformed Themselves into Slick Marketing Machines and Hooked the Nation of Prescription Drugs.* (Picador, 2009).

23 Steve Connor, Glaxo Chief: Our Drugs Do Not Work on Most Patients,. *The Independent,* 8 Dec 2003. https://www.independent.co.uk/news/science/glaxo-chief-our-drugs-do-not-work-on-most-patients-5508670.html. Web 2023 May 23.

24 Gøtzsche PC. Our prescription drugs kill us in large numbers. *Pol Arch Med Wewn,* 2014;124(11):628–34. Doi: 10.20452/pamw.2503. Epub 2014 Oct 30. Accessed at https://pubmed.ncbi.nlm.nih.gov/25355584/.

25 Budnitz DS, Shehab N, Lovegrove MC, Geller AI, Lind JN, Pollock DA. US Emergency Department Visits Attributed to Medication Harms, 2017–2019, *JAMA,* 2021 Oct 5;326(13):1299–1309. Doi: 10.1001/jama.2021.13844. PMID: 34609453; PMCID: PMC8493432. https://pubmed.ncbi.nlm.nih.gov/34609453/.

26 Andreas Kortenkamp, Martin Scholze, Sibylle Ermler, Lærke Priskorn, Niels Jørgensen, Anna-Maria Andersson, Hanne Frederiksen. Combined exposures to bisphenols, polychlorinated dioxins, paracetamol, and phthalates as drivers of deteriorating semen quality. *Environment International,* 2022, 107322, ISSN 0160–4120, https://doi.org/10.1016/j.envint.2022.107322.

27 Patel E, Jones JP 3rd, Bono-Lunn D, Kuchibhatla M, Palkar A, Cendejas Hernandez J, et al. The safety of pediatric use of paracetamol (acetaminophen): a narrative review of direct and indirect evidence. *Minerva Pediatrics,* 2022 Jul 13. DOI: 10.23736/S2724–5276.22.06932–4. https://pubmed.ncbi.nlm.nih.gov/35822581/.

28 Vioxx as well as Celebrex are used as a case in point to emphasize the conflict of interest in setting clinical practice guidelines in John Abramson et al. Effect of Conflict of Interest on Biomedical Research and Clinical Practice Guidelines: Can We Trust the Evidence in Evidence-Based Medicine? *The Journal of the American Board of Family Practice,* Sep 2005, 18 (5) 414–418; DOI: 10.3122/jabfm.18.5.414. https://www.jabfm.org/content/18/5/414.

29 Nagai J, Ishikawa Y. Analysis of anticholinergic adverse effects using two large databases: The US Food and Drug Administration Adverse Event Reporting System database and the Japanese Adverse Drug Event Report database. *PloS One,* 2021 Dec 2;16(12):e0260980. Doi: 10.1371/journal.pone.0260980. PMID: 34855908; PMCID: PMC8638968.

30 Gray SL, Anderson ML, Dublin S, et al. Cumulative Use of Strong Anticholinergics and Incident Dementia: A Prospective Cohort Study. *JAMA Intern Med,* 2015;175(3):401–407. Doi:10.1001/jamainternmed.2014.7663.

31 For a broader discussion on the myths of cholesterol and statin use please see my blog post at https://emmatekstra.com/blog/the-stubborn-myth-of -statins-and-cholesterol/.

32 For a discussion of drug-nutrient interactions with helpful tables documenting known nutrient depletions by different categories of drugs see Karadima V, Kraniotou C, Bellos G, Tsangaris GT. Drug-micronutrient interactions: food for thought and thought for action. *EPMA Journal,* 2016 May 12;7(1):10. Doi: 10.1186/s13167–016-0059–1. PMID: 27182287; PMCID: PMC4866329.

33 You can follow the FDA's investigation into NAC at https://www.fda.gov /food/cfsan-constituent-updates/fda-releases-final-guidance-enforcement -discretion-certain-nac-products.

34 For those interested in learning more about ICD-11 go to https://www.who .int/classifications/classification-of-diseases.

35 WHO Global Report on Traditional and Complementary Medicine 2019 accessed at https://iris.who.int/bitstream/handle/10665/312342/97892415 15436-eng.pdf?sequence=1&isAllowed=y.

36 Nasri H, Baradaran A, Shirzad H, Rafieian-Kopaei M. New concepts in nutraceuticals as alternative for pharmaceuticals. *Int J Prev Med.* 2014 Dec;5(12):1487–99. PMID: 25709784; PMCID: PMC4336979.

37 For a full discussion on the dangers of calcium supplementation and intake of dairy foods read Dr. Thomas Levy's book *Death by Calcium; Proof of the Toxic Effects of Dairy and Calcium Supplements* (Medfox Publishing 2003).

38 See Francis Brinker's excellent compendium called *Herbal Contraindications & Drug Interactions* (Eclectic Medical Publications, 2010).

39 Cohen MM. Tulsi—Ocimum sanctum: A herb for all reasons. *Journal of Ayurveda and Integrative Medicine,* 2014 Oct-Dec;5(4):251–9. Doi: 10.4103/0975–9476.146554. https://pubmed.ncbi.nlm.nih.gov/25624701/.

40 Riaz G, et al. A review on phytochemistry and therapeutic uses of Hibiscus sabdariffa L. *Biomedicine & Pharmacotherapy,* 2018 Jun;102:575–586. Doi: 10.1016/j.biopha.2018.03.023. Epub 2018 Apr 5. https://pubmed.ncbi.nlm .nih.gov/29597091/.

41 Pittler MH, Guo R, Ernst E. Hawthorn extract for treating chronic heart failure. *Cochrane Database Syst Rev,* 2008 Jan 23;(1):CD005312. Doi: 10. 1002/14651858.CD005312.pub2. PMID: 18254076.

42 Darooghegi Mofrad M, Milajerdi A, Koohdani F, Surkan PJ, Azadbakht L. Garlic Supplementation Reduces Circulating C-reactive Protein, Tumor Necrosis Factor, and Interleukin-6 in Adults: A Systematic Review and Meta-

analysis of Randomized Controlled Trials. *The Journal of Nutrition*, 2019 Apr 1;149(4):605–618. Doi: 10.1093/jn/nxy310. PMID: 30949665.

43 Percival SS, Vanden Heuvel JP, Nieves CJ, Montero C, Migliaccio AJ, Meadors J. Bioavailability of herbs and spices in humans as determined by ex vivo inflammatory suppression and DNA strand breaks. *Journal of American College of Nutrition*, 2012 Aug;31(4):288–94. Doi: 10.1080/07315724.2012.10720438. PMID: 23378457.

44 Efferth T, et al. Anti-inflammatory and anti-cancer activities of frankincense: Targets, treatments and toxicities. *Seminars in Cancer Biology*, 2022 May; 80:39–57. Doi: 10.1016/j.semcancer.2020.01.015. Epub 2020 Feb 4. https://pubmed.ncbi.nlm.nih.gov/32027979/.

45 While the scientific literature is light on these types of therapies, Dr. Luc Montagnier, Nobel Prize–winning scientist and virologist best known for discovering the human immunodeficiency virus (HIV), wrote a helpful paper on the electromagnetic frequencies emitted by the DNA of bacteria and viruses. See Montagnier, L., Aïssa, J., Ferris, S. et al. Electromagnetic signals are produced by aqueous nanostructures derived from bacterial DNA sequences. *Interdisciplinary Sciences—Computer Life Sciences*, 1, 81–90 (2009). https://doi.org/10.1007/s12539-009-0036-7. Also see a related paper available in full at https://arxiv.org/PS_cache/arxiv/pdf/1012/1012.5166v1.pdf.

46 For more information on Functional Medicine and to find a practitioner see The Institute for Functional Medicine at IFM.org.

Chapter 3: Don't Blame Grandpa

1 For an interesting overview of the modern science of epigenetics, see Weinhold B. Epigenetics: The Science of Change. *Environmental Health Perspectives*. 2006; 114:A160-A167 at https://ehp.niehs.nih.gov/doi/10.1289/ehp.114-a160.

2 T. Colin Campbell, PhD and Thomas M. Campbell II, MD, *The China Study; Startling Implications for Diet, Weight Loss and Long-Term Health* (BenBella Books, 2006). Also visit www.nutritionstudies.org.

3 Rosenthal T. The effect of migration on hypertension and other cardiovascular risk factors: a review. *Journal of the American Society of Hypertension*, 2014 Mar;8(3):171–91. doi: 10.1016/j.jash.2013.12.007. Epub 2014 Jan 2. https://pubmed.ncbi.nlm.nih.gov/24524887/.

4 Malcolm Gladwell, *Outliers: The Story of Success* (Little, Brown & Company, 2008).

5 You can read about their investigation in the book *The Power of Clan: Influence of Human Relationships on Heart Disease* by Stewart Wolf and John G. Bruhn (Routledge, 1998).

6 There is actually a whole school of science around a sixth sense that might be called consciousness or intuition. We'll look at this briefly in Chapter 8.

You could explore the books of Mark Gober such as *An End to Upside Down Medicine: Contagion, Viruses and Vaccines, and why Consciousness is Needed for a New Paradigm of Health.*

[7]   Rinninella, E.; Raoul, P.; Cintoni, M.; Franceschi, F.; Miggiano, G.A.D.; Gasbarrini, A.; Mele, M.C. What is the Healthy Gut Microbiota Composition? A Changing Ecosystem across Age, Environment, Diet, and Diseases. *Microorganisms*, 2019, 7, 14. https://doi.org/10.3390/microorganisms7010014.

[8]   Maier L, Pruteanu M, Kuhn M, Zeller G, Telzerow A, Anderson EE, Brochado AR, Fernandez KC, Dose H, Mori H, Patil KR, Bork P, Typas A. Extensive impact of non-antibiotic drugs on human gut bacteria. *Nature*, 2018 Mar 29;555(7698):623–628. doi: 10.1038/nature25979. Epub 2018 Mar 19. PMID: 29555994; PMCID: PMC6108420.

[9]   Susan Adams and Will Yakowicz, Drugs from Bugs; Why Gates, Zuck and Benioff Think the Next Blockbusters Will Come from Inside Your Gut. *Forbes Magazine*, Feb 2020. Accessed at https://www.forbes.com/sites /susanadams/2020/02/07/drugs-from-bugs-why-gates-zuck-and-benioff -think-the-next-blockbusters-will-come-from-inside-your-gut/.

[10] For a sense of the sheer volume of information that is currently being generated on the different types of microorganisms that make up our microbiome and their impact on health and disease a good place to start is the MicroPhenoDB database. This article provides a helpful overview. Guocai Yao, Wenliang Zhang, Minglei Yang, Huan Yang, Jianbo Wang, Haiyue Zhang, Lai Wei, Zhi Xie, Weizhong Li, MicroPhenoDB Associates Metagenomic Data with Pathogenic Microbes, Microbial Core Genes, and Human Disease Phenotypes, *Genomics, Proteomics & Bioinformatics*, Volume 18, Issue 6, 2020, Pages 760–772, ISSN 1672–0229, https://doi.org/10.1016/j.gpb.2020.11.001. (https:// www.sciencedirect.com/science/article/pii/S1672022920301698).

[11] Dan Buettner, *The Blue Zones: 9 Lessons for Living Longer from the People Who've Lived the Longest* (National Geographic, 2012). You should also check out https://www.bluezones.com/.

[12] Woolf SH, Schoomaker H. Life Expectancy and Mortality Rates in the United States, 1959–2017. *JAMA*, 2019;322(20):1996–2016. doi:10.1001 /jama.2019.16932.

[13] Xu JQ, Murphy SL, Kochanek KD, Arias E. Mortality in the United States, 2021. NCHS Data Brief, no 456. Hyattsville, MD: National Center for Health Statistics. 2022. DOI: https://dx.doi.org/10.15620/cdc:122516.

[14] These are statistics compiled by the World Health Organization in early 2022 but is based on 2019 data. For more details go to https://www.who.int/data /gho/data/themes/topics/indicator-groups/indicator-group-details/GHO /life-expectancy-and-healthy-life-expectancy.

15 A recent study of the entire Ancestry.com database put the heritability of longevity at a mere 7%: your genetic makeup is 7% of a factor in your ultimate longevity. See J Graham Ruby and others, Estimates of the Heritability of Human Longevity Are Substantially Inflated Due to Assortative Mating. *Genetics*, Volume 210, Issue 3, 1 November 2018, Pages 1109–1124, https://doi.org/10.1534/genetics.118.301613.

16 You can read a brief summary of each location (with photos) at https://www.bluezones.com/exploration/. There is also a new docuseries released in 2023 called *Live to 100: Secrets of the Blue Zones.*

17 This study appeared in *The Lancet* and can be reviewed at https://www.thelancet.com/journals/lancet/article/PIIS0140–6736(12)61031–9/fulltext. Or https://doi.org/10.1016/S0140–6736(12)61031–9.

18 See the study in *Frontiers of Nutrition* (Volume 8, 2021) by Clauss Matthieu, Gérard Philippe, Mosca Alexis, Leclerc Marion Interplay*; Between Exercise and Gut Microbiome in the Context of Human Health and Performance* at https://www.frontiersin.org/articles/10.3389/fnut.2021.637010. Or https://doi.org/10.3389/fnut.2021.637010. Other interesting articles on this topic include Himbert C, Stephens WZ, Gigic B, Hardikar S, Holowatyj AN, Lin T, Ose J, Swanson E, Ashworth A, Warby CA, Peoples AR, Nix D, Jedrzkiewicz J, Bronner M, Pickron B, Scaife C, Cohan JN, Schrotz-King P, Habermann N, Boehm J, Hullar M, Figueiredo JC, Toriola AT, Siegel EM, Li CI, Ulrich AB, Shibata D, Boucher K, Huang LC, Schneider M, Round JL, Ulrich CM. Differences in the gut microbiome by physical activity and BMI among colorectal cancer patients. *American Journal of Cancer Research*, 2022 Oct 15;12(10):4789–4801. PMID: 36381318; PMCID: PMC9641409. https://www.ncbi.nlm.nih.gov/pmc/articles/PMC9641409/ And Dohnalová, L., Lundgren, P., Carty, J.R.E. et al. A microbiome-dependent gut–brain pathway regulates motivation for exercise. Nature 612, 739–747 (2022). https://doi.org/10.1038/s41586–022-05525-z.

19 For a study that actually compares the effect of sedentary behavior on longevity compared to genetic risk see Posis, A. I. B., Bellettiere, J., Salem, R. M., LaMonte, M. J., Manson, J. E., Casanova, R., LaCroix, A. Z., & Shadyab, A. H. (2023). Associations of Accelerometer-Measured Physical Activity and Sedentary Time with All-Cause Mortality by Genetic Predisposition for Longevity, *Journal of Aging and Physical Activity*, *31*(2), 265–275. Retrieved Jun 17, 2023, from https://doi.org/10.1123/japa.2022–0067.

20 Genesis 2:1–3 includes "and on the seventh day God finished his work that he had done, and he rested on the seventh day from all his work . . ." Exodus 23:12 says "Six days you shall do your work, but on the seventh day you shall rest; that your ox and your donkey may have rest, and the son of your servant woman, and the alien, may be refreshed." From the New Testament Jesus

teaches in Mark 6:31 "And he said to them, "Come away by yourselves to a desolate place and rest a while." For many were coming and going, and they had no leisure even to eat" (ESV.org).

21 Matthew Walker, *Why We Sleep: The New Science of Sleep and Dreams* (Penguin Books, 2017), Chapter 6. Also see my detailed review of key themes in the book at https://emmatekstra.com/blog/matthew-walker/.

22 For more information see the book *100 Years of Nobel Prizes* by Baruch Aba Shalev (Americas Group, 2002).

Chapter 4: A Toxic Planet

1 *The Concise Oxford Dictionary*, Ninth Edition (Oxford University Press, 1996).

2 For a deeper understanding of the broad field of toxicology and the different categories of toxic agents of concern to human health see this overview by the Agency for Toxic Substances and Disease (under the department of Health and Human Services) at https://www.atsdr.cdc.gov/training/toxmanual/modules /1/lecturenotes.html.

3 You can read a transcript of the Senate Hearing at https://www.govinfo.gov /content/pkg/CHRG-111shrg21160/html/CHRG-111shrg21160.htm.

4 See this essay in the *British Medical Journal* on the capture of nutrition science by the food industry: Scrinis G. Ultra-processed foods and the corporate capture of nutrition—an essay by Gyorgy Scrinis, *BMJ* 2020; 371:m4601 doi:10.1136/bmj.m4601. For a broader view across other industries also see White J, Bero LA. Corporate manipulation of research: strategies are similar across five industries. *Stanford Law & Policy Review*, 2010;21:105   at   https://heinonline.org/HOL/LandingPage?handle=hein .journals/stanlp21&div=8&id=&page= You can also access it here: https: //www.thefreelibrary.com/Stanford+Law+%26+Policy+Review/2010 /January/1-p51674.

5 Rico-Campà A, et al. Association between consumption of ultra-processed foods and all cause mortality: SUN prospective cohort study. *BMJ*, 2019; 365 :l1949 doi:10.1136/bmj.l1949.

6 UPFs linked to cancer: https://doi.org/10.1016/j.eclinm.2023.101840; UPFs linked to cognitive decline: Gomes Gonçalves N, Vidal Ferreira N, Khandpur N, et al. Association Between Consumption of Ultraprocessed Foods and Cognitive Decline. *JAMA Neurology*, 2023;80(2):142–150. doi:10.1001 /jamaneurol.2022.4397; UPFs linked to cardiovascular disease: Srour B, Fezeu L K, Kesse-Guyot E, AllÃ¨s B, MÃ©jean C, Andrianasolo R M et al. Ultra-processed food intake and risk of cardiovascular disease: prospective cohort study (NutriNet-Santé) BMJ 2019; 365 :l1451 doi:10.1136/bmj .l1451.

[7] Jiang, H., et al. κ-carrageenan induces the disruption of intestinal epithelial Caco-2 monolayers by promoting the interaction between intestinal epithelial cells and immune cells. *Molecular Medicine Reports*, 8, no. 6 (2013): 1635–1642. https://doi.org/10.3892/mmr.2013.1726.

[8] For more information on carrageenan see this helpful consumer report from the Cornucopia Institute at https://www.cornucopia.org/wp-content/uploads/2013/02/Carrageenan-Report1.pdf.

[9] Lerner, Aaron, and Torsten Matthias. Changes in Intestinal Tight Junction Permeability Associated with Industrial Food Additives Explain the Rising Incidence of Autoimmune Disease. *Autoimmunity Reviews*, 14, no. 6 (2015): 479–89. doi:10.1016/J.AUTREV.2015.01.009.

[10] See Zehra Kazmi, et al. Monosodium glutamate: Review on clinical reports. *International Journal of Food Properties*, (2017) 20:sup2, 1807–1815, DOI: 10.1080/10942912.2017.1295260. Accessed at: https://www.tandfonline.com/doi/full/10.1080/10942912.2017.1295260.

[11] Hajihasani MM, et al. Natural products as safeguards against monosodium glutamate-induced toxicity. *Iranian Journal of Basic Medical Sciences*, 2020 Apr;23(4):416–430. doi: 10.22038/IJBMS.2020.43060.10123. PMID: 32489556; PMCID: PMC7239414. Accessed at: https://www.ncbi.nlm.nih.gov/pmc/articles/PMC7239414/pdf/IJBMS-23–416.pdf.

[12] Etemadi A, Sinha R, Ward M H, Graubard B I, Inoue-Choi M, Dawsey S M et al. Mortality from different causes associated with meat, heme iron, nitrates, and nitrites in the NIH-AARP Diet and Health Study: population based cohort study. *BMJ*, 2017; 357 :j1957 doi:10.1136/bmj.j1957.

[13] For an explanation on the dangers of oxidation and free radicals see Lobo V, et al. Free radicals, antioxidants and functional foods: Impact on human health. *Pharmacogn Rev*, 2010 Jul;4(8):118–26. doi: 10.4103/0973–7847.70902. PMID: 22228951; PMCID: PMC3249911.

[14] de Souza R J, et al. Intake of saturated and trans unsaturated fatty acids and risk of all-cause mortality, cardiovascular disease, and type 2 diabetes: systematic review and meta-analysis of observational studies BMJ 2015; 351 :h3978 doi:10.1136/bmj.h3978. Also see Ramsden C E et al. Use of dietary linoleic acid for secondary prevention of coronary heart disease and death: evaluation of recovered data from the Sydney Diet Heart Study and updated meta-analysis *BMJ*, 2013; 346 :e8707 doi:10.1136/bmj.e8707. And https://www.reuters.com/article/us-omega-6/omega-6-fatty-acid-intake-tied-to-breast-cancer-idUSTRE48P70Y20080926.

[15] See Yang Q, Zhang Z, Gregg EW, Flanders WD, Merritt R, Hu FB. Added sugar intake and cardiovascular diseases mortality among US adults. *JAMA Intern Med*, 2014 Apr;174(4):516–24. doi: 10.1001/jamainternmed.2013.13563. PMID: 24493081. And also Softic S, Cohen DE, Kahn CR. Role of Dietary

Fructose and Hepatic De Novo Lipogenesis in Fatty Liver Disease. *Digestive Diseases and Sciences*, 2016 May;61(5):1282–93. doi: 10.1007/s10620–016 -4054–0. Epub 2016 Feb 8. PMID: 26856717; PMCID: PMC4838515.

[16] Lenoir M, Serre F, Cantin L, Ahmed SH. Intense sweetness surpasses cocaine reward. *PLoS One*, 2007 Aug 1;2(8):e698. doi: 10.1371/journal .pone.0000698. PMID: 17668074; PMCID: PMC1931610.

[17] Susan S. Schiffman, Elizabeth H. Scholl, Terrence S. Furey & H. Troy Nagle (2023) Toxicological and pharmacokinetic properties of sucralose-6-acetate and its parent sucralose: in vitro screening assays. *Journal of Toxicology and Environmental Health*, Part B, DOI: 10.1080/10937404.2023.2213903.

[18] Suez J, Korem T, Zeevi D, Zilberman-Schapira G, Thaiss CA, Maza O, Israeli D, Zmora N, Gilad S, Weinberger A, Kuperman Y, Harmelin A, Kolodkin-Gal I, Shapiro H, Halpern Z, Segal E, Elinav E. Artificial sweeteners induce glucose intolerance by altering the gut microbiota. *Nature*, 2014 Oct 9;514(7521):181–6. doi: 10.1038/nature13793. Epub 2014 Sep 17. PMID: 25231862.

[19] Maher TJ, Wurtman RJ. Possible neurologic effects of aspartame, a widely used food additive. *Environmental Health Perspectives*, 1987 Nov;75:53–7. doi: 10.1289/ehp.877553. PMID: 3319565; PMCID: PMC1474447.

[20] Stephanie Seneff, PHD, *Toxic Legacy: How the Weedkiller Glyphosate Is Destroying Our Health and the Environment*, (Chelsea Green, 2021). You can also review her presentation slides at https://people.csail.mit.edu/seneff/2021/ HealthFreedom2021.pdf.

[21] For a study linking the herbicide paraquat to Parkinson's see Tanner CM, et al. *Rotenone, paraquat, and Parkinson's disease. Environmental Health Perspectives*, 2011 Jun;119(6):866–72. doi: 10.1289/ehp.1002839. Epub 2011 Jan 26. PMID: 21269927; PMCID: PMC3114824.

[22] 22 independent researchers around the world have independently studied the effects of atrazine exposure. Their findings were consolidated in this 2011 paper. You can also watch a keynote presentation by Tyrone Hayes at https://www.youtube.com/watch?v=7R8-xC8aj6Q. Read the paper at https://doi.org/10.1016/j.jsbmb.2011.03.015. Tyrone B. Hayes, et al., Demasculinization and feminization of male gonads by atrazine: Consistent effects across vertebrate classes. *The Journal of Steroid Biochemistry and Molecular Biology*, Volume 127, Issues 1–2, 2011, Pages 64–73.

[23] Zhao J, Stockwell T, Naimi T, Churchill S, Clay J, Sherk A. Association Between Daily Alcohol Intake and Risk of All-Cause Mortality: A Systematic Review and Meta-analyses. *JAMA Network Open*, 2023;6(3):e236185. doi:10.1001/jamanetworkopen.2023.6185.

[24] Goding Sauer A, Fedewa SA, Bandi P, Minihan AK, Stoklosa M, Drope J, Gapstur SM, Jemal A, Islami F. Proportion of cancer cases and deaths

attributable to alcohol consumption by US state, 2013–2016. *Cancer Epidemiol*, 2021 Apr;71(Pt A):101893. doi: 10.1016/j.canep.2021.101893. Epub 2021 Jan 19. PMID: 33477084.

25 Again quoting Matthew Walker and *Why We Sleep: The New Science of Sleep and Dreams* (Penguin Books, 2017), Chapter 2.

26 Tucker, L.A. Caffeine consumption and telomere length in men and women of the National Health and Nutrition Examination Survey (NHANES). *Nutrition & Metabolism*, (Lond) 14, 10 (2017). https://doi.org/10.1186/s12986–017-0162-x.

27 See the Environmental Working Group article at https://www.ewg.org/news-insights/news/2022/03/lose-lilial-european-union-ban-shows-risks-chemical-cosmetics.

28 See Chapter 9 and its references from Stephanie Seneff, PhD, *Toxic Legacy: How the Weedkiller Glyphosate Is Destroying Our Health and the Environment*, (Chelsea Green, 2021).

29 For a helpful overview of mechanisms of toxicity for the 5 most problematic heavy metals see the *Frontiers in Pharmacology* article by Balali-Mood Mahdi et al., Toxic Mechanisms of Five Heavy Metals: Mercury, Lead, Chromium, Cadmium, and Arsenic; DOI:10.3389/fphar.2021.643972; Accessed at https://www.frontiersin.org/articles/10.3389/fphar.2021.643972.

30 For a great discussion on the benefits of non-burning sun exposure see Hoel DG, de Gruijl FR. Sun Exposure Public Health Directives. *International Journal of Environmental Research and Public Health*, 2018 Dec 10;15(12):2794. doi: 10.3390/ijerph15122794. PMID: 30544646; PMCID: PMC6313493.

31 Mackie BS, et al. Melanoma and dietary lipids. *Nutrition and Cancer*, 1987;9(4):219–26. doi: 10.1080/01635588709513930. PMID: 3110746.

32 Dorsey ER, et al. Trichloroethylene: An Invisible Cause of Parkinson's Disease? *J Parkinsons Dis*. 2023;13(2):203–218. doi: 10.3233/JPD-225047. PMID: 36938742; PMCID: PMC10041423. You can also access at https://content.iospress.com/download/journal-of-parkinsons-disease/jpd225047?id=journal-of-parkinsons-disease%2Fjpd225047.

33 See Hwang J, et al. An assessment of the toxicity of polypropylene microplastics in human derived cells. *Science of Total Environment*, 2019 Sep 20;684:657–669. doi: 10.1016/j.scitotenv.2019.05.071. Epub 2019 May 17. PMID: 31158627. https://pubmed.ncbi.nlm.nih.gov/31158627/.

34 See Gao H, et al. Bisphenol A and hormone-associated cancers: current progress and perspectives. *Medicine* (Baltimore). 2015 Jan;94(1):e211. doi: 10.1097/MD.0000000000000211. PMID: 25569640; PMCID: PMC4602822. https://pubmed.ncbi.nlm.nih.gov/25569640/.

35 Moon MK. Concern about the Safety of Bisphenol A Substitutes. *Diabetes & Metabolism Journal*, 2019 Feb;43(1):46–48. doi: 10.4093/dmj.2019.0027.

PMID: 30793551; PMCID: PMC6387873. https://www.ncbi.nlm.nih.gov/pmc/articles/PMC6387873/.

[36] Oz K, et al. Volatile Organic Compound Emissions from Polyurethane Mattresses under Variable Environmental Conditions. *Environmental Science and Technology*, 2019 Aug 6;53(15):9171–9180. doi: 10.1021/acs.est.9b01557. Epub 2019 Jul 10. PMID: 31290311. https://pubmed.ncbi.nlm.nih.gov/31290311/.

[37] Jolliet O, et al. High Throughput Risk and Impact Screening of Chemicals in Consumer Products. *Risk Analysis* 2021 Apr;41(4):627–644. doi: 10.1111/risa.13604. Epub 2020 Oct 18. PMID: 33073419; PMCID: PMC8246852. https://pubmed.ncbi.nlm.nih.gov/33073419/.

[38] See this appeal launched in 2018 to the United Nations as an example. https://www.emfcall.org/the-emf-call/ Also see my blog post at https://emmatekstra.com/blog/bravo-france/.

[39] See Anthony B. Miller et al. Cancer epidemiology update, following the 2011 IARC evaluation of radiofrequency electromagnetic fields (Monograph 102), *Environmental Research*, Volume 167, 2018, Pages 673–683, ISSN 0013–9351, https://doi.org/10.1016/j.envres.2018.06.043. Accessed at: https://www.sciencedirect.com/science/article/abs/pii/S0013935118303475.

[40] See Gorpinchenko I, et al. The influence of direct mobile phone radiation on sperm quality. *Central European Journal of Urology*, 2014;67(1):65–71. doi: 10.5173/ceju.2014.01.art14. Epub 2014 Apr 17. PMID: 24982785; PMCID: PMC4074720. Accessed at: https://www.ncbi.nlm.nih.gov/pmc/articles/PMC4074720/.

[41] See Gandhi OP, et al. Exposure limits: the underestimation of absorbed cell phone radiation, especially in children. *Electromagnetic Biology and Medicine*, 2012 Mar;31(1):34–51. doi: 10.3109/15368378.2011.622827. Epub 2011 Oct 14. PMID: 21999884. Accessed at: https://pubmed.ncbi.nlm.nih.gov/21999884/.

[42] See this extensive public letter written by Dr. Martin Pall, professor emeritus from Washington State University, an expert on EMFs. https://s3.amazonaws.com/media.electrosmogrx.com/dr-pall-5g-hazard-letter.pdf. Also see this useful summary with helpful color pictures on the brain effects: https://juniperpublishers.com/aibm/pdf/AIBM.MS.ID.555655.pdf.

[43] For more on the iPhone story see my blog post https://emmatekstra.com/blog/bravo-france/.

Chapter 5: A Body Needs Nourishment

[1] Simona Kitanovska, *Newsweek*, 5 Aug 2022, https://www.newsweek.com/average-american-only-spends-3-dinners-week-loved-ones-poll-shows-1731243.

2   Lesser LI et al. Relationship between funding source and conclusion among nutrition-related scientific articles. *PLoS Med*, 2007 Jan;4(1):e5. doi: 10.1371/journal.pmed.0040005. PMID: 17214504; PMCID: PMC1764435. Access at: https://pubmed.ncbi.nlm.nih.gov/17214504/.

3   Heiman ML, Greenway FL. A healthy gastrointestinal microbiome is dependent on dietary diversity. *Molecular Metabolism*, 2016 Mar 5;5(5):317–320. doi: 10.1016/j.molmet.2016.02.005. https://pubmed.ncbi.nlm.nih.gov/27110483/.

4   Percival SS at al. Bioavailability of herbs and spices in humans as determined by ex vivo inflammatory suppression and DNA strand breaks. *Journal of the American College of Nutrition*, 2012 Aug;31(4):288–94. doi: 10.1080/07315724.2012.10720438.PMID:23378457.https://pubmed.ncbi.nlm.nih.gov/23378457/.

5   AlFadhly, N.K.Z. et al. Trends and Technological Advancements in the Possible Food Applications of Spirulina and Their Health Benefits: A Review. *Molecules*, 2022, *27*, 5584. https://doi.org/10.3390/molecules27175584. Accessed at: https://www.mdpi.com/1420–3049/27/17/5584. Also see https://www.healthline.com/nutrition/10-proven-benefits-of-spirulina.

6   Cerletti, C.; Esposito, S.; Iacoviello, L. Edible Mushrooms and Beta-Glucans: Impact on Human Health. *Nutrients*, 2021, *13*, 2195. https://doi.org/10.3390/nu13072195. https://www.mdpi.com/2072–6643/13/7/2195.

7   See *Advances in Nutrition* article Djibril M Ba et al. Higher Mushroom Consumption Is Associated with Lower Risk of Cancer: A Systematic Review and Meta-Analysis of Observational Studies, Volume 12, Issue 5, 2021, Pages 1691–1704, ISSN 2161–8313, https://doi.org/10.1093/advances/nmab015. https://advances.nutrition.org/article/S2161–8313(22)00464–1/fulltext.

8   McAnulty LS, et al. Effect of blueberry ingestion on natural killer cell counts, oxidative stress, and inflammation prior to and after 2.5 h of running. *Applied Physiology, Nutrition, and Metabolism*, 2011 Dec;36(6):976–84. doi: 10.1139/h11–120. Epub 2011 Nov 23. Accessed at: https://greenmedinfo.com/article/blueberry-ingestion-improves-natural-killer-cell-counts-oxidative-stress-and-i.

9   Abidov M, et al. Effect of Blueberin on fasting glucose, C-reactive protein and plasma aminotransferases, in female volunteers with diabetes type 2: double-blind, placebo controlled clinical study. *Georgian Med News*, 2006 Dec;(141):66–72. Accessed at: https://greenmedinfo.com/article/blueberry-leaf-extract-reduces-fasting-glucose-c-reactive-protein-and-plasma-a.

10 Rubio-Tapia A et al. Increased prevalence and mortality in undiagnosed celiac disease. *Gastroenterology*, 2009 Jul;137(1):88–93. doi: 10.1053/j.gastro.2009.03.059. Epub 2009 Apr 10. PMID: 19362553; PMCID: PMC2704247. https://www.ncbi.nlm.nih.gov/pmc/articles/PMC2704247/#.

[11] Sapkota AR, Lefferts LY, McKenzie S, Walker P. What do we feed to food-production animals? A review of animal feed ingredients and their potential impacts on human health. *Environmental Health Perspectives*, 2007 May;115(5):663–70. doi: 10.1289/ehp.9760. Epub 2007 Feb 8. PMID: 17520050; PMCID: PMC1867957. https://www.ncbi.nlm.nih.gov/pmc/articles/PMC1867957/. Also see this news article about a truckload of red Skittles destined for cattle in Wisconsin, https://www.cnn.com/2017/01/19/health/spilled-skittles-road-trnd/index.html.

[12] One example study of many, Hu FB, at al. A prospective study of egg consumption and risk of cardiovascular disease in men and women. *JAMA*, 1999 Apr 21;281(15):1387–94. doi: 10.1001/jama.281.15.1387. PMID: 10217054. https://pubmed.ncbi.nlm.nih.gov/10217054/.

[13] Bischoff-Ferrari HA et al. Milk intake and risk of hip fracture in men and women: a meta-analysis of prospective cohort studies. *Journal of Bone and Mineral Research*, 2011 Apr;26(4):833–9. doi: 10.1002/jbmr.279. 2017 Nov;32(11):2319. PMID: 20949604. https://pubmed.ncbi.nlm.nih.gov/20949604/.

[14] Aune D, Navarro Rosenblatt DA, Chan DS, Vieira AR, Vieira R, Greenwood DC, Vatten LJ, Norat T. Dairy products, calcium, and prostate cancer risk: a systematic review and meta-analysis of cohort studies. *American Journal of Clinical Nutrition*, 2015 Jan;101(1):87–117. doi: 10.3945/ajcn.113.067157. https://pubmed.ncbi.nlm.nih.gov/25527754/.

[15] Pimpin L, et al. Is Butter Back? A Systematic Review and Meta-Analysis of Butter Consumption and Risk of Cardiovascular Disease, Diabetes, and Total Mortality. *PLoS One*, 2016 Jun 29;11(6):e0158118. doi: 10.1371/journal.pone.0158118. https://pubmed.ncbi.nlm.nih.gov/27355649/.

[16] Deth R, et al. Clinical evaluation of glutathione concentrations after consumption of milk containing different subtypes of β-casein: results from a randomized, cross-over clinical trial. Nutrition Journal, 2016 Sep 29;15(1):82. Doi: 10.1186/s12937–016-0201-x. https://pubmed.ncbi.nlm.nih.gov/27680716/.

[17] Elliott RB et al. Type I (insulin-dependent) diabetes mellitus and cow milk: casein variant consumption. Diabetologia. 1999 Mar;42(3):292–6. Doi: 10.1007/s001250051153. Erratum in: *Diabetologia*, 1999 Aug;42(8):1032. https://pubmed.ncbi.nlm.nih.gov/10096780/.

[18] Mozaffarian D et al. Fish intake, contaminants, and human health: evaluating the risks and the benefits. *JAMA*, 2006 Oct 18;296(15):1885–99. doi: 10.1001/jama.296.15.1885. Erratum in: *JAMA*. 2007 Feb 14;297(6):590. https://pubmed.ncbi.nlm.nih.gov/17047219/ Also see Miles EA, Calder PC. Influence of marine n-3 polyunsaturated fatty acids on immune function and a systematic review of their effects on clinical outcomes in rheumatoid arthritis.

British Journal of Nutrition, 2012 Jun;107 Suppl 2:S171–84. doi: 10.1017/ S0007114512001560. https://pubmed.ncbi.nlm.nih.gov/22591891/.

19 Li F, Liu X, Zhang D. Fish consumption and risk of depression: a meta-analysis. *Journal of Epidemiology and Community Health,* 2016 Mar;70(3):299–304. doi: 10.1136/jech-2015–206278. Epub 2015 Sep 10. https://pubmed.ncbi .nlm.nih.gov/26359502/.

20 There is a lot of detail to the science of fats which is worth digging into but one telling fact is that in 2015 the US Dietary Guidelines Advisory Committee finally eliminated any recommendations to limit dietary fat or cholesterol. Rather than cite many studies here I have recommended useful books in Further Reading that cover the topic well.

21 Read the book *Your Body's Many Cries for Water* by Dr. F. Batmanghelidj who healed fellow prisoners with nothing but water after being jailed for his association with the Shah of Iran.

22 Another interesting book about the intelligence of water is *The Hidden Messages of Water* by Masaru Emoto, who took photographs of frozen water and noticed that pure water forms amazingly beautiful symmetrical crystals each one unique, but when the water is toxic or polluted it fails to form symmetrical crystals instead they appear "tortuous."

23 There is much scientific debate about the pros and cons of water fluoridation. Here's one helpful summary Aoun A, Darwiche F, Al Hayek S, Doumit J. The Fluoride Debate: The Pros and Cons of Fluoridation. *Preventive Nutrition and Food Science,* 2018 Sep;23(3):171–180. doi: 10.3746/pnf.2018.23.3.171. https://www.ncbi.nlm.nih.gov/pmc/articles/PMC6195894/.

Chapter 6: It's Flu Season Again

1 See this interesting article from the Center for Infectious Disease Research and Policy at the University of Minnesota regarding the dire state of the market for antibiotics. https://www.cidrap.umn.edu/report-highlights-fragile-and-failing -antibiotic-pipeline.

2 *UpToDate* article on Antimicrobial stewardship in hospital settings. Accessed at: https://www.uptodate.com/contents/antimicrobial-stewardship-in-hospital -settings.

3 Fecal Microbiota Transplants are being studied for use with other diseases now associated with a damaged microbiome. Read this interesting paper from Korea Fecal Microbiota Transplantation: Current Applications, Effectiveness, and Future Perspectives accessed at https://www.e-ce.org/journal/view.php ?doi=10.5946/ce.2015.117.

4 Ramirez Jaime et al. Antibiotics as Major Disruptors of Gut Microbiota, Frontiers in Cellular and Infection. *Microbiology,* 2020. Accessed at: https: //www.frontiersin.org/articles/10.3389/fcimb.2020.572912 DOI=10.3389 /fcimb.2020.572912 ISSN=2235–2988.

5 Kan WC, Chen YC, Wu VC, Shiao CC. Vancomycin-Associated Acute Kidney Injury: A Narrative Review from Pathophysiology to Clinical Application. *International Journal of Molecular Science*, 2022 Feb 12;23(4):2052. doi: 10.3390/ijms23042052. Accessed at: https://www.ncbi.nlm.nih.gov/pmc /articles/PMC8877514/.

6 Hilton J et al. COVID-19 and Acute Kidney Injury. *Critical Care Clinics*, 2022 Jul;38(3):473–489. doi: 10.1016/j.ccc.2022.01.002. Epub 2022 Jan 10. Accessed at: https://www.ncbi.nlm.nih.gov/pmc/articles/PMC8743571/.

7 Infectious disease specialist Dr. Judy Stone discusses this phenomenon in *Forbes* magazine. https://www.forbes.com/sites/judystone/2016/02/18/common -antibiotics-may-cause-confusion-and-hallucinations/?sh=13de11fa797e.

8 https://www.fda.gov/news-events/press-announcements/fda-updates -warnings-fluoroquinolone-antibiotics-risks-mental-health-and-low-blood -sugar-adverse.

9 Biologist and flagella researcher R.M.McNab describe the conundrum: "Clearly, nature has found two good uses for this sophisticated apparatus. How they evolved is another matter, although it has been proposed that the flagellum is the more ancient device." See Macnab RM. How bacteria assemble flagella. *Annual Review of Microbiology*, 2003;57:77–100. doi: 10.1146/annurev.micro.57.030502.090832.

10 Both bird flu and swine flu are a form of influenza-A. The last H1N1 outbreak was in 1976.

11 Fierce Pharma calls Tamiflu a blockbuster. This term may lead you to believe it must work really well. You'd be wrong. See this article: https://www .fiercepharma.com/pharma/roche-s-1–5b-tamiflu-pandemic-fca-suit-drags -as-federal-judge-allows-case-to-move-forward.

12 See sample studies such as Mark H Ebell et al. Effectiveness of oseltamivir in adults: a meta-analysis of published and unpublished clinical trials, *Family Practice*, Volume 30, Issue 2, April 2013, Pages 125–133, https://doi .org/10.1093/fampra/cms059 and Jefferson T et al. Neuraminidase inhibitors for preventing and treating influenza in adults and children. Cochrane Database of Systematic Reviews 2014, Issue 4. Art. No.: CD008965. DOI: 10.1002/14651858.CD008965.pub4.

13 Hama R, Bennett CL. The mechanisms of sudden-onset type adverse reactions to oseltamivir. *Acta Neurology Scandinavica*, 2017 Feb;135(2):148–160. doi: 10.1111/ane.12629. Epub 2016 Jun 30. Accessed at: https://pubmed.ncbi .nlm.nih.gov/27364959/.

14 Butler, D. Tamiflu report comes under fire. *Nature*, 508, 439–440 (2014). https://doi.org/10.1038/508439a.

15 See https://www.who.int/news-room/fact-sheets/detail/onchocerciasis and https: //www.who.int/teams/control-of-neglected-tropical-diseases/onchocerciasis /prevention-control-and-elimination.

16 For more details on the history of Ivermectin, its safety profile, and its efficacy for Covid-19 and other diseases go to: https://covid19criticalcare.com/ivermectin/.

17 Bohr C, Shermetaro C. *Tonsillectomy and Adenoidectomy*. [Updated 2022 Aug 19]. In: StatPearls [Internet]. Treasure Island (FL): StatPearls Publishing; 2023 Jan-. Available from: https://www.ncbi.nlm.nih.gov/books /NBK536942/.

18 Byars SG et al. Association of Long-Term Risk of Respiratory, Allergic, and Infectious Diseases With Removal of Adenoids and Tonsils in Childhood. *JAMA Otolaryngol Head Neck Surgery*, 2018;144(7):594–603. doi:10.1001/ jamaoto.2018.0614 Accessed at: https://jamanetwork.com/journals/jamaotol aryngology/article-abstract/2683621.

19 https://ashpublications.org/blood/article/133/20/2168/273834/Cross-talk-between-neutrophils-and-the-microbiota and https://www.pnas.org/doi /10.1073/pnas.2211230119.

20 Read the interesting summary by R. Anthony Cox et al., Opinion: The germicidal effect of ambient air (open-air factor) revisited *Atmos. Chemical Physics*, 21, 13011–13018, 2021 https://doi.org/10.5194/acp-21–13011-2021. Accessed at https://acp.copernicus.org/articles/21/13011/2021/acp-21–13011 -2021.pdf.

21 Another description of the open-air method for treating tuberculosis and influenza can be found at Hobday RA, Cason JW. The open-air treatment of pandemic influenza. Am J Public Health. 2009 Oct;99 Suppl 2(Suppl 2):S236–42. doi: 10.2105/AJPH.2008.134627. Epub 2009 May 21.

22 Read this helpful article from the World Council for Health which has links to several published studies. https://worldcouncilforhealth.org/resources/end -mask-mandates/.

23 R. Anthony Cox et al. See note 20.

24 See the website of the International Scientific Committee of Ozone Therapy isco3.org and their tonsils guidelines in particular at https://isco3.org/wp -content/uploads/2015/09/Tonsillitis.pdf.

25 Hobday R, Collignon P (June 20, 2022) An Old Defense Against New Infections: The Open-Air Factor and COVID-19. *Cureus*, 14(6): e26133. doi:10.7759/cureus.26133. Accessed at https://www.cureus.com /articles/97372-an-old-defence-against-new-infections-the-open-air-factor -and-covid-19#!/.

26 Carsten Carlberg, Alberto Muñoz, An update on vitamin D signaling and cancer. *Seminars in Cancer Biology*, Volume 79, 2022, Pages 217–230, ISSN 1044–579X, https://doi.org/10.1016/j.semcancer.2020.05.018.

27 Two example studies which each reviewed multiple studies are: Dissanayake HA et al., Prognostic and Therapeutic Role of Vitamin D in COVID-19: Systematic Review and Meta-analysis. *Journal of Clinical Endocrinology &*

Metabolism, 2022 Apr 19;107(5):1484–1502. doi: 10.1210/clinem/dgab892. And Chiodini I et al. Vitamin D Status and SARS-CoV-2 Infection and COVID-19 Clinical Outcomes. *Front Public Health*. 2021 Dec 22;9:736665. doi: 10.3389/fpubh.2021.736665.

28 For two studies on Vitamin D toxicity levels see Kimball SM et al. Evaluation of vitamin D3 intakes up to 15,000 international units/day and serum 25-hydroxyvitamin D concentrations up to 300 nmol/L on calcium metabolism in a community setting. *Dermatoendocrinol*. 2017 Apr 13;9(1):e1300213. doi: 10.1080/19381980.2017.1300213. And also Hathcock JN, Shao A, Vieth R, Heaney R. Risk assessment for vitamin D. *American Journal of Clinical Nutrition*, 2007 Jan;85(1):6–18. doi: 10.1093/ajcn/85.1.6.

29 Remember the discussion of the chemical nature of the human body and free radicals in Chapter 1? Antioxidants provide electrons to unstable oxygen molecules.

30 Rather than cite many different scientific papers here I would urge you to read the books of Dr. Thomas E. Levy which are each carefully referenced. Start with *Rapid Virus Recovery* and also see *Curing the Incurable: Vitamin C, Infectious Diseases and Toxins*.

31 Marik PE et al. Vitamin C, and Thiamine for the Treatment of Severe Sepsis and Septic Shock: A Retrospective Before-After Study. *Chest*, 2017 Jun;151(6):1229–1238. doi: 10.1016/j.chest.2016.11.036. Epub 2016 Dec 6.

32 *Rapid Virus Recovery* by Dr. Thomas E. Levy lists many studies in its reference. section. You can also go to the website http://orthomolecular.org/resources /omns/index.shtml to see the latest research.

33 Halliwell B, Clement MV, Long LH. Hydrogen peroxide in the human body. *FEBS Lett*. 2000 Dec 1;486(1):10–3. Doi: 10.1016/s0014–5793(00)02197–9. Accessed at: https://febs.onlinelibrary.wiley.com/doi/full/10.1016/S0014 –5793%2800%2902197–9?sid=nlm%3Apubmed.

34 Stein SW, Thiel CG. The History of Therapeutic Aerosols: A Chronological Review. *Journal of Aerosol Medicine and Pulmonary Drug Delivery*, 2017 Feb;30(1):20–41. Doi: 10.1089/jamp.2016.1297. Epub 2016 Oct 17.

35 Te Velthuis AJ et al. Zn(2+) inhibits coronavirus and arterivirus RNA polymerase activity in vitro and zinc ionophores block the replication of these viruses in cell culture. *PloS Pathogens*, 2010 Nov 4;6(11):e1001176. Doi: 10.1371/journal.ppat.1001176.

36 Heggers JP et al. The effectiveness of processed grapefruit-seed extract as an antibacterial agent: II. Mechanism of action and in vitro toxicity. *Journal of Alternative and Complementary Medicine*, 2002 Jun;8(3):333–40. Doi: 10.1089/10755530260128023. Erratum in: *J Altern Complement Med* 2002 Aug;8(4):521.

[37] Vila Domínguez A et al. Antibacterial Activity of Colloidal Silver against Gram-Negative and Gram-Positive Bacteria. *Antibiotics* (Basel). 2020 Jan 19;9(1):36. Doi: 10.3390/antibiotics9010036. Accessed at: https://www.ncbi .nlm.nih.gov/pmc/articles/PMC7167925/.

[38] Data and charts taken from a paper published by CDC researchers in 1999 which only confirmed studies undertaken in previous decades. See Armstrong GL, Conn LA, Pinner RW. Trends in Infectious Disease Mortality in the United States During the 20th Century. *JAMA*, 1999;281(1):61–66. Doi:10.1001/jama.281.1.61.

[39] See the special report prepared by Barbara Loe Fisher and the National Vaccine Information Center at https://www.nvic.org/NVIC/media/LegacySite/pdf /downloads/science-politics-eradicating-measles.pdf.

[40] HOYNE AL. Poliomyelitis problems. *Med Clin North Am.* 1951 Jan;35(1): 175–88. PMID: 14796117.

[41] Dangers in the Manufacture of Paris Green and Scheele's Green (1917). *Monthly Review of the U.S. Bureau of Labor Statistics*, 5(2), 78–83. http://www.jstor.org/stable/41829377.

[42] Putnam JJ. On the Character of the Evidence as to the Injuriousness of Arsenic as a Domestic Poison. Read in the Section of Practice of Medicine and Physiology, at the Forty-second Annual Meeting of the American Medical Association, held at Washington, D. C., May 5–8, 1891. *JAMA*, 1891;XVI(22):778–781. Doi:10.1001/jama.1891.02410740022001e.

[43] van den Berg H. Global status of DDT and its alternatives for use in vector control to prevent disease. *Environmental Health Perspective*, 2009 Nov;117(11):1656–63. Doi: 10.1289/ehp.0900785. Epub 2009 May 29. PMID: 20049114; PMCID: PMC2801202.

[44] See Wesseling C et al. Agricultural pesticide use in developing countries: health effects and research needs. *International Journal of Health Services*, 1997;27(2):273–308. Doi: 10.2190/E259-N3AH-TA1Y-H591. PMID: 9142603. Accessed at https://pubmed.ncbi.nlm.nih.gov/9142603/ And Marx A et al. Differential diagnosis of acute flaccid paralysis and its role in poliomyelitis surveillance. *Epidemiologic Reviews*, 2000;22(2):298–316. Doi: 10.1093/oxfordjournals.epirev.a018041. PMID: 11218380. Accessed at https://pubmed.ncbi.nlm.nih.gov/11218380/.

[45] Hull HF, Ward NA, Hull BP, Milstien JB, de Quadros C. Paralytic poliomyelitis: seasoned strategies, disappearing disease. *Lancet*, 1994 May 28;343(8909):1331–7. Doi: 10.1016/s0140–6736(94)92472–4. PMID: 7910329.

[46] AFP is term first used in the 1950s to attribute to cases of paralysis with no evidence of polio virus detected.

47 For details of the book and access for free to many more charts and graphs go to https://dissolvingillusions.com/.

48 For a quick summary of the lunacies of smallpox vaccination watch the 10min video called Menagerie Roulette at https://dissolvingillusions.com /graphs-images/#Charts.

49 *Turtles all the Way Down: Vaccine Science and Myth*, by anonymous Israeli authors. English version edited by Zoey O'Toole and Mary Holland. The extensive reference document with live links can be accessed at https://tinyurl .com/TurtlesBookEngRef.

50 The older DTP is still administered in many developing countries as a cheaper option than the newer versions.

51 See Lyons-Weiler, J., & Russell L, B. (2022). Revisiting Excess Diagnoses of Illnesses and Conditions in Children Whose Parents Provided Informed Permission to Vaccinate Them. *International Journal of Vaccine Theory, Practice, and Research*, 2(2), 603–618. https://doi.org/10.56098/ijvtpr.v2i2.59. Accessed at https://ijvtpr.com/index.php/IJVTPR/article/view/59/118 Also see Brian S. Hooker and Neil Z. Miller (2021) Health effects in vaccinated versus unvaccinated children with covariates for breastfeeding status and type of birth. *JtranslSci* 7: DOI: 10.15761/JTS.1000459. And the latest book from Brian Hooker and Robert F. Kennedy, Jr., *Vax-Unvax: Let the Science Speak* detailed in Appendix D.

52 See World Health Organization statistics at https://www.who.int/data/stories /leading-causes-of-death-and-disability-2000–2019-a-visual-summary.

53 We'll get into the some of the reasons in Chapter 7 regarding mortality and morbidity related to the Covid-19 vaccinations themselves. Discussion on other ways mortality statistics have been compromised is covered in the Further Reading listed in Appendix D.

Chapter 7: Shedding the Disease

1 Scully JL. What is a disease? *EMBO Reports*, 2004 Jul;5(7):650–3. Doi: 10.1038/sj.embor.7400195. Accessed at: https://www.ncbi.nlm.nih.gov/pmc /articles/PMC1299105/.

2 Raghupathi W, Raghupathi V. An Empirical Study of Chronic Diseases in the United States: A Visual Analytics Approach. *International Journal of Environmental Research and Public Health*, 2018 Mar 1;15(3):431. Doi: 10.3390/ijerph15030431.

3 See Centers for Disease Control and Prevention website at https://www.cdc .gov/chronicdisease/.

4 Data from the Center for Disease Control as summarized in the American Hospital Association piece at https://www.aha.org/system/files /content/00–10/071204_H4L_FocusonWellness.pdf. Also see this article

from *Life Sciences Intelligence* magazine at https://lifesciencesintelligence.com /features/chronic-disease-rates-and-management-strain-the-us-healthcare -system.

5   Kubota Y et al. JACC Study Group. Association of measles and mumps with cardiovascular disease: The Japan Collaborative Cohort (JACC) study. *Atherosclerosis*, 2015 Aug;241(2):682–6. Doi: 10.1016/j.atherosclerosis.2015. 06.026. Epub 2015 Jun 18. PMID: 26122188.

6   Pesonen E et al. Dual role of infections as risk factors for coronary heart disease. *Atherosclerosis*, 2007 Jun;192(2):370–5. Doi: 10.1016/j.atherosclerosis. 2006.05.018. Epub 2006 Jun 15. PMID: 16780845.

7   U.S. Bureau of Labor Statistics, Population—With a Disability, 16 Years and over [LNU00074597], retrieved from FRED, Federal Reserve Bank of St. Louis; https://fred.stlouisfed.org/series/LNU00074597, August 29, 2023.

8   Go to Phinance Technologies which has made the dataset available for study at https://phinancetechnologies.com/HumanityProjects/PIP%20Analysis-Systems .htm.

9   See additional reading recommendations in Appendix D.

10   The actual number is difficult to assess as there is dispute as to which diseases should be categorized as an autoimmune condition. The American college of rheumatology cites 58 million Americans diagnosed with a rheumatic disease which includes rheumatoid arthritis and lupus but not others. See https: //rheumatology.org/press-releases/american-college-of-rheumatology -releases-2022-rheumatic-disease-report-card.

11   Kjetil Bjornevik et al., Longitudinal analysis reveals high prevalence of Epstein-Barr virus associated with multiple sclerosis. *Science*, 375,296– 301(2022). DOI:10.1126/science.abj8222. Accessed at: https://www.science .org/doi/10.1126/science.abj8222.

12   According to FAIR health, an independent nonprofit that analyzes health insurance information. For more information see their infographic at https: //s3.amazonaws.com/media2.fairhealth.org/infographic/asset/Lyme%20 Disease%20Infographic%20-%20Final.pdf and latest news at: https://www .fairhealth.org/press-release/lyme-disease-diagnoses-increased-357-percent -in-rural-areas-over-past-15-years-according-to-private-insurance-claims.

13   Chmielewska-Badora J, Cisak E, Dutkiewicz J. Lyme borreliosis and multiple sclerosis: any connection? A seroepidemic study. *Annals of Agricultural and Environmental Medicine*, 2000;7(2):141–3.

14   This study looks at the connection between the microbiome and autoimmunity. Vieira SM, Pagovich OE, Kriegel MA. Diet, microbiota and autoimmune diseases. *Lupus*, 2014 May;23(6):518–26. Doi: 10.1177/0961203313501401. Accessed at https://www.ncbi.nlm.nih.gov/pmc/articles/PMC4009622/.

15 Theophilus PA et al. Effectiveness of Stevia Rebaudiana Whole Leaf Extract Against the Various Morphological Forms of Borrelia Burgdorferi in Vitro. *European Journal of Microbiology and Immunology*, 2015 Nov 12;5(4):268–80. Doi: 10.1556/1886.2015.00031. Accessed at: https://www.ncbi.nlm.nih.gov/pmc/articles/PMC4681354/.

16 Hadjivassiliou M, Grünewald RA, Davies-Jones GA. Gluten sensitivity as a neurological illness. *Journal of Neurology, Neurosurgery and Psychiatry*, 2002 May;72(5):560–3. Doi: 10.1136/jnnp.72.5.560. Accessed at: https://jnnp.bmj.com/content/jnnp/72/5/560.full.pdf.

17 This detailed case study of a teenager with severe celiac that was reversed through functional medicine includes a great discussion on the topic of gluten and wheat-related disorders. Tom O'Bryan, Aaron Lerner. Nonresponsive Celiac Disease Treated with a Unique Functional Medical Approach. *International Journal of Celiac Disease*, Vol. 9, No. 2, 2021, pp 41–64. http://pubs.sciepub.com/ijcd/9/2/7.

18 For a great summary of how gluten affects the gut and the connection to chronic inflammatory diseases see the work of Dr. Alessio Fasano such as Fasano A. All disease begins in the (leaky) gut: role of zonulin-mediated gut permeability in the pathogenesis of some chronic inflammatory diseases. *F1000Research*, 2020 Jan 31; 9:F1000 Faculty Rev-69. Doi: 10.12688/f1000research.20510.1. Accessed at https://www.ncbi.nlm.nih.gov/pmc/articles/PMC6996528/.

19 Lemke Dirk et al. Vitamin D Resistance as a Possible Cause of Autoimmune Diseases: A Hypothesis Confirmed by a Therapeutic High-Dose Vitamin D Protocol, *Frontiers in Immunology*, Vol. 12, 2021. DOI=10.3389/fimmu.2021.655739 https://www.frontiersin.org/articles/10.3389/fimmu.2021.655739.

20 McCullough PJ et al. Daily oral dosing of vitamin D_3 using 5000 to 50,000 international units a day in long-term hospitalized patients: Insights from a seven year experience. *Journal of Steroid Biochemistry and Molecular Biology*, 2019 May;189:228–239. Doi: 10.1016/j.jsbmb.2018.12.010. Epub 2019 Jan 4. https://pubmed.ncbi.nlm.nih.gov/30611908/.

21 For more tips on improving your microbiome see my blog post at https://emmatekstra.com/blog/a-depleted-microbiome-may-be-the-source-of-your-ailments-10-tips-to-improve-it/.

22 Kostoglou-Athanassiou I et al. The Effect of Omega-3 Fatty Acids on Rheumatoid Arthritis. *Mediterranean Journal of Rheumatology*, 2020 Jun 30;31(2):190–194. Doi: 10.31138/mjr.31.2.190. Accessed at https://www.ncbi.nlm.nih.gov/pmc/articles/PMC7362115/.

23 Schwalfenberg, Gerry K. et al. N-Acetylcysteine: A Review of Clinical Usefulness (an Old Drug with New Tricks), *Journal of Nutrition and*

Metabolism, 2021, https://doi.org/10.1155/2021/9949453, accessed at https://www.hindawi.com/journals/jnme/2021/9949453/.

[24] *The LDN Book*, edited by Linda Elsegood (Chelsea Green Publishing, 2016). Also see https://ldnresearchtrust.org/.

[25] See latest stats at https://www.who.int/news-room/fact-sheets/detail/diabetes.

[26] There are many studies going back more than a decade showing that diabetes medications have very little benefit. They do not reduce the risk of heart attacks or strokes (in some cases they increase the risk), nor reduce the risk of other complications like kidney failure, blindness, or neuropathy. For example: René Rodríguez-Gutiérrez et al. Glycemic Control for Patients With Type 2 Diabetes Mellitus: Our Evolving Faith in the Face of Evidence. *Circulation: Cardiovascular Quality and Outcomes*, Aug 2016 https://doi.org/10.1161/CIRCOUTCOMES.116.002901. https://www.ahajournals.org/doi/full/10.1161/CIRCOUTCOMES.116.002901. Also Boussageon R et al. Effect of intensive glucose lowering treatment on all cause mortality, cardiovascular death, and microvascular events in type 2 diabetes: meta-analysis of randomized controlled trials. *BMJ*, 2011; 343 :d4169 doi:10.1136/bmj.d4169; https://www.bmj.com/content/343/bmj.d4169.

[27] A great study showing that being overweight or obese is not in itself a good predictor of mortality risk. Orpana HM et al. BMI and mortality: results from a national longitudinal study of Canadian adults. *Obesity*, 2010 Jan; 18(1):214–8. Doi: 10.1038/oby.2009.191. Epub 2009 Jun 18. https://pubmed.ncbi.nlm.nih.gov/19543208/.

[28] Chobot A, Górowska-Kowolik K, Sokołowska M, Jarosz-Chobot P. Obesity and diabetes-Not only a simple link between two epidemics. *Diabetes/Metabolism Research and Reviews*, 2018 Oct;34(7):e3042. Doi: 10.1002/dmrr.3042. Epub 2018 Jul 17. https://www.ncbi.nlm.nih.gov/pmc/articles/PMC6220876/.

[29] See https://www.ema.europa.eu/en/news/ema-statement-ongoing-review-glp-1-receptor-agonists.

[30] See this explanation from FLCCChttps://covid19criticalcare.com/protocol/eat-well-guide-to-fasting-and-healthy-eating/.

[31] Jun Yin et al. Efficacy of Berberine in Patients with Type 2 Diabetes. *Metabolism*, 2008 May ; 57(5): 712–717. https://europepmc.org/backend/ptpmcrender.fcgi?accid=PMC2410097&blobtype=pdf.

[32] Somlak Chuengsamarn et al. Curcumin Extract for Prevention of Type 2 Diabetes. *Diabetes Care* 1 November 2012; 35 (11): 2121–2127. https://doi.org/10.2337/dc12–0116; Accessed at: https://diabetesjournals.org/care/article/35/11/2121/30921/Curcumin-Extract-for-Prevention-of-Type-2-Diabetes.

33 Chowdhury AI et al. Effect of stevia leaves (Stevia rebaudiana Bertoni) on diabetes: A systematic review and meta-analysis of preclinical studies. *Food Science & Nutrition*, 2022 Apr 24;10(9):2868–2878. Doi: 10.1002/fsn3.2904. PMID: 36171777; Accessed at: https://www.ncbi.nlm.nih.gov/pmc/articles/PMC9469865/.

34 Bobiş O et al. Honey and Diabetes: The Importance of Natural Simple Sugars in Diet for Preventing and Treating Different Type of Diabetes. *Oxidative Medicine and Cellular Longevity*, 2018 Feb 4;2018:4757893. Doi: 10.1155/2018/4757893.

35 A new study just published in the magazine *Cell Metabolism* shows how insulin resistance, diabetes, and excess sugar leads to pancreatic cancer. Anni M.Y. Zhang, et al. Hyperinsulinemia acts via acinar insulin receptors to initiate pancreatic cancer by increasing digestive enzyme production and inflammation. *Cell Metabolism*, Vol 35, Issue 12, 2023, Pages 2119–2135. e5,ISSN 1550–4131, https://doi.org/10.1016/j.cmet.2023.10.003. https://www.sciencedirect.com/science/article/pii/S1550413123003728.

36 Tate JG et al. COSMIC: the Catalogue Of Somatic Mutations In Cancer. *Nucleic Acids Research*, 2019 Jan 8;47(D1):D941-D947. Doi: 10.1093/nar/gky1015. Accessed at: https://www.ncbi.nlm.nih.gov/pmc/articles/PMC6323903/.

37 For more about Gerson Therapy go to https://gerson.org/how-it-works/.

38 Seyfried TN et al. Press-pulse: a novel therapeutic strategy for the metabolic management of cancer. *Nutrition & Metabolism*, 2017 Feb 23;14:19. Doi: 10.1186/s12986–017-0178–2. Accessed at: https://www.ncbi.nlm.nih.gov/pmc/articles/PMC5324220/ Also see Seyfried Thomas N. et al. Consideration of Ketogenic Metabolic Therapy as a Complementary or Alternative Approach for Managing Breast Cancer. *Frontiers in Nutrition* Vol 7 2020; https://www.frontiersin.org/articles/10.3389/fnut.2020.00021; DOI=10.3389/fnut.2020.00021.

39 See government fact sheet at https://www.whitehouse.gov/ostp/news-updates/2023/03/09/fact-sheet-cancer-fy24/.

40 For a wonderful explanation on what causes cardiovascular disease, how it couldn't possibly be cholesterol or saturated fat in the diet, and what to do about it, read *The Clot Thickens* by Dr. Malcolm Kendrick. He brings levity and engagement to this complex topic.

41 Ma H et al. Association of habitual glucosamine use with risk of cardiovascular disease: prospective study in UK Biobank. *BMJ*, 2019 May 14;365:l1628. Doi: 10.1136/bmj.l1628. PMID: 31088786; https://pubmed.ncbi.nlm.nih.gov/31088786/ And also see Melgar-Lesmes P, Garcia-Polite F, Del-Rey-Puech P, Rosas E, Dreyfuss JL, Montell E, Vergés J, Edelman ER, Balcells M. Treatment with chondroitin sulfate to modulate inflammation and atherogenesis in obesity. *Atherosclerosis*, 2016 Feb;245:82–7. Doi: 10.1016/j

.atherosclerosis.2015.12.016. Epub 2015 Dec 13. https://pubmed.ncbi.nlm
.nih.gov/26714044/.

42 See my blog article https://emmatekstra.com/blog/my-knee-pain-gone-two
-simple-remedies-that-really-work/.

43 Bachi K, et al. Vascular disease in cocaine addiction. *Atherosclerosis*, 2017
Jul;262:154–162. Doi: 10.1016/j.atherosclerosis.2017.03.019. Epub 2017
Mar 14. https://www.ncbi.nlm.nih.gov/pmc/articles/PMC5757372/.

44 Talarico GP, et al. Cocaine and coronary artery diseases: a systematic review
of the literature. *Journal of Cardiovasc Medicine* (Hagerstown), 2017 May;
18(5):291–294. Doi: 10.2459/JCM.0000000000000511. https://pubmed.ncbi
.nlm.nih.gov/28306693/.

45 Go to https://qrisk.org/ to see the twenty-plus factors that help a clinician
assess whether the person sitting in front of them is likely to have a heart
attack in the next ten years. You can play around with it to see how little
difference it makes if you adjust cholesterol levels or even body mass index.

46 See my blog article https://emmatekstra.com/blog/the-stubborn-myth-of
-statins-and-cholesterol/.

47 Harcombe, Zoë, Baker, Julien S. 2014. Plant Sterols Lower Cholesterol
but Increase Risk for Coronary Heart Disease, *OnLine Journal of Biological
Sciences*, Vol 14, DOI: 10.3844/ojbsci.2014.167.169, https://thescipub.com
/abstract/ojbsci.2014.167.169. Also see Ramsden, C.E. et al. (2013), The
Sydney Diet Heart Study: a randomized controlled trial of linoleic acid for
secondary prevention of coronary heart disease and death. *The FASEB Journal*,
27: 127.4–127.4. https://doi.org/10.1096/fasebj.27.1_supplement.127.4.

Chapter 8: Mind Your Body to Heal Your Brain

1 Kathleen Davis. What is Takotsubo cardiomyopathy? *Medical News Today*,
June 28, 2018. https://www.medicalnewstoday.com/articles/309547.

2 Andrew Goliszek Ph.D, Is There a Cancer-Prone Personality? How You
Think May Put You at Risk. *Psychology Today*, Nov 13, 2014. https://www
.psychologytoday.com/us/blog/how-the-mind-heals-the-body/201411/is
-there-cancer-prone-personality.

3 Read Matthew Walker, *Why We Sleep: The New Science of Sleep and Dreams*
(Penguin Books, 2017). Also see my detailed review of key themes in the
book at https://emmatekstra.com/blog/matthew-walker/.

4 Nguyen TT et al. Type 3 Diabetes and Its Role Implications in Alzheimer's
Disease. *International Journal of Molecular Sciences*, 2020 Apr 30;21(9):3165.
Doi: 10.3390/ijms21093165. Accessed at https://www.ncbi.nlm.nih.gov/pmc
/articles/PMC7246646/.

5 Zhuo Wang et al. Analyses Reveal Microbiome–Gut–Brain Crosstalk Centered
on Aberrant Gamma-Aminobutyric Acid and Tryptophan Metabolism

in Drug-Naïve Patients with First-Episode Schizophrenia. *Schizophrenia Bulletin*, 2023, sbad026, https://doi.org/10.1093/schbul/sbad026.

6   For a more extensive discussion on consciousness and its relevance to our health read Mark Gober's interesting book *An End to Upside Down Medicine: Contagion, Viruses and Vaccines, and Why Consciousness is Needed for a New Paradigm of Health* (2023).

7   Allen Frances, MD was previously the chair of the DSM-IV task force and had grave concerns at the damage DSM-5 was going to do to psychiatry as a profession and the millions of patients it was going to needlessly medicate. Read his insightful book *Saving Normal: An Insider's Revolt against Out-of-Control Psychiatric Diagnosis, DSM-5, Big Pharma, and the Medicalization of Ordinary Life* (William Morrow, 2014).

8   Allsopp K, et al. Heterogeneity in psychiatric diagnostic classification. *Psychiatry Research*, 2019 Sep;279:15–22. Doi: 10.1016/j.psychres.2019.07.005. Epub 2019 Jul 2. Accessed at: https://pubmed.ncbi.nlm.nih.gov/31279246/.

9   Taken from the helpful video on the Institute for Functional Medicine website explaining the difference between conventional treatment for depression and a functional medicine approach. Watch the video at https://www.ifm.org/functional-medicine/.

10 Moore TJ et al. Adult Utilization of Psychiatric Drugs and Differences by Sex, Age, and Race. *JAMA Internal Medicine*, 2017;177(2):274–275. Doi:10.1001/jamainternmed.2016.7507.

11 See Philip Smith, When Meth was Medicine: Big Pharma Amphetamine ads from the days of better living through chemistry. https://www.alternet.org/2016/10/when-meth-medicine-big-pharma-amphetamine-ads Also Erin Blakemore, A Speedy History of America's Addiction to Amphetamines, *Smithsonian Magazine*. https://www.smithsonianmag.com/history/speedy-history-americas-addiction-amphetamine-180966989/.

12 See the 2022 World Drug Report from the United Nations. Booklet 4. https://www.unodc.org/res/wdr2022/MS/WDR22_Booklet_4.pdf.

13 Watch the documentary *Speed Demons: Killing for Attention* by Andrew Thibault. Also watch out for his new series in post-production at the time of writing called *Prescription to Kill*.

14 It's not just ADHD drugs implicated in mass shootings and homicides. See the website madinamerica.com for more information. Start with the 2016 article by Andrew Thibault, The FSA is Hiding Reports Linking Psych Drugs to Homicides at https://www.madinamerica.com/2016/05/the-fda-is-hiding-reports-linking-psych-drugs-to-homicides/.

15 Peter Wehrwein, Astounding increase in use of antidepressants by Americans, https://www.health.harvard.edu/blog/astounding-increase-in-antidepressant-use-by-americans-201110203624.

[16] CDC National Center for Health Statistics, https://www.cdc.gov/nchs /products/databriefs/db76.htm.

[17] Moncrieff, J., et al. The serotonin theory of depression: a systematic umbrella review of the evidence. *Molecular Psychiatry*, July 2022. https://doi .org/10.1038/s41380–022-01661–0. Accessed at https://www.nature.com /articles/s41380–022-01661–0. Also see their follow up paper at https: //www.madinamerica.com/2022/07/response-criticism-serotonin-paper/.

[18] Jakobsen JC et al. Should antidepressants be used for major depressive disorder? *BMJ Evidence-Based Medicine*, 2020;25:130. Accessed at https: //ebm.bmj.com/content/25/4/130.

[19] Kang, S., Han, M., Park, C.I. et al. Use of serotonin reuptake inhibitors and risk of subsequent bone loss in a nationwide population-based cohort study. *Scientific Reports*, 11, 13461 (2021). https://doi.org/10.1038/s41598–021 -92821–9.

[20] Nevels RM, Gontkovsky ST, Williams BE. Paroxetine—The Antidepressant from Hell? Probably Not, But Caution Required. *Psychopharmacology Bulletin*, 2016 Mar 1;46(1):77–104. https://www.ncbi.nlm.nih.gov/pmc /articles/PMC5044489/.

[21] Food and Drug Administration. https://www.fda.gov/drugs/postmarket-drug -safety-information-patients-and-providers/suicidality-children-and-adolescents -being-treated-antidepressant-medications.

[22] Uçok A, Gaebel W. Side effects of atypical antipsychotics: a brief overview. *World Psychiatry*, 2008 Feb;7(1):58–62. Doi: 10.1002/j.2051–5545.2008. tb00154.x. Accessed at https://www.ncbi.nlm.nih.gov/pmc/articles/PMC2327229/.

[23] Ray WA, et al. Association of Antipsychotic Treatment With Risk of Unexpected Death Among Children and Youths. *JAMA Psychiatry*, 2019;76(2):162–171. Doi:10.1001/jamapsychiatry.2018.3421 https://jamanetwork.com/journals /jamapsychiatry/fullarticle/2717966#:~:text=Among%20study%20 children%20and%20youths,increased%20risk%20of%20unexpected%20 deaths.

[24] How the FDA approved an antipsychotic that failed to show a meaningful benefit but raised the risk of death, *BMJ*, 2023; 382 doi: https://doi .org/10.1136/bmj.p1801 (Published 17 August 2023) https://www.bmj.com /content/382/bmj.p1801.

[25] You can read about my thoughts on evil at my blog post https://emmatekstra .com/blog/how-can-there-be-a-god-with-so-much-evil-in-the-world/.

[26] For a thorough understanding of trauma's effect on the body and ways to heal read the wonderful book by Dr. Bessel van der Kolk called *The Body Keeps the Score: Brain, Mind, and Body in the Healing of Trauma*.

[27] Logue MW et al. Smaller Hippocampal Volume in Posttraumatic Stress Disorder: A Multisite ENIGMA-PGC Study: Subcortical Volumetry Results

From Posttraumatic Stress Disorder Consortia. *Biological Psychiatry*, 2018 Feb 1;83(3):244–253. Doi: 10.1016/j.biopsych.2017.09.006. Epub 2017 Sep 20. Accessed at https://www.ncbi.nlm.nih.gov/pmc/articles/PMC5951719/.

28 Zaninotto AL et al. Updates and Current Perspectives of Psychiatric Assessments after Traumatic Brain Injury: A Systematic Review. *Front Psychiatry*, 2016 Jun 14;7:95. Doi: 10.3389/fpsyt.2016.00095. Accessed at https://www.ncbi.nlm.nih.gov/pmc/articles/PMC4906018/.

29 Fujii D et al. Psychotic Disorder Due to Traumatic Brain Injury: Analysis of Case Studies in the Literature. *The Journal of Neuropsychiatry*, 1 Jul 2012, https://doi.org/10.1176/appi.neuropsych.11070176, Accessed at https://neuro.psychiatryonline.org/doi/10.1176/appi.neuropsych.11070176.

30 Schachar RJ et al. Mental Health Implications of Traumatic Brain Injury (TBI) in Children and Youth. *Journal of Canadian Academy of Child Adolescent Psychiatry*, 2015 Fall;24(2):100–8. Epub 2015 Aug 31. Accessed at https://www.ncbi.nlm.nih.gov/pmc/articles/PMC4558980/.

31 Nordstrom A et al. (2018) Traumatic brain injury and the risk of dementia diagnosis: A nationwide cohort study. *PloS Med*, 15(1): e1002496. https://doi.org/10.1371/journal. pmed.1002496 Accessed at https://journals.plos.org/plosmedicine/article?id=10.1371/journal.pmed.1002496.

32 Go to MoldyMovie.com to watch for free.

33 Story taken from *The End of Mental Illness* by Dr. Daniel G. Amen.

34 Shinohara M, Yamada M. [Drug-induced Cognitive Impairment]. *Brain Nerve*, 2016 Apr;68(4):421–8. Japanese. Doi: 10.11477/mf.1416200415. https://pubmed.ncbi.nlm.nih.gov/27056860/.

35 University of Rochester Medical Center, Chemotherapy's Damage to the Brain Detailed. *ScienceDaily*, April 22, 2008. Accessed at: https://www.sciencedaily.com/releases/2008/04/080422103947.htm.

36 Bittner EA et al. Brief review: anesthetic neurotoxicity in the elderly, cognitive dysfunction and Alzheimer's disease. *Canadian Journal of Anesthesia*, 2011 Feb;58(2):216–23. Doi: 10.1007/s12630–010-9418-x. Epub 2010 Dec 21. Accessed at https://www.ncbi.nlm.nih.gov/pmc/articles/PMC4248669/ Also see Chen CW et al. Increased risk of dementia in people with previous exposure to general anesthesia: a nationwide population-based case-control study. *Alzheimer's & Dementia*, 2014 Mar;10(2):196–204. Doi: 10.1016/j.jalz.2013.05.1766. Epub 2013 Jul 27. https://pubmed.ncbi.nlm.nih.gov/23896612/.

37 Bruning J et al. Gut Microbiota and Short Chain Fatty Acids: Influence on the Autonomic Nervous System. *Neuroscience Bulletin*, 2020 Jan;36(1):91–95. Doi: 10.1007/s12264–019-00410–8. Epub 2019 Jul 12. https://www.ncbi.nlm.nih.gov/pmc/articles/PMC6940411/.

38 Silva YP et al. The Role of Short-Chain Fatty Acids From Gut Microbiota in Gut-Brain Communication. *Front Endocrinology* (Lausanne), 2020 Jan 31;11:25. Doi: 10.3389/fendo.2020.00025. Accessed at https://www.frontiersin.org/articles/10.3389/fendo.2020.00025/full.

39 Radjabzadeh, D et al. Gut microbiome-wide association study of depressive symptoms. *Nature Communications*, 13, 7128 (2022). https://doi.org/10.1038/s41467-022-34502-3.

40 There is much research connecting gluten to neurological conditions. Two of the most prolific researchers are Professor Marios Hadjivassilou in the UK and Dr. Alessio Fasano in the US.

41 Taken from the book *Grain Brain* by Dr. David Perlmutter which provides an in-depth look at gluten, brain health and neurological conditions with an extensive reference section to scientific studies.

42 See the work of Dr. Andrew Saul and the late Dr. Abram Hoffer as summarized in the helpful book *Niacin: The Real Story* (2nd edition) or through a PubMed search of Dr. Hoffer's many published articles.

43 Lahoda Brodska, H. et al. The Role of Micronutrients in Neurological Disorders. *Nutrients*, 2023, 15, 4129. https://doi.org/10.3390/nu15194129.

44 Castellano-Guerrero AM et al. Prevalence and predictors of depression and anxiety in adult patients with type 1 diabetes in tertiary care setting. *Acta Diabetologica*, 2018 Sep;55(9):943-953. doi: 10.1007/s00592-018-1172-5. Epub 2018 Jun 13. https://pubmed.ncbi.nlm.nih.gov/29948408/.

45 Niwa H et al. Clinical analysis of cognitive function in diabetic patients by MMSE and SPECT. *Diabetes Research and Clinical Practice*, 2006 May;72(2):142-7. doi: 10.1016/j.diabres.2005.10.012. Epub 2005 Dec 1. https://pubmed.ncbi.nlm.nih.gov/16325958/.

46 McGaffee J, Barnes MA, Lippmann S. Psychiatric presentations of hypothyroidism. *American Family Physician*, 1981 May;23(5):129-33.

47 See https://emmatekstra.com/blog/a-thyroid-saga/.

48 Santos NC, et al. Revisiting thyroid hormones in schizophrenia. *Journal of Thyroid Research*, 2012;2012:569147. doi: 10.1155/2012/569147. Epub 2012 Mar 26. https://www.ncbi.nlm.nih.gov/pmc/articles/PMC3321576/ . Also see Identifying Hypothyroidism in Psychiatric Presentations by David Baxter PhD at https://forum.psychlinks.ca/threads/identifying-hyperthyroidism-s-psychiatric-presentations.4690/.

49 Benros ME et al. Autoimmune diseases and severe infections as risk factors for mood disorders: a nationwide study. *JAMA Psychiatry*, 2013 Aug;70(8):812-20. doi: 10.1001/jamapsychiatry.2013.1111. https://pubmed.ncbi.nlm.nih.gov/23760347/ Also see *The End of Mental Illness* by Dr. Daniel Amen, Chapter 12 with many more references.

50 Brown JS Jr. Geographic correlation of schizophrenia to ticks and tick-borne encephalitis. *Schizophrenia Bulletin*, 1994;20(4):755–75. doi: 10.1093/schbul /20.4.755. https://pubmed.ncbi.nlm.nih.gov/7701281/.

51 Landry, R.L.; Embers, M.E. Does Dementia Have a Microbial Cause? *NeuroSci*, 2022, *3*, 262–283. https://doi.org/10.3390/neurosci3020019.

52 See *The End of Mental Illness* by Dr. Daniel Amen, Chapter 15 for several references.

53 Kripke DF, et al. Hypnotics' association with mortality or cancer: a matched cohort study. *BMJ Open*, 2012;2:e000850. doi: 10.1136/bmjopen-2012–000850 https://bmjopen.bmj.com/content/2/1/e000850 Also see Ambien Side Effects by Nitara Osbourne at https://americanaddictioncenters.org/ambien-treatment /side-effects.

54 You can read more in-depth strategies and about sleep at https://emmatekstra .com/blog/sleep-deserves-way-more-respect-than-were-giving-it-12-tips-to -improve-yours/.

55 For a broader overview of the many critical functions of cholesterol in the body read my blog article https://emmatekstra.com/blog/the-stubborn-myth -of-statins-and-cholesterol/.

56 For a detailed understanding of the role of statins and a low-fat diet in causing Alzheimer's read Dr. Stephanie Seneff's essay at https://people.csail.mit.edu /seneff/alzheimers_statins.html.

57 Read Dr. David Perlmutter's book *Grain Brain*, Chapter 3, for an extensive discussion of fat in brain health and the associated scientific studies referenced.

58 Pauling L. Orthomolecular psychiatry. Varying the concentrations of substances normally present in the human body may control mental disease. *Science*, 1968 Apr 19;160(3825):265–71. Doi: 10.1126/science.160.3825.265. Accessed at https://pubmed.ncbi.nlm.nih.gov/5641253/.

59 For detailed information on niacin and its therapeutic use in not only for mental health but many conditions read the work of Dr. Andrew Saul and the late Dr. Abram Hoffer as summarized in the helpful book *Niacin: The Real Story* (2nd edition).

60 For more on niacin see my blog post at https://emmatekstra.com/blog/the -many-benefits-of-niacin-b3-supplementation/.

61 A very interesting recent article provides a comprehensive overview of melatonin and its many uses. Minich DM et al., Is Melatonin the "Next Vitamin D"?: A Review of Emerging Science, Clinical Uses, Safety, and Dietary Supplements. *Nutrients*, 2022 Sep 22;14(19):3934. doi: 10.3390/ nu14193934. https://www.ncbi.nlm.nih.gov/pmc/articles/PMC9571539/.

62 Williams, J.L. et al., The Effects of Green Tea Amino Acid L-Theanine Consumption on the Ability to Manage Stress and Anxiety Levels: a Systematic

Review. *Plant Foods for Human Nutrition*, 75, 12–23 (2020). https://doi.org/10.1007/s11130–019-00771–5.

63   Mashayekh A, Pham DL, Yousem DM, Dizon M, Barker PB, Lin DD. Effects of Ginkgo biloba on cerebral blood flow assessed by quantitative MR perfusion imaging: a pilot study. *Neuroradiology*, 2011 Mar;53(3):185–91. doi: 10.1007/s00234–010-0790–6.

64   Biernacka P et al. The Potential of Ginkgo biloba as a Source of Biologically Active Compounds—A Review of the Recent Literature and Patents. *Molecules*, 2023 May 9;28(10):3993. doi: 10.3390/molecules28103993. Accessed at https://www.ncbi.nlm.nih.gov/pmc/articles/PMC10222153/.

65   Linde K et al. St John's wort for major depression. *Cochrane Database of Systematic Reviews*, 2008 Oct 8;2008(4):CD000448. doi: 10.1002/14651858. CD000448.pub3. Accessed at https://pubmed.ncbi.nlm.nih.gov/18843608/.

66   Singh B, et al Effectiveness of physical activity interventions for improving depression, anxiety and distress: an overview of systematic reviews. *British Journal of Sports Medicine*, 2023;57:1203–1209. Accessed at https://bjsm.bmj.com/content/57/18/1203.

67   Joseph Firth et al., Effect of aerobic exercise on hippocampal volume in humans: A systematic review and meta-analysis, *NeuroImage*, Volume 166, 2018, https://doi.org/10.1016/j.neuroimage.2017.11.007.

68   Mandolesi L et al. Effects of Physical Exercise on Cognitive Functioning and Wellbeing: Biological and Psychological Benefits. *Frontiers in Psychology*, (2018). doi: 10.3389/fpsyg.2018.00509. Accessed at https://www.frontiersin.org/articles/10.3389/fpsyg.2018.00509/.

69   Dossett ML, et al. A New Era for Mind-Body Medicine. *New England Journal of Medicine*, 2020 Apr 9;382(15):1390–1391. doi: 10.1056/NEJMp1917461.

70   Bach D et al. Clinical EFT (Emotional Freedom Techniques) Improves Multiple Physiological Markers of Health. *Journal of Evidence-Based Integrative Medicine*, 2019 Jan–Dec;24:2515690X18823691. doi: 10.1177/2515690X 18823691.

71   Read James Nestor's *Breath: The New Science of a Lost Art*, Riverhead Books, 2020.

72   See https://www.wimhofmethod.com/practice-the-method.

73   Marzbani H et al. Neurofeedback: A Comprehensive Review on System Design, Methodology and Clinical Applications. *Basic Clinical Neuroscience*, 2016 Apr;7(2):143–58. doi: 10.15412/J.BCN.03070208. Accessed at https://www.ncbi.nlm.nih.gov/pmc/articles/PMC4892319/.

74   Shapiro F. The role of eye movement desensitization and reprocessing (EMDR) therapy in medicine: addressing the psychological and physical symptoms stemming from adverse life experiences. *Permanente Journal*, 2014

Winter;18(1):71–7. doi: 10.7812/TPP/13–098. Accessed at https://www
.ncbi.nlm.nih.gov/pmc/articles/PMC3951033/.

[75] See resources on the website MAPS.org (Multidisciplinary Association for
Psychedelic Studies).

[76] Go to https://thestellateinstitute.com/stellate-ganglion-block-for-ptsd/ for more
information and link to scientific studies.

[77] George, M. et al. Noninvasive techniques for probing neurocircuitry and
treating illness: vagus nerve stimulation (VNS), transcranial magnetic
stimulation (TMS) and transcranial direct current stimulation (tDCS).
Neuropsychopharmacology, 35, 301–316 (2010). https://doi.org/10.1038/npp
.2009.87.

[78] Christopher Berglund, *Psychology Today*, 2022 https://www.psychologytoday
.com/us/blog/the-athletes-way/202201/how-does-vagus-nerve-stimulation
-reduce-ptsd-symptoms.

[79] For other ideas read *Accessing the Healing Power of the Vagus Nerve: Self-help
exercises for anxiety, depression, trauma and autism* by Stanley Rosenberg with
a foreword by Stephen Porges PhD, the developer of polyvagal theory.

[80] Tal S, et al. Hyperbaric Oxygen Therapy Can Induce Angiogenesis and
Regeneration of Nerve Fibers in Traumatic Brain Injury Patients. *Frontiers in
Human Neuroscience*, 2017 Oct 19;11:508. doi: 10.3389/fnhum.2017.00508.
https://www.ncbi.nlm.nih.gov/pmc/articles/PMC5654341/.

[81] Harch PG, et al. A phase I study of low-pressure hyperbaric oxygen therapy
for blast-induced post-concussion syndrome and post-traumatic stress
disorder. *Journal of Neurotrauma*, 2012 Jan 1;29(1):168–85. doi: 10.1089/
neu.2011.1895. Epub 2011 Nov 22. https://pubmed.ncbi.nlm.nih.gov/22026588/.

[82] Efrati S et al. Hyperbaric oxygen therapy can diminish fibromyalgia syndrome
—prospective clinical trial. *PLoS One*, 2015 May 26;10(5):e0127012.
doi: 10.1371/journal.pone.0127012. https://pubmed.ncbi.nlm.nih.gov/26010952/.

[83] Löndahl, M. et al. Relationship between ulcer healing after hyperbaric oxygen
therapy and transcutaneous oximetry, toe blood pressure and ankle–brachial
index in patients with diabetes and chronic foot ulcers. *Diabetologia*, 54, 65–
68 (2011). https://doi.org/10.1007/s00125–010-1946-y. Accessed at https:
//link.springer.com/article/10.1007/s00125–010-1946-y.

[84] Dulai PS et al. Systematic review: The safety and efficacy of hyperbaric
oxygen therapy for inflammatory bowel disease. *Alimentary Pharmacology
Therapeutics*, 2014 Jun;39(11):1266–75. doi: 10.1111/apt.12753. Epub
2014 Apr 16. Accessed at https://pubmed.ncbi.nlm.nih.gov/24738651/.

Chapter 9: Aging Well

[1] See https://www.vitaminrush.com/6378/dr-abram-hoffer-natural-treatment
-mental-health-vitamin-b3-niacin-feed-your-head-2010/.

[2] François Robin-Champigneul, Jeanne Calment's Unique 122-Year Life Span: Facts and Factors; Longevity History in Her Genealogical Tree. *Rejuvenation Research*, 2020 23:1, 19–47, https://www.liebertpub.com/doi/abs/10.1089 /rej.2019.2298.

[3] Fries JF. Aging, natural death, and the compression of morbidity. *New England Journal of Medicine*, 1980 Jul 17;303(3):130–5. doi: 10.1056/ NEJM198007173030304. https://pubmed.ncbi.nlm.nih.gov/7383070/.

[4] For a discussion on aging clocks see: Fedor Galkin et al. Stress, diet, exercise: Common environmental factors and their impact on epigenetic age. *Ageing Research Reviews*, Volume 88, 2023, 101956, ISSN 1568–1637, https://doi .org/10.1016/j.arr.2023.101956. https://www.sciencedirect.com/science/article /pii/S1568163723001150.

[5] Tian, Y.E., et al. Heterogeneous aging across multiple organ systems and prediction of chronic disease and mortality. *Nature Medicine*, 29, 1221–1231 (2023). https://doi.org/10.1038/s41591–023-02296–6.

[6] You might be interested in this simple heart age calculator as an example: https://www.nyc.gov/site/doh/health/health-topics/heart-age-calculator.page.

[7] Ferrucci, L., Fabbri, E. Inflammageing: chronic inflammation in ageing, cardiovascular disease, and frailty. *Nature Reviews Cardiology*, 15, 505–522 (2018). https://doi.org/10.1038/s41569–018-0064–2. Accessed at https: //www.nature.com/articles/s41569–018-0064–2.

[8] You can read more about DEXA here https://courses.washington.edu /bonephys/opbmd.html.

[9] Järvinen TL et al. Osteoporosis: the emperor has no clothes. *Journal of Internal Medicine*, 2015 Jun;277(6):662–73. doi: 10.1111/joim.12366. PMID: 25809279; https://pubmed.ncbi.nlm.nih.gov/25809279/.

[10] See FDA letter to the *New England Journal of Medicine* at https://www.nejm .org/doi/full/10.1056/NEJMc0808738.

[11] Heckbert SR, et al. Use of alendronate and risk of incident atrial fibrillation in women. *Arch Intern Med*, 2008 Apr 28;168(8):826–31. doi: 10.1001 /archinte.168.8.826.

[12] Wright J. Marketing disease: is osteoporosis an example of 'disease mongering'? *British Journal of Nursing*, 2009 Sep 24–Oct 7;18(17):1064–7. doi: 10.12968 /bjon.2009.18.17.44163.

[13] Eichwald J, et al. Survey of Teen Noise Exposure and Efforts to Protect Hearing at School—United States, 2020. *Morbidity and Mortality Weekly Report*, 2020;69:1822–1826. https://www.ncbi.nlm.nih.gov/pmc/articles/PMC 7714025/.

[14] Curhan SG, et al. Adherence to Healthful Dietary Patterns Is Associated with Lower Risk of Hearing Loss in Women. *Journal of Nutrition*, 2018 Jun

1;148(6):944–951. doi: 10.1093/jn/nxy058. https://www.ncbi.nlm.nih.gov /pmc/articles/PMC6481387/.

15 Fiorini AC, et al. Can you hear me now? The quest for better guidance on omega-3 fatty acid consumption to combat hearing loss. *Clinics* (Sao Paulo), 2016 Aug;71(8):420–2. doi: 10.6061/clinics/2016(08)01. https://www.ncbi .nlm.nih.gov/pmc/articles/PMC4975785/#b1-cln_71p420.

16 Curhan SG, et al. Carotenoids, vitamin A, vitamin C, vitamin E, and folate and risk of self-reported hearing loss in women. *American Journal of Clinical Nutrition*, 2015 Nov;102(5):1167–75. doi: 10.3945/ajcn.115.109314. Epub 2015 Sep 9. https://www.ncbi.nlm.nih.gov/pmc/articles/PMC4625586/.

17 Yong RJ, et al. Prevalence of chronic pain among adults in the United States. *Pain*, 2022 Feb 1;163(2):e328-e332. doi: 10.1097/j.pain.0000000000002291. https://pubmed.ncbi.nlm.nih.gov/33990113/.

18 Darrell J. Gaskin et al. The Economic Costs of Pain in the United States. *Journal of Pain*, 18 May 2012, https://doi.org/10.1016/j.jpain.2012.03.009 https://www.jpain.org/article/S1526–5900(12)00559–7/fulltext#articleInformation.

19 Manchikanti L, et al. Therapeutic use, abuse, and nonmedical use of opioids: a ten-year perspective. *Pain Physician*, 2010 Sep-Oct;13(5):401–35. https://pubmed.ncbi.nlm.nih.gov/20859312/.

20 See the National Center for Drug Abuse Statistics website at https://drugabusestatistics.org/drug-overdose-deaths/.

21 See a Stanford Medicine summary at https://stanfordhealthcare.org/medical -treatments/g/general-surgery/complications.html.

22 Geoffrey P. Dobson, Trauma of major surgery: A global problem that is not going away. *International Journal of Surgery*, Volume 81, 2020, Pages 47–54, ISSN 1743–9191, https://doi.org/10.1016/j.ijsu.2020.07.017. https://www .sciencedirect.com/science/article/pii/S1743919120305525.

23 James JT. Patient Harms Associated with Hospital Care. *Journal of Patient Safety*, 2013 Sept;9(3) https://journals.lww.com/journalpatientsafety/fulltext /2013/09000/a_new,_evidence_based_estimate_of_patient_harms.2.aspx.

24 Henson, K., et al. Radiation-related mortality from heart disease and lung cancer more than 20 years after radiotherapy for breast cancer. *British Journal of Cancer*, 108, 179–182 (2013). https://doi.org/10.1038/bjc.2012.575.

25 Jørgensen KJ, et al. Overdiagnosis in publicly organised mammography screening programmes: systematic review of incidence trends. *BMJ*, 2009 Jul 9;339:b2587. doi: 10.1136/bmj.b2587.

26 See https://oncoblotlabs.com/how-it-works/.

27 See https://rgcc-international.com/about-rgcc-tests/.

28 Note this Johns Hopkins article on infection rates https://www.hopkins medicine.org/news/newsroom/news-releases/2018/05/infection-rates

-after-colonoscopy-endoscopy-at-us-specialty-centers-are-far-higher-than
-previously-thought.

29 Check out one option at https://www.cologuard.com/.

30 Lee, JWL et al. Association of distinct microbial signatures with premalignant
colorectal adenomas. *Cell Host & Microbe*, Volume 31, Issue 5, 30 April 2023,
doi: https://doi.org/10.1016/j.chom.2023.04.007.

31 Fenton JJ, Robbins JA, Amarnath ALD, Franks P. Osteoporosis Overtreatment
in a Regional Health Care System. *JAMA Intern Med,* 2016;176(3):391–393.
doi:10.1001/jamainternmed.2015.6020   https://jamanetwork.com/journals
/jamainternalmedicine/fullarticle/2478896.

32 Mandrola J. et al. The Case Against Coronary Artery Calcium Scoring for
Cardiovascular Disease Risk Assessment, *American Family Physician*, 2019;
100(12):734–735 https://www.aafp.org/pubs/afp/issues/2019/1215/p734.html.

33 Radiation Risk from medical Imaging, Harvard Medical School, https:
//www.health.harvard.edu/cancer/radiation-risk-from-medical-imaging.

34 Prostate Cancer Screening, *American Family Physician*, https://www.aafp
.org/pubs/afp/issues/2015/1015/p683.html#:~:text=31-,Screening%20
Recommendations,treatment%20outweigh%20the%20limited%20benefits.

35 Wright JD, et al. Overuse of Cervical Cancer Screening Tests Among Women
With Average Risk in the United States From 2013 to 2014. *JAMA Netw
Open*, 2021;4(4):e218373. doi:10.1001/jamanetworkopen.2021.8373.

36 Sirovich BE, Welch HG. Cervical cancer screening among women without a
cervix. *JAMA*, 2004 Jun 23;291(24):2990–3. doi: 10.1001/jama.291.24.2990.
https://pubmed.ncbi.nlm.nih.gov/15213211/.

37 Go to https://www.choosingwisely.org/.

38 Jessica Y. Ho; Life Course Patterns of Prescription Drug Use in the United
States. *Demography*, 1 October 2023; 60 (5): 1549–1579. doi: https://doi
.org/10.1215/00703370–10965990. Accessed at https://read.dukeupress.edu
/demography/article/60/5/1549/382305/Life-Course-Patterns-of
-Prescription-Drug-Use-in.

39 Covarrubias AJ, Perrone R, Grozio A, Verdin E. NAD+ metabolism and its
roles in cellular processes during ageing. *Nature Reviews Molecular Cell Biology*,
2021 Feb;22(2):119–141. doi: 10.1038/s41580–020-00313-x. Epub 2020
Dec 22. https://www.ncbi.nlm.nih.gov/pmc/articles/PMC7963035/.

40 See my blog article https://emmatekstra.com/blog/the-many-benefits-of
-niacin-b3-supplementation/.

41 Ge M, et al. Senolytic targets and new strategies for clearing senescent
cells. *Mechanisms of Ageing and Development*, 2021 Apr;195:111468. doi:
10.1016/j.mad.2021.111468. Epub 2021 Mar 16.

42 Kirkland JL, Tchkonia T. Senolytic drugs: from discovery to translation. *Journal of Internal Medicine*, 2020 Nov;288(5):518–536. doi: 10.1111/joim.13141. Epub 2020 Aug 4. https://pubmed.ncbi.nlm.nih.gov/32686219/.

43 Matthew Walker, *Why We Sleep: The New Science of Sleep and Dreams* (Penguin Books, 2017), Chapter 5. Also see my detailed review of key themes in the book at https://emmatekstra.com/blog/matthew-walker/.

44 Twohig-Bennett C, Jones A. The health benefits of the great outdoors: A systematic review and meta-analysis of greenspace exposure and health outcomes. *Environmental Research*, 2018 Oct;166:628–637. doi: 10.1016/j.envres.2018.06.030. Epub 2018 Jul 5. https://www.ncbi.nlm.nih.gov/pmc/articles/PMC6562165/.

45 One recent example is AIB Posis et al., Associations of Accelerometer-Measured Physical Activity and Sedentary Time With All-Cause Mortality by Genetic Predisposition for Longevity. *Journal of Aging and Physical Activity*, 2023, 31, 265–275, https://doi.org/10.1123/japa.2022–0067. Also see Dong Hoon Lee et al. Long-Term Leisure Time Physical Activity Intensity and All-Cause and Cause-Specific Mortality: A Prospective Cohort of US Adults. Circulation, 25 Jul 2022. 2022;146:523–534. https://doi.org/10.1161/CIRCULATIONAHA.121.058162.

46 Jennifer L. Kraschnewski, et al., Is strength training associated with mortality benefits? A 15-year cohort study of US older adults. *Preventive Medicine*, Volume 87, 2016, Pages 121–127, ISSN 0091–7435, https://doi.org/10.1016/j.ypmed.2016.02.038. https://www.sciencedirect.com/science/article/pii/S0091743516300160.

47 Gaser C, et al. Brain structures differ between musicians and non-musicians. *Journal of Neuroscience*, 2003 Oct 8;23(27):9240–5. doi: 10.1523/JNEUROSCI.23-27-09240.2003. Erratum in: *Journal of Neuroscience*, 2013 Sep 4;33(36):14629. https://www.jneurosci.org/content/23/27/9240.

48 Belleville S, et al. Training-related brain plasticity in subjects at risk of developing Alzheimer's disease. *Brain*, 2011 Jun;134(Pt 6):1623–34. doi: 10.1093/brain/awr037. Epub 2011 Mar 22. https://pubmed.ncbi.nlm.nih.gov/21427462/.

49 For some insight into the incredible monarch butterfly check out https://monarchjointventure.org/monarch-biology/life-cycle.

50 You can read about my pickleball conversion on my blog post https://emmatekstra.com/blog/my-knee-pain-gone-two-simple-remedies-that-really-work/.

51 Davidson RJ, McEwen BS. Social influences on neuroplasticity: stress and interventions to promote well-being. *Nature Neuroscience*, 2012 Apr 15;15(5):689–95. doi: 10.1038/nn.3093. https://www.ncbi.nlm.nih.gov/pmc/articles/PMC3491815/.

[52] Terracciano A, et al. Loneliness and Risk of Parkinson Disease. *JAMA Neurol,* Published online October 02, 2023. doi:10.1001/jamaneurol.2023.3382.

[53] Cacioppo, S., et al. Loneliness: Clinical Import and Interventions. *Perspectives on Psychological Science,* (2015) 10(2), 238–249. https://doi.org/10.1177/1745691615570616.

[54] Start with John 15:12 and also see Proverbs 27:10, 1 Samuel 18:1, Colossians 3:12–14, 1 John 3:16 as a small sample.

[55] Patricia A Thomas et al. Lost Touch? Implications of Physical Touch for Physical Health. *The Journals of Gerontology: Series B,* Volume 76, Issue 3, March 2021, Pages e111–e115, https://doi.org/10.1093/geronb/gbaa134.

[56] Robert D. Putnam, *Bowling Alone; The Collapse and Revival of American Community* (Simon & Schuster 2000). Also see *Habits of the Heart,* Robert N. Bellah et al.

[57] Shakya HB, Christakis NA. Association of Facebook Use With Compromised Well-Being: A Longitudinal Study. *American Journal of Epidemiology,* 2017 Feb 1;185(3):203–211. doi: 10.1093/aje/kww189. https://pubmed.ncbi.nlm.nih.gov/28093386/.

[58] Tristen K Inagaki, et al. Support-Giving Is Associated With Lower Systemic Inflammation. *Annals of Behavioral Medicine,* Volume 57, Issue 6, June 2023, Pages 499–507, https://doi.org/10.1093/abm/kaac059.

[59] Sonja Hilbrand, et al. Caregiving within and beyond the family is associated with lower mortality for the caregiver: A prospective study. *Evolution and Human Behavior,* Volume 38, Issue 3, 2017, Pages 397–403, ISSN 1090–5138, https://doi.org/10.1016/j.evolhumbehav.2016.11.010.

[60] Kovaleva M, et al. Chronic Stress, Social Isolation, and Perceived Loneliness in Dementia Caregivers. *Journal of Psychosocial Nursing and Mental Health Services,* 2018 Oct 1;56(10):36–43. doi: 10.3928/02793695–20180329-04. Epub 2018 Apr 19. https://pubmed.ncbi.nlm.nih.gov/29667698/.

[61] Barbara L. Fredrickson et al. A functional genomic perspective on human well-being. *PNAS,* Vol. 110. No. 33, July 29, 2013, 110 (33) 13684–13689. https://doi.org/10.1073/pnas.1305419110.

[62] Boyle PA, et al. Effect of a purpose in life on risk of incident Alzheimer disease and mild cognitive impairment in community-dwelling older persons. *Archives of General Psychiatry,* 2010 Mar;67(3):304–10. doi: 10.1001/archgenpsychiatry.2009.208. https://www.ncbi.nlm.nih.gov/pmc/articles/PMC2897172/.

[63] See Ellen Langer's book *Counterclockwise: Mindful Health and the Power of Possibility.* And the recent published study: Pagnini F, et al. Ageing as a mindset: a study protocol to rejuvenate older adults with a counterclockwise psychological intervention. *BMJ Open,* 2019 Jul 9;9(7):e030411. doi: 10.1136/bmjopen-2019–030411. https://www.ncbi.nlm.nih.gov/pmc/articles/PMC6615788/.